THE POISONING OF PARADISE: CRYSTAL METHAMPHETAMINE IN HAWAII

HEARING

BEFORE THE

SUBCOMMITTEE ON CRIMINAL JUSTICE,
DRUG POLICY AND HUMAN RESOURCES

OF THE

COMMITTEE ON
GOVERNMENT REFORM

HOUSE OF REPRESENTATIVES

ONE HUNDRED EIGHTH CONGRESS

SECOND SESSION

AUGUST 2, 2004

Serial No. 108–276

Printed for the use of the Committee on Gover...

Available via the World Wide Web: http://www.gpo.gov/congress/house
http://www.house.gov/reform

U.S. GOVERNMENT PRINTING OFFICE

98–604 PDF WASHINGTON : 2005

For sale by the Superintendent of Documents, U.S. Government Printing Office
Internet: bookstore.gpo.gov Phone: toll free (866) 512–1800; DC area (202) 512–1800
Fax: (202) 512–2250 Mail: Stop SSOP, Washington, DC 20402–0001

COMMITTEE ON GOVERNMENT REFORM

TOM DAVIS, Virginia, *Chairman*

DAN BURTON, Indiana
CHRISTOPHER SHAYS, Connecticut
ILEANA ROS-LEHTINEN, Florida
JOHN M. McHUGH, New York
JOHN L. MICA, Florida
MARK E. SOUDER, Indiana
STEVEN C. LATOURETTE, Ohio
DOUG OSE, California
RON LEWIS, Kentucky
JO ANN DAVIS, Virginia
TODD RUSSELL PLATTS, Pennsylvania
CHRIS CANNON, Utah
ADAM H. PUTNAM, Florida
EDWARD L. SCHROCK, Virginia
JOHN J. DUNCAN, Jr., Tennessee
NATHAN DEAL, Georgia
CANDICE S. MILLER, Michigan
TIM MURPHY, Pennsylvania
MICHAEL R. TURNER, Ohio
JOHN R. CARTER, Texas
MARSHA BLACKBURN, Tennessee
PATRICK J. TIBERI, Ohio
KATHERINE HARRIS, Florida

HENRY A. WAXMAN, California
TOM LANTOS, California
MAJOR R. OWENS, New York
EDOLPHUS TOWNS, New York
PAUL E. KANJORSKI, Pennsylvania
CAROLYN B. MALONEY, New York
ELIJAH E. CUMMINGS, Maryland
DENNIS J. KUCINICH, Ohio
DANNY K. DAVIS, Illinois
JOHN F. TIERNEY, Massachusetts
WM. LACY CLAY, Missouri
DIANE E. WATSON, California
STEPHEN F. LYNCH, Massachusetts
CHRIS VAN HOLLEN, Maryland
LINDA T. SANCHEZ, California
C.A. "DUTCH" RUPPERSBERGER, Maryland
ELEANOR HOLMES NORTON, District of Columbia
JIM COOPER, Tennessee
BETTY McCOLLUM, Minnesota

BERNARD SANDERS, Vermont (Independent)

MELISSA WOJCIAK, *Staff Director*
DAVID MARIN, *Deputy Staff Director/Communications Director*
ROB BORDEN, *Parliamentarian*
TERESA AUSTIN, *Chief Clerk*
PHIL BARNETT, *Minority Chief of Staff/Chief Counsel*

SUBCOMMITTEE ON CRIMINAL JUSTICE, DRUG POLICY AND HUMAN RESOURCES

MARK E. SOUDER, Indiana, *Chairman*

NATHAN DEAL, Georgia
JOHN M. McHUGH, New York
JOHN L. MICA, Florida
DOUG OSE, California
JO ANN DAVIS, Virginia
JOHN R. CARTER, Texas
MARSHA BLACKBURN, Tennessee
PATRICK J. TIBERI, Ohio

ELIJAH E. CUMMINGS, Maryland
DANNY K. DAVIS, Illinois
WM. LACY CLAY, Missouri
LINDA T. SANCHEZ, California
C.A. "DUTCH" RUPPERSBERGER, Maryland
ELEANOR HOLMES NORTON, District of Columbia
BETTY McCOLLUM, Minnesota

EX OFFICIO

TOM DAVIS, Virginia
HENRY A. WAXMAN, California

J. MARC WHEAT, *Staff Director*
NICHOLAS COLEMAN, *Professional Staff Member and Counsel*

CONTENTS

THE POISONING OF PARADISE: CRYSTAL METHAMPHETAMINE IN HAWAII

MONDAY, AUGUST 2, 2004

HOUSE OF REPRESENTATIVES,
SUBCOMMITTEE ON CRIMINAL JUSTICE, DRUG POLICY AND HUMAN RESOURCES,
COMMITTEE ON GOVERNMENT REFORM,
Kailua-Kona, HI.

The subcommittee met, pursuant to notice, at 9:20 a.m., at Kealakehe Intermediate School, 74–5062 Onipaa Street, Kailua-Kona, HI, Hon. Mark E. Souder (chairman of the subcommittee) presiding.

Present: Representatives Souder and Case.

Staff present: Nicholas P. Coleman, professional staff member/counsel; David Thomasson, congressional fellow; and Alena Guagenti, legislative assistant.

Mr. SOUDER. Come to order. Good morning and thank you all for coming. This hearing continues our subcommittee's work on the problem of methamphetamine abuse—a problem that is ravaging the State of Hawaii and the entire Nation. I'd like to thank Congressman Ed Case for inviting us here to the Big Island, and for his support for a bipartisan approach to confronting the meth epidemic.

In 2003, Congressman Case testified before our subcommittee about the meth problem in Hawaii, and since then we have frequently discussed ways to help communities like this one to reduce drug abuse.

Meth is one of the most powerful and dangerous drugs available. A recent study of the effects of meth abuse using MRI scans of addicts revealed what one expert called a forest fire of brain damage. Addicts' brains lose 11 percent of the tissue in the limbic region, controlling mood and emotion, and 8 percent of the hippocampus region, responsible for forming new memories, comparable to the brain deficits created by Alzheimer's disease. Here in Hawaii the form of meth called crystal or ice is increasing in popularity. It is highly pure and extremely addictive.

Sadly, meth is also one of the easiest drugs to make. It can be cooked using common household or agricultural chemicals and simple cold medicines, following recipes easily available on the Internet.

The meth here in Hawaii and other States comes from two major sources of supply. First, meth comes from the so-called superlabs in California and northern Mexico. By the end of the 1990's these superlabs produced over 70 percent of the Nation's supply of meth.

The superlabs are operated by large Mexican drug trafficking organizations that have used their established distribution and supply networks to transport meth throughout the country.

The second major source of meth comes from small, local labs that are generally unaffiliated with major trafficking organizations. These labs have proliferated throughout the country. The total amount of meth actually supplied by these labs is relatively small; however, the environmental damage and health hazard they create make them a serious problem for local communities, particularly the State and local law enforcement agencies charged with the duty to uncover and clean them up. In my home State of Indiana, for example, more than 20 percent of the labs raided by police were discovered only after they had exploded and started fires. Children are often found at meth labs and have frequently suffered from severe health problems as a result of the hazardous chemicals used in drug manufacturing.

Our hearings during the 107th Congress were mostly held in Washington and looked at this problem from a national perspective. This year, however, we have taken a different approach. We have instead been holding hearings in specific regions that have been hardest-hit by meth trafficking and abuse. In February we held a hearing in northeastern Indiana, followed by a hearing in Detroit, Michigan, where large quantities of meth precursor chemicals like pseudoephedrine, which comes predominantly from Belgium and Holland, were being smuggled in until very recently. In June we held a hearing in Bentonville, Arkansas where the use of crystal meth is also growing rapidly.

Everywhere we go we hear about many of the same issues; the environmental damage caused by the labs; the high costs and long hours required for law enforcement agencies to process lab sites; the heartbreaking stories of children exposed to drugs and chemicals and in need of emergency medical care and a safe place to go. We hear about how addictive and deadly this drug is and how difficult it is to provide treatment and get meth users off of drugs.

The Bush administration, and especially the Office of National Drug Control Policy [ONDCP], has pushed for strong and effective action against meth abuse. We will need to take action at every level, Federal, State, and local, to respond to this problem. Let me briefly mention three issues that need to be addressed.

First, what do we need to do to reduce the supply of meth? In the late 1990's the Federal Government responded to the meth problem both here and elsewhere with stricter laws against the precursor chemical trade and tougher enforcement. The proliferation of smaller meth labs, however, means that we probably will have to further restrict the ability of meth cooks to get precursor chemicals—especially pseudoephedrine. Already many States have acted to restrict sales of cold medicines and other pseudoephedrine sources. A major question Congress must address is whether to enact a national standard for these sales, and if so, what form should it take?

Second, how should we deal with the environmental issues created in the wake of a meth lab seizure? We have to ensure that the toxic chemicals produced and dumped by lab operators are cleaned up, but these criminals rarely have enough money to compensate the government for those costs. If we impose the costs on unsuspecting landowners or landlords, however, we may give them a disincentive to monitor their property and report suspicious activity to the police. In California, for example, some farmers prefer to bury the remains of meth labs they find on their property because if they report them, they will be liable for the clean-up costs. We will have to carefully consider how we assign the responsibility for the difficult and expensive task.

Finally, how do we get meth addicts into treatment and how do we keep young people from starting on meth in the first place? We can all agree that education and outreach are vital, but the hard part is figuring out what works best. What works for marijuana, ecstasy or cocaine may not work as well for meth.

This hearing will address these difficult questions and hopefully bring us closer to some answers. Again, I thank Congressman Case for inviting us here, and for the assistance that he and his staff provided to our subcommittee in setting up this hearing. Our first panel of witnesses begins with the distinguished Lieutenant Governor of Hawaii, James R. Duke Aiona who together with Governor Linda Lingle has provided strong leadership in this State on drug abuse issues.

We next welcome three witnesses who have joined us to discuss the Federal Government's response to the meth problem: Mr. Larry D. Burnett, Director of the Hawaii High Intensity Drug Trafficking Area [HIDTA], administered by the White House Office of National Drug Control Policy [ONDCP]; Mr. Charles Goodwin, Special Agent in Charge of the FBI's Honolulu division; and Mr. Briane Grey, Assistant Special Agent in Charge of the Drug Enforcement Administration's Honolulu office.

At a hearing like this, it is vitally important for us to hear from the State and local agencies forced to fight on the front lines against meth and other illegal drugs. We welcome Mayor Harry Kim of the County of Hawaii; Mr. Keith Kamita, Chief of the Narcotics Enforcement Division of the Hawaii County Police Department; and Mr. Richard Botti, Executive Director of the Hawaii Food Industry Association.

We also welcome four witnesses whose work in the field of drug treatment and prevention is of vital importance here in Hawaii: Dr. Kevin Kunz of Kona Addiction Services; Mr. Wesley Margheim of the Big Island Substance Abuse Council; Mr. Allen Salavea of the Hawaii County Prosecutor's Office's Youth Builder's Program; and Dr. Jamal Wasan of the Lokahi Treatment Program. We thank everyone for taking the time to join us this morning and look forward to your testimony. Now to Congressman Case for an opening statement.

[The prepared statement of Hon. Mark E. Souder follows:]

Opening Statement
Chairman Mark Souder

"The Poisoning of Paradise: Crystal Methamphetamine in Hawaii"

Subcommittee on Criminal Justice, Drug Policy, and Human Resources
Committee on Government Reform

August 2, 2004

Good morning, and thank you all for coming. This hearing continues our Subcommittee's work on the problem of methamphetamine abuse – a problem that is ravaging the state of Hawaii and the entire nation. I'd like to thank Congressman Ed Case for inviting us here to the Big Island, and for his support for a bi-partisan approach to confronting the meth epidemic. In 2003, Congressman Case testified before our Subcommittee about the meth problem in Hawaii, and since then we have frequently discussed ways to help communities like this one to reduce drug abuse.

Meth is one of the most powerful and dangerous drugs available. A recent study of the effects of meth abuse using M.R.I. scans of addicts revealed what one expert called a "forest fire of brain damage." Addicts' brains lost 11 percent of the tissue in the limbic region (controlling mood and emotion), and 8 percent of the hippocampus region (responsible for forming new memories) – comparable to the brain deficits created by Alzheimer's disease.[1] Here in Hawaii, the form of meth called "crystal" or "ice" is increasing in popularity; it is highly pure and extremely addictive.

Sadly, meth is also one of the easiest drugs to make. It can be "cooked" using common household or agricultural chemicals and simple cold medicines, following recipes easily available on the Internet. The meth here in Hawaii and in other states comes from two major sources of supply. First, most meth comes from the so-called "superlabs" in California and northern Mexico. By the end of the 1990's these superlabs produced over 70 percent of the nation's supply of meth. The superlabs are operated by large Mexican drug trafficking organizations that have used their established distribution and supply networks to transport meth throughout the country.

The second major source of meth comes from small, local labs that are generally unaffiliated with major trafficking organizations. These labs have

---

[1] See "This Is Your Brain On Meth: A 'Forest Fire' of Damage," New York Times, Page F-1, July 20, 2004.

proliferated throughout the country. The total amount of meth actually supplied by these labs is relatively small; however, the environmental damage and health hazard they create make them a serious problem for local communities, particularly the state and local law enforcement agencies charged with the duty to uncover and clean them up. In my home state of Indiana, for example, more than 20% of the labs raided by police were discovered only after they had exploded and started fires. Children are often found at meth labs, and have frequently suffered from severe health problems as a result of the hazardous chemicals used in drug manufacturing.

Our hearings during the 107th Congress were mostly held in Washington, and looked at this problem from a national perspective. This year, however, we have taken a different approach. We have instead been holding hearings in specific regions that have been hardest-hit by meth trafficking and abuse. In February, we held a hearing in northeastern Indiana, followed by a hearing in Detroit, Michigan, where large quantities of meth precursor chemicals like pseudoephedrine were being smuggled until very recently. In June, we held a hearing in Bentonville, Arkansas, where the use of crystal meth is also growing rapidly.

Everywhere we go, we hear about many of the same issues: the environmental damage caused by the labs; the high costs and long hours required for law enforcement agencies to process lab sites; the heartbreaking stories of children exposed to drugs and chemicals and in need of emergency medical care and a safe place to go. We hear about how addictive and deadly this drug is, and how difficult it is to provide treatment and get meth users off of drugs.

The Bush Administration, and especially its Office of National Drug Control Policy (ONDCP), has pushed for strong and effective action against meth abuse. We will need to take action at every level – federal, state and local – to respond to this problem. Let me briefly mention three issues that need to be addressed:

First, what do we need to do to reduce the supply of meth? In the late 1990's, the federal government responded to the meth problem both here and elsewhere with stricter laws against the precursor chemical trade and tougher enforcement. The proliferation of smaller meth labs, however, means that we probably will have to further restrict the ability of meth cooks to get precursor chemicals – especially pseudoephedrine. Already many states have acted to restrict sales of cold medicines and other pseudoephedrine sources. A major question Congress must address is whether to enact a national standard for these sales, and if so, what form should it take?

Second, how should we deal with the environmental issues created in the wake of a meth lab seizure? We have to ensure that the toxic chemicals produced and dumped by lab operators are cleaned up, but these criminals rarely have enough money to compensate the government for those costs. If we impose the costs on unsuspecting landowners or landlords, however, we may give them a disincentive to monitor their property and report suspicious activity to the police. In California, for example, some farmers prefer to bury the remains of meth labs they find on their property, because if they report them they will be liable for the clean-up costs. We will have to carefully consider how we assign the responsibility for this difficult and expensive task.

Finally, how do we get meth addicts into treatment, and how do we keep young people from starting on meth in the first place? We can all agree that education and outreach are vital, but the hard part is figuring out what works best. What works for marijuana, ecstasy or cocaine may not work as well for meth.

This hearing will address these difficult questions and hopefully bring us closer to some answers. Again, I thank Congressman Case for inviting us here, and for the assistance that he and his staff provided to our Subcommittee in setting up this hearing. Our first panel of witnesses begins with the distinguished Lieutenant Governor of Hawaii, James R. "Duke" Aiola, who together with Governor Linda Lingle has provided strong leadership in this state on drug abuse issues. We next welcome three witnesses who have joined us to discuss the federal government's response to the meth problem: Mr. Larry D. Burnett, Director of the Hawaii High Intensity Drug Trafficking Area (HIDTA), administered by the White House Office of National Drug Control Policy (ONDCP); Mr. Charles Goodwin, Special Agent in Charge of the FBI's Honolulu division; and Mr. Briane Grey, Assistant Special Agent in Charge of the Drug Enforcement Administration's Honolulu office.

At a hearing like this, it is vitally important for us to hear from the state and local agencies forced to fight on the "front lines" against meth and other illegal drugs. We welcome Mayor Harry Kim of the County of Hawaii; Mr. Keith Kamita, Chief of the Narcotics Enforcement Division of the Hawaii Department of Public Safety; Captain Sam Thomas of the Hawaii County Police Department; and Mr. Richard Botti, Executive Director of the Hawaii Food Industry Association.

We also welcome four witnesses whose work in the field of drug treatment and prevention is of vital importance here in Hawaii: Dr. Kevin Kunz of Kona Addiction Services; Mr. Wesley Margheim of the Big Island Substance Abuse Council; Mr. Alan Salavea of the Hawaii County Prosecutor's Office's "Youth Builders" program; and Dr. Jamal Wasan of the Lokahi Treatment Program. We thank everyone for taking the time to join us this morning, and look forward to your testimony.

Mr. CASE. Thank you very much, Mr. Chair. Good morning and aloha to all of you. It's good to be back home on my home island. Even under these difficult circumstances it's good to be here and to be with you and to address the crisis that we all face together.

I want to tell you just a little bit about what is actually going on here today. This is the U.S. House Committee on Government Reform's Subcommittee on Criminal Justice, Drug Policy and Human Resources. Now, that's a fancy way of saying that this is the subcommittee, in all subcommittees in the U.S. House, is the subcommittee responsible for criminal justice and drug policy. It's kuleana is all of our Federal Government's law enforcement efforts, especially as they deal with drugs. So we have right here the subcommittee, the place in the U.S. House that's responsible for formulating overall policy.

And it's a tremendous opportunity for us to say to the U.S. House and to the U.S. Congress and to our Federal Government both what our problems are, what our needs are, and what we offer to the rest of our country much less to our State. And it's a very great pleasure for me to introduce my colleague Congressman Mark Souder from Indiana. And I want to tell you just a little bit about him so he's more than just Mr. Chair here today.

Congressman Mark Souder was born and raised in Ft. Wayne, Indiana. He is the chair of this subcommittee so he's the guy, he's the guy that's responsible for this stuff and is going to be making decisions in conjunction with his colleagues. He still represents Indiana's great Third District, which is headquartered right around Ft. Wayne, so he's born and raised and representing exactly the district that he grew up in just like I am. He attended Notre Dame so if you want to talk football with him, I'm sure he'd be happy to do that.

He went to work in Congress just like me, caught the bug, was a business person in his other life, and he is now finishing his 10th year in the U.S. House and has been very, very involved in the drug policy. You will see that in some of his questions, some of his testimony, he knows what he's talking about. He worked in this area, he cares, he is the best that Congress has to offer to our country.

He also serves on some other committees as most of us in Congress do and he's out here working in many different hats. Congressman Souder also serves on the Natural Resources Committee. He has a special interest in our country's national parks and national wildlife, fisheries and is on those subcommittees.

Yesterday, he spent the entire day touring our national parks and national historic areas. I guess I can say this. He's going up and spending some time at Hawaii Volcanos National Park and maybe, if there's time, he's going to spend some time in the rest of our beautiful island.

He also serves on the U.S. House Select Committee on Homeland Security which is a crucial topic of discussion in Congress today, especially with the issuance of the 9/11 Commission report and the President's endorsement of many of his recommendations this morning.

So he has spent time with our military, he's spent time with homeland security. He's wearing many hats. Today he's wearing the hat trying to help us with ice. So I really want to recognize and send a very warm aloha to Congressman Souder. I do have a little present for him here and he can open it later, but it's a very nice aloha shirt to go with the one he has on right here for the remainder of his time out here in Hawaii. Thank you very much, Congressman.

I also want to recognize the ranking minority member on the subcommittee Elijah Cummings of Maryland who has demonstrated an equal interest in this and this is a bi-partisan/non-partisan effort. You know ice and other drugs don't care what party you're in. They don't care what district you represent, from whatever parties. We all work together on this.

Thank you very much, Chairman Souder.

On behalf of all of my over 600,000 constituents of Hawaii's great Second Congressional District, and for all of the people of Hawaii, I am especially pleased that my home island of Hawaii is hosting this hearing today.

We in Hawaii share many of the same concerns as others in our Nation in regard to the urgent need to support drug control, education, prevention, and treatment efforts, especially those dealing directly with the scourge of crystal methamphetamine or ice. However, our geographic isolation, not only from the contiguous United States, but also just in terms of the isolation of the "Neighbor Islands" from Oahu, as well as a number of other unique factors, not the least of which are our ethnic and cultural diversity, create unique challenges that we need to address here. So we deal with the big picture of ice with everybody else in our country, but we also deal with unique circumstances that we face right here.

Of course, general drug abuse has plagued many of our communities for decades. And to target what is needed to prevent this abuse now and in the future, we have to first understand what causes it and then focus our efforts on overcoming those causes. And uniquely, it is, in fact, up to our Federal Government to take the lead on this issue as it is the only effective entity with the resources and the scope and ability to coordinate the indispensable multi-pronged approach to stamping out drug abuse. So I commend this subcommittee for taking the lead.

Let's be clear first. We know that the roots of drug abuse lie largely where educational and economic opportunity are lacking and the social and community fabric are torn. Thus, in the big picture and long term, our best overall efforts to stamp out drug abuse lie in fixing our economies and improving our schools and strengthening our families and communities.

But where drug abuse has taken hold there are four basic causes. First, insufficient education of our young people on the danger of drugs before they start. Second, law enforcement's inability, often because of lack of resources to catch, prosecute, and lock up the worst offenders, the dealers and the manufacturers. Third, a community's lack of community-wide involvement in prevention and elimination. We cannot do this alone. It takes a community. And fourth, a lack of sufficient social local rehabilitation programs to give abusers a second chance and bring them back into society. If we do not rehabilitate abusers, keep up with them, we keep on creating the significant consequences of ice abuse.

All of this is true in spades with the drug we face most directly and critically today, ice. It is truly poisoning paradise as we know it.

Hawaii was one of the first places in our country where the drug made its appearance back in the mid 1980's so it is not a new drug here. Due to its highly addictive properties, as it is almost 90 percent pure in this form, Hawaii now has the Nation's highest rate of adults who have tried ice. There are many other statistics and they're in my testimony, but we can see the link between ice and homicides, ice and child abuse, ice and property crime. Perhaps one of the most alarming statistics is the reach of ice down to our young people.

I spent time with the police, local police, on the Island of Lanai, just three, 4 days ago. What I try to do is get out and spend time. And we were hanging out at the end of the day, talking on the front porch of the Island of Lanai's police station which is about the size of one-fifth of this room.

And basically, they said they've seen it down to 12-year-olds on the Island of Lanai. That is unbelievable.

So this scourge is an absolute top priority in Hawaii's immediate drug elimination efforts. On education, our schools and communities are increasingly focusing on working with our youth to show the devastation that ice can cause and is causing. Our law enforcement community is starting to focus much more on attacking ice dealers. All of our needs now include some elements of rehabilitation.

Most encouraging, we now see our communities standing up and saying no to ice. This is happening on all of our islands. Kahaluu on the Island of Oahu was the first community to hold ice breaker meetings, a drug response plan formed on the county of Kauai to implement a community-wide approach, the Coalition for a Drug-Free Lanai with its recent second year grant from the Office of National Drug Control Policy. Over in Wailuku on Maui, Thursday we will be visiting a fantastic effort over there to take on ice at the community level.

And here on the Big Island Mayor Kim, with his great assistant, Billy Kenoi, who is here with us today spearheaded a unique coordinated islandwide attack on ice. And we see many of our communities sign waving on Hugs Not Drugs. That's what it's going to take, but we do need much more.

The FBI and the DEA who are with us today and care very much about this need, I believe, to station a permanent agent on each of our counties on the ground where we do not have a Federal presence in order to focus Federal law enforcement efforts on ice.

With our congressional delegation, we've advocated for increased funding for the High Intensity Drug Trafficking Area which we will hear from today. The Weed and Seed Program is so successful throughout our country and through the First Congressional District. And general coordination is always welcome.

To sum up, we in Hawaii, one of the hardest hit areas of our country with this incredible ice epidemic do, in fact, face a crisis. We have the will to address it, but we need help from our Federal Government. We need more Federal law enforcement at the county and local level. We need preventative education, and we need effective rehabilitation.

Chair Souder, I thank you, again, for bringing the subcommittee here. I thank all of the witnesses for your participation. I thank the audience for your participation and for many of you in the audience, in fact, all of you for your hard work, we will, in fact, accomplish this together. Mahalo.

[The prepared statement of Hon. Ed Case follows:]

WASHINGTON OFFICE:
128 CANNON HOUSE OFFICE BUILDING
WASHINGTON, DC 20515
(202) 225-4906
FAX: (202) 225-4987
HAWAI'I OFFICE:
5104 PRINCE KUHIO FEDERAL BUILDING
HONOLULU, HI 96850-4974
(808) 541-1986
FAX: (808) 538-0233
NEIGHBOR ISLAND TOLL FREE NUMBERS:
BIG ISLAND 935-3756
KAUA'I / NI'IHAU 245-1951
MAUI 242-1818
LANA'I 565-7199
MOLOKA'I 552-0160

ed.case@mail.house.gov
www.house.gov/case

U.S. HOUSE OF REPRESENTATIVES

CONGRESSMAN ED CASE
SECOND DISTRICT, HAWAI'I
ISLANDS OF HAWAI'I, MAUI, KAHO'OLAWE, LANA'I, MOLOKA'I, O'AHU (WINDWARD, NORTH SHORE, CENTRAL, LEEWARD), KAUA'I AND NI'IHAU, AND NORTHWESTERN HAWAIIAN ISLANDS

COMMITTEES:
EDUCATION AND THE WORKFORCE
EDUCATION REFORM
EMPLOYER-EMPLOYEE RELATIONS
AGRICULTURE
CONSERVATION, CREDIT, RURAL DEVELOPMENT AND RESEARCH
GENERAL FARM COMMODITIES AND RISK MANAGEMENT
SMALL BUSINESS
RURAL ENTERPRISES, AGRICULTURE AND TECHNOLOGY
WORKFORCE EMPOWERMENT AND GOVERNMENT PROGRAMS
REGULATORY REFORM AND OVERSIGHT

THE POISONING OF PARADISE: CRYSTAL METHAMPHETAMINE IN HAWAI'I

TESTIMONY OF CONGRESSMAN ED CASE
BEFORE THE HOUSE GOVERNMENT REFORM COMMITTEE
SUBCOMMITTEE ON CRIMINAL JUSTICE, DRUG POLICY, AND HUMAN RESOURCES

August 2, 2004

Chairman Souder, Ranking Member Cummings, and members of this Subcommittee, good morning and aloha! On behalf of all of my over 600,000 constituents of Hawai'i's great Second Congressional District, and for all of the people of Hawai'i, I would like to welcome you to our great Aloha State. I am especially pleased that my home island, the Big Island of Hawai'i, is hosting this hearing today.

We in Hawai'i share many of the same concerns as others in our nation in regard to the urgent need to support drug control, education, prevention, and treatment efforts, especially those targeted at the spreading scourge of crystal methamphetamine, or "ice." However, our geographic isolation, not only from the contiguous United States, but also just from these "Neighbor Islands," which comprise the bulk of the 2nd District, to the Island of O'ahu, our urban center, as well as a host of other unique factors like our ethnic and cultural diversity, create equally unique needs and solutions as we all work to wipe out ice.

General drug abuse, of course, has plagued many of our communities for decades. To target what is needed to prevent this abuse now and in the future, we must first understand what causes it and then focus our efforts on overcoming those causes. And uniquely, it is up to our federal government to take the lead on the issue as it is the only entity with the resources and ability to coordinate the indispensable multi-pronged approach to stamping out drug abuse. I commend Chairman Souder and Ranking Member Cummings for your leadership on this issue.

First, let's be clear. We know that the roots of drug abuse lie largely where educational and economic opportunity are lacking and the social and community fabric are torn. Thus, in the big picture and long term, our best efforts to stamp out drug abuse lie in fixing our economies, improving our schools, and strengthening our families and communities.

But where drug abuse has taken hold, there are four basic causes. The first is insufficient education of our young people on the danger of drugs before they start. The second is law enforcement's inability, usually because of lack of resources, to catch, prosecute, and lock up the worst offenders, mainly the dealers. The third is a community's lack of community-wide involvement in prevention and elimination. The fourth is a lack of sufficient local rehabilitation programs to give abusers a second chance and bring them back into society.

All of this is true in spades with the drug we face most directly and critically today: ice. It is truly poisoning paradise as we know it.

Hawai'i was one of the first places in our country where the drug made its appearance; ice began arriving in Hawai'i in large amounts in 1985. Due to its highly addictive properties, as it is almost 90% pure in this form, Hawai'i now has the nation's highest rate of adults who have tried ice.

Deaths in Hawai'i attributed to ice have almost doubled in two years. In our state, 44% of the homicides and 90% of the child abuse cases are reportedly related to drug abuse, including in particular ice. Property crime rates have also experienced similar increases. The saddest and most alarming statistics are from the year 2000, when 6% of 12th graders, 5% of 10th graders, 2% of 8th graders, and 1% of 6th graders reported that they have tried a form of methamphetamine at least once. These same trends and experiences of our state are now spreading throughout our nation.

The scourge of ice is an absolute top priority in Hawai'i's immediate drug elimination efforts. On education, our schools and communities are increasingly focusing on working with our youth to show the devastation that ice can cause and is causing. Our law enforcement community is starting to focus much more on attacking ice dealers. All of our needs now include some elements of rehabilitation.

Most encouraging, whole communities are rising up across our state to say: yes, ice is our problem, and we must all be part of the solution. Kahalu'u on the Island of O'ahu was the first community to hold "ice breaker" meetings and start sign-waving efforts. After holding five regional drug summits, a drug response plan has been formulated for communities on the Island of Kaua'i with the goal of reducing drug use over the next two years. The Coalition for a Drug-Free Lana'i recently received its second-year grant from the Office of National Drug Control Policy and will continue its work to enhance public awareness, train teachers to lead drug-free programs, and increase the number of students enrolled in drug prevention classes. This Thursday, we will be visiting Ka Hale A Ke Ola Homeless Resource Center in Wailuku on Maui to discuss and review its successful chemical dependency program.

Here, on the Big Island of Hawai'i, Mayor Kim, together with his great assistant, Billy Kenoi, who is here with us today, have spearheaded a unique coordinated islandwide attack on ice that continues to this day. In our communities, several islandwide "Hugs Not Drugs" sign-waving campaigns have been held with over one thousand citizens from twenty-three communities and neighborhoods participating in the very first event alone.

But so much more needs to be done to support these community efforts. I believe that the Federal Bureau of Investigation and Drug Enforcement Administration need to station a permanent agent on each island that currently does not have a federal presence in order to focus federal law enforcement efforts and assist in coordination with county law enforcement agencies.

I have worked with the members of our Congressional delegation to advocate for an increase in funding for the High Intensity Drug Trafficking Area program in Hawai'i in order to expand its current jurisdiction and support its effective programs. I have also testified before the Commerce-Justice-State Appropriations Subcommittee to highlight the importance of increased funding for the successful Weed and Seed Program, which has benefited many of our troubled communities and needs funding for sustainability and expansion. And general coordination efforts, which are indispensable, are severely underfunded.

In closing, Mr. Chairman, I want to reiterate my full-fledged support and the support of our state for the campaign to end drug abuse, and in particular to address the ice epidemic in Hawai'i. Many of Hawai'i's political leaders and members of our law enforcement community have long worked on this issue, and we will hear from many of these individuals today, but additional federal resources and support are needed in this fight so we can overcome the plague of ice and work to eliminate the abuse of other harmful drugs as well.

Mahalo, Mr. Chairman; we all truly appreciate your willingness to understand firsthand the unique challenges we face, to hear of our efforts to keep drugs out of our homes and communities, and to see our successes in our fight against the scourge of ice. I look forward to continuing to work with you on this issue of critical importance to individuals, families and communities across our nation.

###

Mr. SOUDER. Let me explain a little bit about the process of how we do our hearings. As Congressman Case mentioned, this is a part of the Government Reform Oversight, which is historically what's known as the Oversight Committee. We've changed the name of the reform because when we do oversight, it isn't just to have a hearing. It's trying to figure out what we're going to change in the administrative capacity.

What's unusual about this subcommittee is we also have authorization over narcotics issues including the Drug Czar's office, and so we need both legislative and oversight and also share the speakers drug task force.

Each witness will have 5 minutes.

We have a light that's supposed to work that will be green for four, yellow for one, red a little more generous, meaning another 60 seconds to a few minutes, if your statement doesn't work within the 5 minutes. It gives us a chance to ask questions, get some interaction.

Each witness, as you'll hear when we go through the procedures, has the ability to submit additional information. We want anything you make a reference to to get into the hearing record because ultimately this will be a hearing book. And in the process of doing this, there is a series of hearings in Washington and California and other places over the last couple years.

People can look through it and say, OK, how are they tackling the meth issue and what information is there. So if you refer to something, it will be good to get a copy of it later to put into the hearing record. Also, we may submit additional questions as we review it and as we look at some things to you to put into the hearing record. If any individuals have something they want to submit, either submit to our staff here today or Congressman Case's office, we can get that into the record as well.

Let me first go to procedural matters. I ask consent that all Members have 5 legislative days to submit written statements and questions to the hearing director. Any answers to written questions provided by the witnesses are also included in the record. No objections, so ordered.

Second, I ask that all Members present be permitted to participate in the hearing. Without objection, so ordered. Now, because we're an oversight committee, the oversight being Congress, we're the only one that actually swears in its witnesses. Historically, we haven't had to do much with that, but we had a few hearings where, in fact, we did.

This committee has heard everything from Whitewater to China investigations to Waco to all of those kind of things, and it's important that each witness understands that it's not just testifying, this is actually oversight to see the laws are there so we swear in each witness. So if you would each raise your right hand.

[Witnesses sworn.]

Mr. SOUDER. Let the record show that each of the witnesses responded in the affirmative. We appreciate your willingness to come and we're going to start with the distinguished Lieutenant Governor of Hawaii, the Honorable James Aiona, and we appreciate your long-time leadership.

STATEMENT OF JAMES R. "DUKE" AIONA, LIEUTENANT GOVERNOR, STATE OF HAWAII

Mr. AIONA. Thank you, Chairman Souder, and of course, Congressman Case for this opportunity to address you on this matter. I have submitted testimony in this case and if you don't mind, I'm going to supplement that. I'm not going to read my testimony. I'm going to supplement it.

I do want to give you a little perspective, and for the record, my background, so you'll understand where I'm coming from when I make my comments.

First of all, I'm a father of four children. My oldest is 21, my youngest is 12. I've been a coach in the community, both on the high school level and on the youth level for the past 20, 25 years.

I was a prosecutor when I first came out of law school in 1980 and I was a prosecutor in the career criminal unit for about 3 years. I then went to the city Attorney's Office. Then in 1990 I was appointed to the Family Court bench and served for about 2½ years, was elevated to the Circuit Court bench and served on the criminal calendar for about 4 years and about 1½ to 2 years of that I was the first administrative judge to the Drug Court Program here in Hawaii.

I then went back to Family Court and I've been a lifelong resident, except for my studies up in Stockton, California, for all of my life. So I think I understand the community and where we're at at this point in time in regards to this problem methamphetamine.

When I was a prosecutor in 1980, methamphetamine was first making its move into the island, so to speak, in a powder form known as crank. And subsequently, it has now materialized into what we now call ice or "batu" and there are many names for its form right now.

But what I have seen is I have seen the proliferation of it, not only in the courtroom, but also in the community, I think, simply, because of a couple of things.

First and foremost in the 1980's when cocaine was the No. 1 drug of choice in Hawaii, 1970's and 1980's, we saw what law enforcement did in choking off the supply, not necessarily arresting people and putting them in jail and making that a deterrent, but basically attacking the supply. And it really choked it out to a significant degree. And this same high that people had been getting in cocaine they were now seeing it happen in methamphetamine and I saw the proliferation happen.

I think as a result of the fact that methamphetamine is something that's manufactured, it's very difficult to eradicate simply by attacking the supply. So as such, what I've seen in the courtroom has been devastating. As you stated and as Congressman Case stated, we've seen the devastation of families and children and everything else that could possibly happen.

I think it all lined up in the stars for me. It was truly God's blessing that I was elected to this office and as such Governor Lingle has charged me with the task of addressing this issue. And as such what we did repeatedly was we went out to the communities to get their input. And what really happened with that was basically two-fold. At that point in time when we got elected back in 2002, I think the community at that point in time had really seen enough of what was happening with methamphetamine.

So the level of awareness and making it known to everyone in the community had risen to, I would say, beyond belief. And we had community meetings, as Congressman Case noted, in certain communities where they would go out and wave signs, they had rallies, etc., just kind of slow hauled to approaching the whole island.

So we went out to the community, the administration did, in talk story events such as this, and just got feedback from them. And then in September last year we had for the first time ever what we called a Drug Summit in which we brought as many participants as possible in the provider field, in law enforcement, in the community, etc., to basically come up with some recommendations that they felt were needed. And we adopted at that point in time a drug control strategy which basically is similar to the national policy which is prevention and intervention. So we basically adopted that, we got the recommendations from the community and right now we are in the middle of our working groups, we're calling them ad hoc committees, in which they are developing action plans for the prevention, for treatment, for law enforcement, for what we call community mobilization and also a coordinating branch.

Now, that's very important because probably the biggest feedback we got from the community was the fact that there was a lack of collaboration and coordination amongst our various, not only State agencies but also our Federal agencies. People were duplicating services, there were gaps in the services, money was being ineffectively used and deficiently used. And so as such a big recommendation was to have some kind of coordinating committee or person to deal with all of these issues. And we did that in January of this year by appointing what we've called a drug liaison in the Lt. Governor's office.

So we are on the verge right now of basically bringing together all of the people I had mentioned, the ad hoc committees, with their—what we're calling, their action plans and having them submitted to us for implementation.

I would also note that what had happened is we've stepped up our efforts with regards to youth programs. We've stepped up our efforts with our underage drinking because we really believe that leads to it. We've stepped up our efforts in regards to educating not only our children but also the public.

I think you're going to hear testimony of how our Narcotics Enforcement Division has gone out and educated a lot of people in regards to the meth labs and the effect that it has and the harm it has done in the community. And so what we've done is we've really brought it out.

I've been fortunate to be appointed to the National Advisory Committee of SAMHSA, which you well know has been a great partner with us. They have provided technical assistance at almost every request that we've made, whether it be in grants, whether it be in setting up these ad hoc committees that we've now set up. During our Summit they've given us some support in regards to educating our public with meth labs and I can't say enough what SAMHSA has done for us.

I do want to put a plug in, though, for something that is a tremendous breakthrough in regards to treatment; and that is this new initiative called Access to Recovery. I know that the Bush administration had requested about $200,000,000 and Congress had only appropriated $100,000,000. Nevertheless, I think it's something that needs to be looked at very carefully. I can see nothing but good things coming out of it, and I really hope that Congress when that budget comes up again, that they will give them a real hard look and really support that effort.

If you talk to the people in the community, people in the profession, I should say, they're going to tell you that Access to Recovery really is revolutionary in regards to what it's going to do and what SAMHSA is doing. SAMHSA is, and I agree wholeheartedly with what they're doing, they are now basically going out and coordinating with the States, going from the executive office, and not putting money out there for various treatment programs, but more or less building systems, working the interagency relationships between service providers, nonprofits and then, of course, on the law enforcement side working it that route.

At our last council meeting we found out that they have now partnered with various branches within the Federal Government which would includes ONDCP, Justice, Department of Health and Human Services.

I know I've gone over my time, I thank you very much, and, of course, I'm open for questions.

[The prepared statement of Mr. Aiona follows:]

OFFICE OF THE LIEUTENANT GOVERNOR
State Capitol, Fifth Floor
Honolulu, Hawaii 96813
Phone: (808)586-0255
Fax: (808)586-0231
email: ltgov@hawaii.gov
www.hawaii.gov/ltgov

JAMES R. AIONA, JR.
LIEUTENANT GOVERNOR

Statement of
JAMES R. AIONA, JR.
Lieutenant Governor
State of Hawaii

Before the

U. S. House Committee on Government Reform
Subcommittee on Criminal Justice, Drug Policy and Human Resources
"The Poisoning of Paradise: Crystal Methamphetamine in Hawaii"

Chairman Souder and distinguished members of the Subcommittee, thank you for allowing me to testify on the pervasive problem of substance abuse in Hawaii.

For many people, Hawaii conjures up images of a tropical paradise with pristine beaches, beautiful flowers, and warm, friendly people. While the beauty of our State is indisputable, we are not immune to the devastation caused by the use and abuse of illegal substances.

Crystal methamphetamine or "ice" is the most abused illicit drug in the State of Hawaii, and Hawaii tops the nation in ice use. Hawaii users prefer the higher purity of imported smokable ice. This highly addictive, intense stimulant has reached epidemic proportions with devastating impact on families, communities, and the fabric of life in the islands. Its effects are seen in increased drug arrests, treatment admissions, child abuse reports, domestic violence, prison admissions, and health care costs. Ice and other illicit substances pose a tremendous burden on our economy with increasing challenges for federal, state, and local government, and most importantly, on our communities.

You will hear representatives from the law enforcement community testifying about the quantities of drugs seized, and the number of people arrested for drug-related crimes. You will also hear about the relationship between substance abuse and the State's inordinately high property crime rate and the relationship between substance abuse and violence. Mr. Keith Kamita of the Department of Public Safety's Narcotics Enforcement Division will brief you on Hawaii's experience with clandestine drug laboratories. Moreover, you will hear about the substantial disruption that substance abuse has on our families, communities, and the workplace.

Although attempts have been made to address the problem, all too often organizations worked within their own boundaries. Despite the best efforts of the individual entities, the abuse of illegal substances, in particular crystal methamphetamine, escalated.

To draw on the wisdom of our citizens, I have listened to their concerns and ideas during 13 community forums held throughout the State last summer, during a September 2003 youth summit held in collaboration with Mothers Against Drunk Driving, the Coalition for a Drug-Free Hawaii, and the Department of Health, and at the first statewide drug summit in September 2003.

Family breakdown and family violence, drug houses, and drug dealing were identified as primary concerns for communities. These same communities believed that more organized youth activities and community action groups were necessary to reduce illicit substance use and underage drinking. Youth summit participants echoed similar preventive measures: implement more youth activities in the community and schools, develop recreational centers, and create a cutting-edge media campaign aimed at youth.

What else can we in Hawaii do to change the drug statistics and lives of families devastated by substance abuse?

Participants at the drug summit unequivocally called for better coordination in the delivery of services in order to avoid duplication and to maximize resources. To address the problem in its totality, partnerships, including federal partnerships, are critical. Most importantly, the drug summit attendees felt that communities must be equal partners in designing, developing, and deciding on strategies.

Because no community has all the answers, however, we often look to our federal partners for direction, guidance, and resources. One example of a successful partnership between Hawaii and the federal government is the High Intensity Drug Trafficking Area program, which has mobilized county, state, and federal law enforcement agencies to collectively disrupt the distribution of drugs into, within, and out of Hawaii. Another welcome partner is the Substance Abuse and Mental Health Administration (SAMHSA), whose vision of "a life in the community for everyone" is being fulfilled by building resilience and facilitating recovery.

We concur with SAMHSA's direction of engaging in immediate and long-term strategies to address the highly complex issues surrounding substance and alcohol abuse. With assistance from SAMHSA, the State is currently undergoing an action planning process with key partners to focus on issues surrounding prevention, treatment, community mobilization, legal changes, and collaboration. It is intended that the plan, which will guide our efforts in the years to come, be flexible and ever-evolving to be responsive to various circumstances and opportunities.

I commend the Subcommittee on Criminal Justice, Drug Policy and Human Resources for focusing attention on this problem and for venturing across the continent to hear about Hawaii's experience. I appreciate the opportunity to provide a brief overview of the approach that the State is taking to ensure the health and safety of the citizens of Hawaii. As we seek a comprehensive yet balanced approach to dealing with not only crystal methamphetamine but all illegal substances and underage drinking, we look forward to working collaboratively with our federal partners.

Mr. SOUDER. Thank you. Second witness will be Mr. Burnett, head of the HIDTA Hawaii.

STATEMENT OF LARRY D. BURNETT, DIRECTOR, HAWAII HIGH INTENSITY DRUG TRAFFICKING AREA

Mr. BURNETT. Chairman Souder, I would like to take this opportunity to recognize you and Congressman Case for your outstanding work in the area of drug law enforcement. As HIDTA director, I've had the opportunity to work with you and your staffs on drug issues, both, domestically and internationally.

You're untiring efforts are greatly appreciated.

The commitment of Congressman Case to the methamphetamine epidemic in Hawaii is evident today by holding this hearing in your home State. Congratulations.

Mr. Chairman, as I mentioned in my written statement, the State of Hawaii and U.S. territories of the Pacific are currently under attack from crystal methamphetamine, commonly called ice. The rampant abuse of crystal methamphetamine along with the violence and dangers associated with the drug is the single most significant drug problem affecting the State. That's a point that cannot be overemphasized.

As you're aware, based on the crystal methamphetamine epidemic and other criteria, Hawaii was designated a HIDTA in 1999. HIDTA designation brings with it and it provides a catalyst for genuine coordination and cooperation among Hawaii's law enforcement community. Resources donated by participating agencies are formed into investigation and interdiction strike forces, intelligence gathering groups, and support initiatives. By sharing strategic and tactical information, the Hawaii HIDTA provides a comprehensive response to illicit drug activity by bringing together all available law enforcement resources in a united front.

For our purposes here today Hawaii's drug abuse problem can be categorized probably in three tiers and that's how HIDTA looks at it. In the first tier are the two drugs that are causing the most serious problems, that's crystal methamphetamine and marijuana. Arrest and seizure data for both these drugs indicate that availability is high. Demand data suggests that use of both drugs, along with the consequences of that use, is high and increasing.

The second-tier drugs are cocaine, which is usually crack cocaine here, and heroin.

Cocaine-related arrests and seizures are on an upswing but demand data suggests the opposite, the declining prevalence and consequences of use. At the same time heroin distribution and abuse appears to be diminishing as indicated by the declines in arrests, seizures, and reports that we see.

And the third tier are drugs such as MDMA, GHB, steroids, ecstasy, and diverted pharmaceuticals. They are available and abused in Hawaii but to a much lesser extent. The focus of third-tier drugs appears to be among young party club goers and the younger members of our military.

Hawaii is both a destination and transiting point for the West Coast, the mainland United States, Canada, Mexico, and Asia. Hawaii is also a source of high potency marijuana to the U.S. mainland, Canada, and, even to a lesser extent, for Mexico.

International and local drug trafficking organizations have ample opportunity to traffic drugs to, through, and from the area because of Hawaii's high volume of international and domestic air and sea traffic. The Hawaii HIDTA's primary goal is to disrupt and dismantle these organizations.

For fiscal year 2005 law enforcement organizations will contribute a total of 311 full- and part-time law enforcement personnel to this effort. I would also like to comment that regrettably there remain at this time legal and legislative barriers that sometimes impede the ability of law enforcement to effectively combat the drug problem. For example, evidence obtained from Federal wiretap and consensual encounters remain, at this time, inadmissible in Hawaii courts, in the State courts. As a result many lower level drug distributors who do not meet Federal guidelines, they go unprosecuted in the State system. It is not uncommon to find individuals with 30-plus arrests still free on the streets.

Our outlook, I think you will find that coordination and cooperation among Hawaii's law enforcement agencies is at an all time high. Hawaii remains a target rich environment. We believe the maritime seizures of illicit drugs will increase with the implementation of the Maritime Transportation Security Act. And although its primary purpose is to counter terrorism, it will have a fall-out effect on the drugs.

We are hopeful that proposed legislation will be enacted to bring State wiretap laws into line with the rest of the country. The Hawaii HIDTA's and its participating member agencies will continue to devote resources to identify, investigate, disrupt, and dismantle the organizations responsible for the spread of methamphetamine across Hawaii and our country.

Thank you for this opportunity to testify before the subcommittee. I will be happy to answer questions at the appropriate time.

[The prepared statement of Mr. Burnett follows:]

Statement of
Larry D. Burnett – Director
Hawaii High Intensity Drug Trafficking Area

Before the

House Committee on Government Reform
Subcommittee on Criminal Justice, Drug Policy
and Human Resources

August 2, 2004

"The Poisoning of Paradise: Crystal Methamphetamine in Hawaii"

Executive Summary

The state of Hawaii and U.S. Territories of the Pacific are currently under attack from crystal methamphetamine, commonly called "ICE".[i] The rampant abuse of crystal methamphetamine, along with the violence and dangers associated with the drug, is the single most significant drug problem afflicting the state, *a point that cannot be overemphasized.* This problem, which threatens the well-being of Hawaii's citizens and challenges its law enforcement personnel, could not have reached such epidemic proportions if not for the constant pressure of Drug Traffickers supplying crystal methamphetamine, as well as other illicit drugs, to the region. This constant pressure fuels a market that generates larceny, theft, burglary, homicides, domestic abuse, and child endangerment.

To this end, based on the crystal methamphetamine epidemic and other criteria, Hawaii was designated a High Intensity Drug Trafficking Area (HIDTA) in 1999: "....to prioritize and focus national and local resources on Hawaii's regional drug threats."

HIDTA designation provides a catalyst for genuine law enforcement partnership, coordination, and cooperation among Hawaii's counterdrug stakeholders. The Hawaii HIDTA functions through an Executive Board comprised of an equal number of (8) federal and (8) state/local law enforcement **agency heads that have decision-making authority for the department or agency.** This Executive Board provides direction and oversight. Membership is selected based on an agency's committed resources and ability to have an effect on the regional drug threat. Three additional non-voting members provide an advisory function. The Chair and Vice-Chair alternate between state/local and federal law enforcement each year. The Executive Board provides a coordination umbrella for HIDTA task forces, the Investigative Support and Intelligence Center (ISC), and any single-agency task forces and narcotics units operating within the Hawaii HIDTA region.

By design, significant effort is made to collocate and commingle Hawaii HIDTA personnel and resources. These resources, donated by participating agencies, are formed into Task/Strike Forces, Interdiction Groups, Intelligence Gathering Subsystems, and Support/Administrative Initiatives.

By fostering interagency cooperation and sharing of strategic and tactical information, the Hawaii HIDTA provides a comprehensive response to illicit drug activity by bringing together all available law enforcement resources in a united front. Success of the Hawaii HIDTA is measured in part by its ability to facilitate greater efficiency, effectiveness and cooperation among external participating agencies, thereby yielding tangible, measurable results. This goal is supported by intelligence driven drug task forces aimed at eliminating or reducing domestic drug trafficking and its harmful consequences, through enhancement and coordination of drug trafficking control efforts among federal, state and local law enforcement agencies.

Introduction

High Intensity Drug Trafficking Areas (HIDTA) are regions in the country that have severe drug trafficking problems. HIDTA's receive their designation from the Executive Office of the President through the Office of National Drug Control Policy (ONDCP). The Anti-Drug Abuse Act of 1988 (P. L. 100-690), and the ONDCP Re-authorization Act of 1998 (P.L. 105-277) empower the Director of ONDCP, upon consultation with the Attorney General, Secretary of the Treasury, heads of national drug control agencies, and the Governor of each applicable state, to designate any specified area of the United States as a HIDTA.

Geographic Area of Responsibility:

State of Hawaii- Hawaii, Honolulu, Kauai & Maui counties

Mission Statement:

As the crossroad of the Pacific and gateway into the continental United States, the Hawaii HIDTA's participating agencies work together through enhanced coordination and integrated initiatives to disrupt and dismantle illicit drug distribution, production, money laundering, transportation, & trafficking within the region.

The Hawaii HIDTA is a partnership between Federal, State, and Local Law Enforcement that consists of the following member agencies:

Bureau of Alcohol, Tobacco and Firearms
City and County of Honolulu Prosecutor
Drug Enforcement Administration
Federal Bureau of Investigation
Hawaii National Guard
Hawaii County Police Department
Hawaii State Department Public Safety
Honolulu Police Department
Immigration and Customs Enforcement
Internal Revenue Service
Kauai Police Department
Maui Police Department
U. S. Attorney's Office
U. S. Marshal's Service
U. S. Postal Inspection Service
Western States Information Network
Bureau of Prisons*
U. S. Coast Guard*
Naval Criminal Investigative Service*

(* indicates advisory non-voting Executive Board members.)

Threat

Hawaii and the U.S. Territories of the Pacific are beset with a myriad of illicit drug challenges. Illegal use and trafficking of crystal methamphetamine, commonly referred to as ICE, has reached epidemic proportions straining resources to the breaking point. State Legislators are holding hearings to explore the problem. The Governor and Lieutenant Governor crisscrossed the state in a series of town hall meetings. Communities fed up with the problems, violence, and crime associated with crystal methamphetamine addiction waved signs and demonstrated.

A multitude of illicit drugs are available to varying degrees in Hawaii, as in any populated area; however, these drugs can be categorized in three tiers based on the severity of the problems they pose to Hawaii's law enforcement and citizens.

1. In the first tier are the two drugs causing the most serious problems—crystal methamphetamine and marijuana. Arrest and seizure data for both these drugs indicate that availability is high. Demand data suggest that use of both drugs, along with the consequences of that use, is high and increasing.

Nonetheless, the magnitude of the crystal methamphetamine problem in Hawaii—a far more socially disruptive problem—overshadows marijuana, which has seen an increase in associated violence, but not nearly to the same extent.

2. The second-tier drugs are cocaine (usually crack cocaine) and heroin which, although they remain problems in Hawaii, appear to rank well behind crystal methamphetamine and marijuana in contributing to the state's drug troubles. Cocaine-related arrests and seizures are on an upswing, but demand data suggest declining prevalence and consequences of use. At the same time, heroin distribution and abuse appear to be diminishing in light of indicators suggesting declines in arrests, seizures, reported use, and treatment.

3. In the third tier are drugs such as MDMA, GHB, steroids, and diverted pharmaceuticals, which are available and abused in Hawaii but to a much lesser extent. The focus of third tier drugs appears to be among young club goers and younger members of the military. While it is imperative to continue combating these drugs and thus preventing them from becoming a larger problem in the future, it is the trafficking and abuse of primarily crystal methamphetamine as well as marijuana, cocaine, and heroin that currently pose the most viable drug threats to Hawaii.

International and local DTOs have ample opportunity to traffic drugs to, through, and from the area because of Hawaii's high volume of international and domestic air and sea traffic including passengers, cargo, and mail. Hawaii is a destination for crystal methamphetamine, cocaine, and heroin supplied from the West Coast and Mexico by Mexican Consolidated Priority Organization Targets (CPOTs) and DTOs; for crystal methamphetamine and heroin transported from Asia, Canada, and the West Coast by Asian DTOs; and for marijuana transported from Canada and the Pacific Northwest by local DTOs. Hawaii is a trans-shipment point for methamphetamine transported from the West Coast to locations in the Pacific Basin, such as Guam, by local DTOs supplied by Mexican DTOs. It also is a transshipment point for methamphetamine transported from the West Coast or Asia to locations in the Pacific Basin by Asian DTOs. Finally, Hawaii is the source of high potency marijuana transported to the U.S. mainland, Canada and, to a lesser extent, Mexico by local DTOs.

In addition to the threat posed by the presence of international and local DTOs, drug fugitives, armed violent drug offenders smuggling, money laundering, and the use of public lands for cannabis cultivation plague the counties. Because of the way Hawaii's drug laws are written, a significant number of drug traffickers are identified but not prosecuted.

Strategy

The Hawaii HIDTA's primary goal is to dismantle, disrupt, arrest, and prosecute drug trafficking organizations, drug gangs and organized crime groups involved in drug distribution, drug manufacturing, money laundering, and other drug related crimes. The team and task force concepts advance the National Drug Control Strategy and the National Gang Strategy, emphasize collocated/commingled, multi-agency investigations, and promote cooperative efforts among HIDTA participants.

The process utilized by the Executive Board to develop a counter strategy to illicit drug trafficking and abuse includes:

1) Identifying primary threats by geographic area;

2) Developing desired goals to counter the threats;

3) Assigning responsibility to accomplish the desired goals;

4) Evaluating effectiveness of the program's outcomes;

5) Providing oversight and implementing changes as necessary.

The Hawaii HIDTA strategy has each subsystem, intelligence/operational initiative, task force, and support group target one or more of the identified threats and needs that are listed in the current Hawaii HIDTA Threat Assessment Matrix. For FY2005 law enforcement organizations will contribute a total of 311 (full and/or part time) law enforcement personnel and support staff, organized into 12 initiatives. Two additional far reaching initiatives will be implemented should supplemental funding become available.

Each HIDTA initiative develops a mission statement to focus their efforts on one or more of the goals, which are designed to reduce drug availability and its harmful consequences. The initiatives work to accomplish these goals through a clearly defined strategy fostered by examination of the region's threats and needs.

Results

Through its initiatives the Hawaii HIDTA and its participating agencies are disrupting and dismantling the DTOs responsible for trafficking illicit drugs in Hawaii through the interdiction of crystal methamphetamine, marijuana, cocaine, heroin, and other illicit drugs as they are transported throughout the state and region. The Hawaii HIDTA is also disrupting these DTOs by seizing the money they use to operate and the assets they acquire with illicit drug proceeds.

The Hawaii HIDTA and its federal and state/local law enforcement partners are removing weapons from the street and bringing drug offenders and fugitives to justice in its effort to cripple the drug trade and reduce drug-related crime in Hawaii. The future impact of Hawaii HIDTA initiatives will be measured in the continuing and increasing seizures of illicit drugs and proceeds as well as the arrests and successful prosecutions of those responsible for transporting drugs and drug proceeds through Hawaii's airports, parcel facilities, and ports.

The investigative subsystem consists of eight investigative groups, two interdiction groups, one fugitive task force, and one safe neighborhoods strike force. The investigative task forces are most closely aligned with law enforcement goals of impacting the crime rate through arrests, seizures, and reducing drug availability.

COMBINED HAWAII HIDTA GOALS	Investigation Results - Operations	Goal	Actual	%
	TARGET DRUG DISTRIBUTION ORGANIZATIONS AND DISMANTLE OR DISRUPT THOSE TARGETED	10	34	340%
	TARGET DRUG MANUFACTURING ORGANIZATIONS AND DISMANTLE OR DISRUPT THOSE TARGETED	4	4	100%
	CLEAR WARRANTS FOR DRUG CHARGES	100	290	290%
	ARREST ARMED VIOLENT OFFENDERS WITH A NARCOTICS NEXUS	45	95	211%
	ARREST INDIVIDUALS WHO SMUGGLE NARCOTICS THROUGH AIRPORTS	50	47	94%
	INSPECT PARCELS	1000	10,000	1000%
	SEIZE PARCELS	100	60	60%
	TARGET DTOs FOR MONEY LAUNDERING CHARGES	1	1	100%
	SEIZE ILLICIT DRUG RELATED ASSETS	$1,000,000	2,510,906	251%
	ERADICATE MARIJUANA PLANTS	50,000	392,276	784.5%
	SEIZE FIREARMS	110	162	147.2%
	CLEAR WARRANTS FOR DRUG CHARGES	100	290	290%
	FORFEIT $1,000,000 IN ILLICIT DRUG RELATED ASSETS	$1,000,000	$1,237,740	123.7%

Section 3 HIDTA Matrix – consolidated goals and outcomes for all Investigative Initiatives

COMBINED HAWAII HIDTA GOALS	Coordination Results	Goal	Actual	%
	ACHIEVE AND MAINTAIN 100% PARTICIPATION BY LAW ENFORCEMENT AGENCIES IN THE WSIN DECONFLICTION SERVICES	100%	100%	100%
	SUBMIT CASE/SUBJECT DECONFLICTIONS AMONG HIDTA INITIATIVES AND PARTICIPATING AGENCIES	9000	9393	104.3%
	SUBMIT EVENT DECONFLICTIONS AMONG HIDTA INITIATIVES AND PARTICIPATING AGENCIES	1400	1333	95.2%

Section 3 HIDTA Matrix- consolidated goals and outcomes for Oversight and Support Initiatives

COMBINED HAWAII HIDTA GOALS	Intelligence Results	Goal	Actual	%
	ACHIEVE AND MAINTAIN 100% PARTICIPATION BY LAW ENFORCEMENT AGENCIES IN THE WSIN DECONFLICTION SERVICES	100%	100%	100%
	SUBMIT CASE/SUBJECT DECONFLICTIONS AMONG HIDTA INITIATIVES AND PARTICIPATING AGENCIES	9000	9393	104.3%
	ISC TO CONDUCT DATABASE QUERIES	4000	3202	80%
	ISC TO PROVIDE INTELLIGENCE PROFILES	100	390	390%
	COMPLETE REQUESTS FOR CASE ASSISTANCE	20	24	120%
	PROVIDE ANALYTICAL PRODUCTS (TOLL ANALYSES, LINK ANALYSES, GRAPHS, CHARTS, PROFILES, ETC)	3,000	4030	134.3%
	DEVELOP AN ACTIVE MEANS OF COMMUNICATING WITH PACIFIC BASIN/RIM LAW ENFORCEMENT	100%	25%	25%
	PROVIDE ELECTRONIC LINK FROM ISC TO NEIGHBOR ISLANDS VIA WSIN SECURE INTRANET	100%	100%	100%
	SHARE INTELLIGENCE WITH HIDTAS/LEAS OUTSIDE OF HAWAII	*	*	*

Section 3 HIDTA Matrix – consolidated goals and outcomes for Intelligence Initiatives

Barriers to Effective Prosecution

Regrettably, there remain, at this time, legal and legislative barriers to the effective prosecution of drug offenders in Hawaii.

Hawaii state law sometimes impedes the ability of law enforcement to effectively combat drug offenders. For example, evidence obtained from federal wiretap and consensual encounters remain, at this time, inadmissible in Hawaii state courts. While evidence found during a federal investigation can be used in federal court, federal thresholds for drug possession are higher than at the state level, and arrested offenders not meeting federal thresholds are released without prosecution. As a result, many lower level drug distributors who do not meet federal thresholds go unprosecuted in state courts. It is not uncommon to find individuals with 30-plus arrests still free on city streets in Hawaii.

Two of the larger barriers to effective prosecution of drug offenders in the state involve the (1) "challenger provision" to Hawaii's electronic surveillance law and (2) the state law governing consensual encounters.

The challenger provision, which is not in federal statutes, requires that an in-camera adversarial hearing be held before a judge. A defense attorney is appointed to the hearing and is provided with the application for the wiretap as well as all supporting documents. Moreover, at the hearing, the defense attorney has the right to cross-examine all witnesses. The requirements for dissemination of information regarding potential targets, witnesses, and evidence create many problems for local law enforcement. This not only increases the risk that the target of an investigation will find out about the investigation but also increases the potential danger to any informants and witnesses.

Consensual encounters commonly referred to as "walk and talks," are not permited under the Hawaii State Constitution. In 1996 the Hawaii Supreme Court ruled that simply approaching someone in the airport violated the state constitution. Even if an investigator informs the person being approached that a drug investigation is being conducted, that he or she is talking to a police officer, and that he or she is free to leave at any time, that person cannot be prosecuted in Hawaii courts for any drugs discovered.

Despite the state law governing consensual encounters, they are conducted at Hawaii airports because local law enforcement officers are cross-designated with federal authority to conduct such encounters. Unfortunately, any evidence of an offense discovered through this technique can be used only in a federal court—evidence obtained from federal consensual encounters is inadmissible in Hawaii courts.

Outlook

Coordination and cooperation among Hawaii's law enforcement agencies is at an all time high. We believe in the integration of neighborhood activism, education/prevention, and effective treatment in our overall strategy. Recognition of the dangers crystal methamphetamine poses to public health and safety has caused many in Hawaii to realize that reducing the problems associated with crystal methamphetamine and other illicit drugs requires action by all members of our communities.

Hawaii remains a target rich environment. Seizures of methamphetamine laboratories will increase in Hawaii as training of law enforcement results in the identification of laboratories previously unrecognized as such.

Maritime seizures of illicit drugs will increase following the July 1, 2004, deadline given to U.S. and global ports to implement all measures required by the Maritime Transportation Security Act. Although the act is designed to counter terrorism, a collateral effect will be an increase in drug seizures in the near term as it will necessitate a rise in the rate inspections and help identify high-risk containers, thus facilitating seizures without the need for specific intelligence.

Successful prosecutions of drug distributors will increase provided that a proposed bill that would make it easier for law enforcement to use wiretaps against suspected criminals becomes law.

The Hawaii HIDTA and its participating member agencies will continue to devote resources to identify, investigate, and dismantle the organizations responsible for the spread of methamphetamine across Hawaii and our country.

Thank you for the opportunity to testify before the Subcommittee.

---

[i] Ice methamphetamine, also known as glass, shabu, or batu, is a pure, highly addictive form of methamphetamine resembling shards of ice. It is the product of the process of recrystallizing powdered methamphetamine in a solvent such as water, methanol, ethanol, isopropanol, or acetone to remove impurities. Ice typically is smoked using either a glass pipe, an empty aluminum can, a piece of aluminum foil, or a light bulb. NDIC, *National Drug Threat Assessment 2004*, April 2004. Definition supplied by the Drug Enforcement Administration.

Mr. SOUDER. Thank you very much. Our next witness is Mr. Charles Goodwin, special agent-in-charge, Honolulu office, for the FBI.

STATEMENT OF CHARLES GOODWIN, SPECIAL AGENT-IN-CHARGE, HONOLULU DIVISION, FEDERAL BUREAU OF INVESTIGATION

Mr. GOODWIN. Good morning, Chairman Souder, Congressman Case. Thank you for inviting here today to speak to you on the problem of crystal methamphetamine trafficking and abuse here in Hawaii.

I also appreciate the opportunity to comment on the FBI's efforts in partnership with other Federal Government agencies and State and local authorities to address the battle against drugs and ice here in Hawaii.

First, I want to emphasize that the FBI remains committed to the fight against illegal drugs in Hawaii and working with you to put the drug trafficking organizations out of business. As you're all aware, though, through law enforcement reports and the news media, ice continues to rank as the most widely abused illicit drug in Hawaii. Much of the ice abuse in Hawaii is attributed to the drug trafficking organizations which have strong ties to both domestic and international organized crime enterprises.

Although the FBI Honolulu Division continues to investigate drug trafficking organizations using the Enterprise Theory of Investigation; that is, to seek the dismantlement of the entire criminal organization and not just individual members, we are doing so with a lot less manpower resources.

After September 11, 2001 the FBI with the blessing of Congress reallocated several hundred Special Agents working drug investigations to counterterrorism and other investigative programs.

This decision was done clearly out of necessity and it provided the Counterterrorism Program with some of the best investigators in the FBI. In response to this move, the FBI Drug Program bolstered its presence in Hawaii on the High Intensity Drug Trafficking Area, Organized Crime Drug Enforcement Task Force and other task forces as a force-multiplier.

Part of the reasoning behind the reallocation of FBI drug investigative resources was the realization that there are thousands of other highly committed, qualified, experienced State and local law enforcement officials engaged in drug investigations. At the Federal level, the DEA, Immigration and Customs Enforcement, IRS, ATF, U.S. Coast Guard are all valuable assets in the war on drugs.

The FBI, however, is not abdicating its commitment to drug investigations. In the meantime the FBI continues to concentrate the vast majority of our FBI drug agents on dismantling the largest drug trafficking organization and criminal enterprises, those identified by the Attorney General's list of 41 Consolidated Priority Organization Targets. We also remain committed to the national programs, OCDETF and HIDTA, as well as major joint intelligence efforts in Hawaii. Bottom line, the FBI remains committed to working with you in this fight against illegal drugs.

Ice is the drug of choice in Hawaii. The sale and use and transportation of ice in Hawaii has had a devastating impact on all of

Hawaiian society. As we are acutely aware, ice tears away at the inner fabric of Hawaii. It brings violence to our streets, wastes young lives, wreaks havoc on families, saps millions of dollars from our economy, and drains the resources of our criminal justice and health care systems.

Drugs such as ice make criminal enterprises across the country and around the world richer, stronger, and more formidable.

The specific statistics on how crystal methamphetamine affects the overall crime issues is staggering. An estimated 90 percent of property crime in Hawaii is believed to be drug-related. In addition, many homicides and other violent crimes, including hostage situations, have been associated with ice. In 2002, U.S. Attorney, Ed Kubo stated that ice had been associated with over 90 percent of the confirmed child abuse cases. Recently, news articles in Hawaii have reported that assaults on police officers have increased fivefold over the past 5 years and that the violence associated with ice abuse is a contributing factor to that increase.

The widespread use of ice has also deeply hurt the economy and social image of Hawaii. Several studies done by universities have reported that Hawaii authorities have spent close to half a billion dollars per year on corrections, education, and counselling, and other programs relative to the ice problem. There are as many as 30,000 ice users in Hawaii who spend between $540 million to $1.8 billion annually on their habits. Many researchers also believe the manufacturing and usage of ice is having a detrimental effect on the environment.

Here in Hawaii the problems with ice transcends beyond the typical street dealers. The FBI, in cooperation with other law enforcement agencies, has determined that the ice problem extends to international boundaries and have strong organized crime ties. In Hawaii, traditional Asian organized crime organizations distribute ice. Today, Mexican drug trafficking organizations and other criminal organizations are becoming increasingly more involved in the production and distribution of ice.

In fact, our intelligence indicates that most of the ice in Hawaii appears to be produced in Mexico and California. Mexican drug trafficking organizations transport ice to Honolulu, Maui, and other Hawaiian counties from California and to a lesser extent, Las Vegas. Some Asian trafficking organizations, such as Filipino, Vietnamese, and Korean organizations transport ice to Hawaii via Canada and California to avoid potential customs and border patrol inspections conducted at Hawaii ports of entry such as the Honolulu International Airport. Hawaii law enforcement estimates a large percentage of the ice in Hawaii is smuggled through the airport via mailed parcels and couriers on commercial flights. We've also intercepted shipments arriving by shipping containers from the mainland which are not searched.

I'm going to jump ahead here because I've clearly run out of my time, but the main thing the FBI, the strategies that we use to fight drugs here in Hawaii, continue to direct appropriate investigative and analytical resources to address the threats posed by priority targets; encourage the use of Title IIIs, criminal pen registers, and subpoenas; encourage the use of complex undercover operations; maximize the use of specialized drug intelligence sources to fully develop investigations of drug trafficking enterprises; consult with respective counterparts in DEA to confirm investigative efforts are not being duplicated and to identify opportunities for joint initiatives and investigations.

We want to ensure that appropriate deconfliction is shared through data bases; ensure initiation and coordination of multi-jurisdictional investigations; ensure investigations are initiated against priority targets posing the greatest threat to the Honolulu Division and Hawaii which are multi-jurisdictional, regional, and national significance. We want to actively participate in ad hoc task forces such as HIDTA initiatives. And with that I'll conclude my testimony and certainly be available for questioning.

[The prepared statement of Mr. Goodwin follows:]

STATEMENT OF

CHARLES L. GOODWIN

SPECIAL AGENT IN CHARGE

HONOLULU DIVISION

FEDERAL BUREAU OF INVESTIGATION

BEFORE THE

HOUSE GOVERNMENT REFORM SUBCOMMITTEE ON CRIMINAL JUSTICE, DRUG POLICY, AND HUMAN RESOURCES

AThe Poisoning of Paradise: Crystal Methamphetamine in Hawaii@

August 2, 2004

Good morning Chairman Souder and members of the Committee. Thank you for inviting me here today to speak to you on the problem of crystal methamphetamine trafficking and abuse in Hawaii. I also appreciate the opportunity to comment on the Federal Bureau of Investigation=s efforts in partnership with other federal government agencies and state and local authorities to address the battle against drugs and crystal methamphetamine in Hawaii.

Introduction

First, I want to emphasize that the Federal Bureau of Investigation (FBI) remains committed to fighting the fight against illegal drugs in Hawaii and working with you to put the drug trafficking organizations out of business. As you are all aware through law enforcement reports and the news media, crystal methamphetamine continues to rank as the most widely abused illicit drug in Hawaii. Much of the crystal methamphetamine abuse in Hawaii is attributed to the drug trafficking organizations which have strong ties to both domestic and international organized crime enterprises.

Although the FBI Honolulu Division continues to investigate drug trafficking organizations using the Enterprise Theory of Investigation- that is, to seek the dismantlement of the entire criminal organization and not just individual members, we are doing so with a lot less manpower resources. After September 11, 2001, the FBI, with the blessing of Congress, reallocated several hundred Special Agents working drug investigations to counterterrorism and other investigative programs. This decision was done clearly out of necessity, and it provided the Counterterrorism Program with some of the best investigators in the FBI. In response to this move, the FBI Drug Program bolstered its presence in Hawaii on the High Intensity Drug Trafficking Area (HIDTA), Organized Crime Drug Enforcement Task Force (OCDETF) and other joint task forces as a force-multiplier.

Part of the reasoning behind the reallocation of FBI drug investigative resources was the realization that there are thousands of other highly committed, experienced, state and local law enforcement officials engaged in drug investigations. At the federal level, the DEA, ICE, IRS, ATF, and U.S. Coast Guard are all valuable assets in the war on drugs. The FBI, however, is not abdicating its commitment to drug investigations. In the meantime, the FBI continues to concentrate the vast majority of our FBI drug agents on dismantling the largest drug trafficking organizations and criminal enterprises, those identified in the Attorney General's list of 41 Consolidated Priority Organization Targets. We also remain committed to the national programs -- OCDETF and HIDTA -- as well as major joint intelligence efforts in Hawaii. Bottom line: the FBI remains committed to working with you in this fight against illegal drugs.

Crystal Methamphetamine in Hawaii BTrends and Abuses

Crystal methamphetamine, commonly known as ice, is the drug of choice in Hawaii. The sale, use and transportation of crystal methamphetamine in Hawaii has had a devastating impact on all of Hawaiian society. As we all are acutely aware, crystal methamphetamine tears away at the inner fabric of Hawaii. Crystal methamphetamine brings violence to our streets. Crystal methamphetamine wastes young lives and wreaks havoc on families. Crystal methamphetamine saps millions of dollars out of our economy every year. Crystal methamphetamine drains the resources of our criminal justice and health care systems. And drugs such as crystal methamphetamine make criminal enterprises across the country and around the world -- richer, stronger, and more formidable.

The specific statistics on how crystal methamphetamine affects the overall crime issues is staggering. An estimated 90 percent of property crime in Hawaii is believed to be drug-related. In addition, many homicides and other violent crimes, including hostage situations, have been associated with crystal methamphetamine. In 2002, U.S. Attorney Ed Kubo stated that crystal methamphetamine had been associated with over 90 percent of confirmed child abuse cases. Recently, news articles in Hawaii have reported that assaults on police officers have increased fivefold over the past five years and that the violence associated with crystal methamphetamine abuse is a contributing factor to that increase.

The wide-spread use of crystal methamphetamine has also deeply hurt the economy and social image of Hawaii. Several studies done by universities have reported that Hawaii authorities spend close to half a billion dollars per year on corrections, education, counseling , and other related programs relative to the crystal methamphetamine problem. News reports have noted that there are as many as 30,000 crystal methamphetamine users in Hawaii who spend between $540 million to 1.8 billion annually based on a $50 to $170 per day habit. In addition, the crystal methamphetamine also has a negative impact on the natural environment in Hawaii. Many researchers believe that the manufacturing and usage of crystal methamphetamine may be having a detrimental impact on the environment.

Crystal Methamphetamine in Hawaii B Deeper Ties to International & Organized Crime Connections

Here in Hawaii, the problems with crystal methamphetamine transcends beyond the typical street dealer. The FBI in cooperation with other law enforcement agencies has determined that the crystal methamphetamine problems extend to international boundaries and strong organized crime connections. For example, in Hawaii, traditional Asian criminal organizations distributed crystal methamphetamine. Lately, Mexican drug trafficking organizations and other criminal organizations are becoming increasingly more involved in the production and distribution of crystal methamphetamine.

Recent law enforcement reports indicate that most of the crystal methamphetamine in Hawaii appears to be produced in Mexico and California. Mexican drug trafficking organizations transport crystal methamphetamine to Honolulu, Maui and other Hawaiian counties via California and to a lesser extent Las Vegas. Some Asian drug trafficking organizations, such as Filipino, Vietnamese, and Korean, transport crystal methamphetamine to Hawaii via Canada and California to avoid strict Customs and Border Patrol inspections conducted at Hawaii ports of entry such as the Honolulu International Airport (HIA). Hawaii law enforcement estimates that approximately 80-90 percent of the crystal methamphetamine seized in Hawaii is smuggled through the HIA via mailed parcels and couriers on commercial flights.

Once the crystal methamphetamine is successfully smuggled into Hawaii, the local drug trafficking organizations generally distribute the drug throughout the islands via independent distributors. Some of these distribution sites may be local night clubs or simply street corners or beach-front sites. However, the line between the international drug traffickers and the local Hawaiian drug traffickers is becoming more blurred as the locals are participating in more complex international operations. Some of the local, as well as the international drug trafficking organizations, are expanding their drug business to other U.S. territories such as Guam and Saipan. The FBI, with resident agencies in Guam and Saipan, bolstered its resources to fight the spread of the crystal methamphetamine traffickers in these islands.

To address these international, domestic, and organized crime connections, the FBI developed the FBI Drug Program Plan (DPP). The FBI DPP is designed to dismantle and disrupt Drug Trafficking Criminal Enterprises (DTCE) which pose the greatest threats to the economic and national security of the United States. Specifically, the FBI and its partner agencies in Hawaii are attempting to identify the primary targets and crystal methamphetamine-related organizations involved in the manufacture and distribution of this drug. These goals will be accomplished through task forces and other joint initiatives with other agencies.

<u>Multi-Jurisdictional Approach and the Use of Sophisticated Techniques to Fight the Crystal Methamphetamine Problem</u>

In support of the FBI=s DP to disrupt and dismantle the DTCEs, the FBI Honolulu Division utilizes a multi-jurisdiction, interagency approach to its investigations. Coordination with other law enforcement agencies, especially the DEA, is vital to the success of the federal counter-drug effort. In cooperation with other agencies, the FBI will also utilize the following sophisticated investigative techniques and strategies to fight illegal drugs:

(1) Direct appropriate investigative and analytical resources to address the threats posed by priority targets;

(2) Encourage the use of Title III=s, criminal pen registers, and subpoenas;

(3) Encourage the use of complex undercover operations;

(4) Maximize the use of specialized drug intelligence sources to fully develop investigations of drug trafficking enterprises;

(5) Consult with respective counterparts in DEA to confirm investigative efforts are not being duplicated and to identify opportunities for joint initiatives and investigations;

(6) Ensure appropriate deconfliction through shared databases such as DRUGX;

(7) Ensure initiation and coordination of multi-jurisdictional investigations through office leads and referrals;

(8) Ensure investigations are initiated against priority targets posing the greatest threat to the Honolulu Division, and which are multi-jurisdictional and of regional/and or national significance and influence; and

(9) Actively participate in ad hoc task forces High Intensity Drug Trafficking Area (HIDTA) initiatives.

Besides the sophisticated techniques listed above, the FBI in cooperation with other partners continues to work closely with the Hawaiian communities through programs such as the U.S. Department of Justice initiative AWeed and Seed@. The Weed and Seed Program is designed to support the community involvement in the fight against illegal drugs. The Weed and Seed program is a multi-faceted proactive approach to fight crime by weeding out the criminal element and seeding the community with services that support the neighborhood revitalization. Because of the program=s success, the Hawaii HIDTA is joining forces with the Honolulu Weed and Seed. Through this cooperation, the HIDTA hopes to reduce the harmful consequences associated with crystal methamphetamine.

Task Force Approach in Action: OCDETF and HIDTA

Pursuant to the Organized Crime Drug Enforcement Task Force (OCDETF), the FBI has joined forces with other federal government and local agencies through HIDTA to investigate and neutralize drug trafficking in Hawaii. OCDETF and HIDTA permit law enforcement to use a multi-faceted approach to cull various expertise and resources to the table to address the drug problems. With the expertise and knowledge of ICE officials, IRS officials, ATF officials, DEA officials, Customs and Border Protection (BCP) officials, local/state police, and the FBI, a full throttle attack on drugs has become commonplace in Hawaii.

FBI Honolulu Special Agents are collocated with other agents in HIDTA to address the drug problems in Hawaii in a timely and accurate fashion. As a result of this close cooperation, law enforcement has been very successful in carrying out its mission to arrest and neutralize drug trafficking organizations in Hawaii. For example, in October of 2003 under the codename AOperation Shave Ice@, law enforcement arrested nearly 60 people on drug charges in Oahu, the Big Island of Hawaii, Las Vegas, Nevada, Los Angeles, California, and Phoenix, Arizona. The arrests and searches of businesses and homes were a coordinated effort by federal, state, and local law enforcement officers in the war on crystal methamphetamine. Operation Shave Ice, an OCDETF investigation, dismantled five loosely affiliated crystal methamphetamine rings in Hawaii. U.S. Attorney Ed Kubo for the District of Hawaii noted that Operation Shave Ice ranked among the top 10 drug ring shutdowns in Hawaii history. Over $200,000 from the ring was confiscated with 12 firearms. The arrests also revealed a complex import system that used commercial airliners, shipping companies and the U.S. Postal Service.

Expansion in the FBI=s Intelligence Component

In addition to the multi-jurisdictional approach as evidenced by the FBI=s participation in HIDTA, the FBI will enhance its intelligence sharing efforts to enable it to more effectively target and pursue these drug trafficking organizations. The FBI realizes that to dismantle the most significant DTCEs requires an intelligence capability which can accomplish the following: identify existing or emerging drug activities, determine associations between individuals and groups engaged in drug trafficking, and provide strategic intelligence in support of drug investigations.

FBI drug investigations will maximize the use of intelligence resources such as the National Drug Intelligence Center (NDIC), the multi-agency Special Operations Division (SOD), the U.S. Department of Justice=s Criminal Intelligence Section (CIS), the El Paso Intelligence Center (EPIC), the Financial Crimes Enforcement Network (FINCEN), the OCDETF Fusion Center, and other specialized drug intelligence resources to insure the sharing of information, collection of intelligence, and analysis of that information to state and local partners and to drive our own investigations. This process enables the FBI to identify the most worthy targets.

The FBI Honolulu Division has also created the Field Intelligence Group (FIG), a new squad designed to collect, analyze, and disseminate raw intelligence information to relevant agencies to address the fight against drugs, terrorism, and hostile intelligence organizations in a more timely manner.

DOD=s Joint Interagency Task-Force

In July 2004, the Department of Defense=s (DOD) Joint Interagency Task Force-West moved from the San Francisco area to Honolulu. The FBI will be partnering with this task force to intercept drugs coming from the Far East. The FBI believes this joint coordination will flush out human smuggling, money laundering, and narcoterrorism investigations.

The FBI, in coordination with the DOD Joint Interagency Task-Force, is keen to maintain vigilance over the investigation of major drug trafficking cartels who have established successful smuggling routes into the United States, whether overland via Points of Entry (POEs) in Mexico and Canada, by sea through commercial ports on either coast, or by air. It is clear that narcotics traffickers are exploiting smuggling routes into the United States as hundreds of tons of cocaine as well as thousands of illegal aliens find their way across our borders each year. The FBI, in conjunction with all our law enforcement partners, especially the DEA and the Department of Homeland Security, must remain committed to identifying and eliminating these smuggling routes, which could easily be adopted for other, even more catastrophic purposes- like to import a weapon of mass destruction.

The FBI is instituting major initiatives against special interest aliens (SIA) as a means to identify, dismantle, and prevent sleeper terrorist cells from operating in the United States. The FBI's continuing commitment against major drug cartels is a natural extension of this effort, as the same smuggling routes and smuggling organizations used to import illegal drugs are also used to move SIAs into the country.

Conclusion

I do not see the fight against illegal drugs in Hawaii ending anytime soon. We are in this for the long haul.

The FBI Honolulu Division, despite our limited resources available for drug investigations, will continue to partner with all agencies to attack the crystal methamphetamine problem in Hawaii.

Thank you for giving me the opportunity to testify before the Subcommittee today. I will be happy to answer any questions you may have.

Mr. SOUDER. Thank you very much. Our last witness on the first panel is Mr. Briane Grey, Special Agent in Charge, Honolulu Office, Los Angeles Field Division of DEA.

STATEMENT OF BRIANE GREY, ASSISTANT SPECIAL AGENT IN CHARGE, HONOLULU OFFICE, DRUG ENFORCEMENT ADMINISTRATION

Mr. GREY. Chairman Souder, Congressman Case, and distinguished members of the subcommittee, it is a pleasure to appear before you today. On behalf of the DEA Administrator Karen P. Tandy and Los Angeles Field Division Special Agent in Charge Stephen C. Delgado, I would like to thank this subcommittee for your continued support of the DEA and its mission.

While Hawaii has always been viewed as a paradise destination, it currently has the distinction of being No. 1 per capita for crystal methamphetamine use in the United States. The spread of crystal methamphetamine use has long been a problem for the Hawaiian islands and the user population continues to grow due to its highly addictive nature.

Crystal methamphetamine, commonly known as ice, is the No. 1 drug threat in Hawaii, Guam, and Saipan. In the last 2 years Hawaii has seen a significant increase in the amount of crystal methamphetamine being distributed and seized.

According to the Substance Abuse and Mental Health Services Administration's Treatment Episode Data Sets, treatment admissions for methamphetamine abuse in Hawaii increased from 1,243 in 1998 to 2,238 in 2002. This rate has steadily increased. In 2003, Hawaii was the only State to have crystal methamphetamine treatment admissions exceed alcohol abuse treatment admissions.

In Hawaii ice abusers have been linked to violent crimes including child abuse, hostage situations, and homicides. Ice abusers are also linked to Hawaii's high property crime rate which is one of the worst in the Nation. Methamphetamine and the violence associated with the drug threaten the well-being of all of Hawaii's citizens, continue to challenge all law enforcement, health care, and social services entities within the State. This epidemic is fueled by the ever increasing number of drug trafficking organizations associated with larger organizations in Mexico and the U.S. West Coast.

Ice production and distribution first appeared in Hawaii in 1985 and is associated with Asian drug trafficking organizations. To avoid Hawaii's strict U.S. Customs and Border Protection inspections, Asian organizations routinely transported drugs from source countries such as Korea, Thailand, and the Philippines through Canada to Hawaii via California. In the 1990's the trend shifted. Mexican organizations became the principal ice suppliers in Hawaii.

The DEA has recently and successfully emphasized investigations targeting the flow of precursor chemicals used to produce methamphetamine. Due to the successes of OCDETF investigations Operations Mountain Express III and Northern Star between 2002 and 2003, U.S. importation of bulk pseudoephedrine from Canada dramatically dropped. These enforcement successes at the Northern border have forced traffickers to import pseudoephedrine to Mexico from Hong Kong, increased methamphetamine manufacturing in Mexico.

Presently, Mexican organizations are producing ice in Mexico, California, and southwestern States and use their established transportation networks to distribute the drug throughout the United States and the Hawaiian islands. Clandestine superlabs located in Mexico and the southwestern United States are responsible for most of the ice distributed in Hawaii.

Through DEA's State and Local Task Force Program and the HIDTA program, the DEA Honolulu District Office has joined forces with our State and local partners to address methamphetamine-related trends from large Mexican trafficking organizations down to small-time producers operating out of their homes. In March 2004, an investigation with the Bureau of Customs and Border Protection, the DEA Airport Task Force seized 20 pounds of crystal methamphetamine concealed inside aluminum pipes sent from an individual in Mexico to Honolulu, as well as $200,000 in proceeds. At the other end of the chain, in February 2004, the Maui Post of Duty arrested an individual with 15 grams of ice who was prosecuted federally who allegedly supplied high school students and was the source for other dealers on Lanai since July 2003.

The Honolulu District Office has DEA Task Forces in Maui and Hilo and at the Honolulu Airport. This team effort has led to significant investigations allowing law enforcement to jointly attack crystal methamphetamine trafficking.

A joint investigation between the DEA and Honolulu Office of Immigration and Customs Enforcement led to the February seizure of five gallons of red phosphorous in the possession of a Canadian citizen. The subsequent investigation identified the individual as a methamphetamine chemist who was responsible for the distribution of the approximately 30 to 40 pounds of ice per month in 2002 and early 2003. This investigation eliminated a clandestine manufacturing operation based in Canada.

More recently, the DEA with State and local officers seized 1.8 kilograms of ice shipped from California to Kihei, Maui and 1.44 kilograms of ice from two individuals arriving in Honolulu from Las Vegas, Nevada. Our Guam office also seized 200 grams of liquid methamphetamine sent from the Philippines to Guam.

The DEA is committed to protecting the American public's safety from the serious consequences resulting from the methamphetamine threat. The DEA has had a significant impact on the trafficking of precursor chemicals and continues to target Mexican trafficking organizations controlling the majority of the methamphetamine produced and distributed in our country.

Thank you again for the opportunity to testify before the subcommittee today. I will be happy to answer any questions at the appropriate time.

[The prepared statement of Mr. Grey follows:]

Statement of

Briane M. Grey
Assistant Special Agent in Charge
Honolulu District Office
Drug Enforcement Administration

Before the

House Government Reform Committee
Subcommittee on Criminal Justice, Drug Policy
and Human Resources

August 2, 2004

"The Poisoning of Paradise: Crystal Methamphetamine in Hawaii"

Introduction

Chairman Souder and distinguished members of the Subcommittee it is a pleasure to appear before you. My name is Briane M. Grey and I am the Assistant Special Agent in Charge of the Honolulu District Office. On behalf of the DEA Administrator Karen P. Tandy and Los Angeles Field Division Special Agent in Charge Stephen C. Delgado, I would like to thank this subcommittee for your continued support of the DEA and its mission.

While Hawaii has always been viewed as a paradise destination, it currently has the distinction of being number one per capita for crystal methamphetamine use in the United States. The spread of crystal methamphetamine use has been a longstanding problem in the Hawaiian Islands and the user population continues to grow due to crystal methamphetamine's highly addictive nature.

Current trafficking of crystal methamphetamine in Hawaii is similar to the overall trends experienced throughout the entire Pacific Rim. Crystal methamphetamine, also known as "Ice", "Batu", and "Speed" is the number one drug threat in Hawaii, Guam and Saipan. The "Ice" situation in Hawaii is a twofold challenge: Combating the proliferation of Mexican and Asian organizations that are expanding their wholesale and retail distribution in Hawaii and disrupting or dismantling the growing "Ice" retail networks in our areas of operation. As the most isolated island chain in the world, Hawaii presents a unique challenge for federal, state, and local law enforcement officials. The DEA in conjunction with the High Intensity Drug Trafficking Area (HIDTA) has joined forces with our state and local law enforcement counterparts to identify, investigate, disrupt and dismantle drug organizations operating in our area.

In the last two years, Hawaii has seen a significant increase in the amount of crystal methamphetamine being distributed and seized. The majority of recent "Ice" seizures have been linked to Mexican organizations, a significant departure from "Ice" traditionally supplied by Asian criminal organizations.

The profitability of dealing "Ice" in Hawaii has attracted Mexican organizations that now control the majority of the wholesale methamphetamine distribution to Hawaii. Mexican organizations transport multi-pound quantities from clandestine methamphetamine "superlabs" located on the Southwest border and Mexico to Hawaii for distribution.

Hawaii in the Grip of Crystal Methamphetamine

According to the Substance Abuse and Mental Health Services Administration's Treatment Episode Data Sets, treatment admissions for amphetamine abuse in Hawaii increased from 1,243 in 1998 to 2,238 in 2002. This rate has increased steadily, and in 2003, Hawaii was the only State to have crystal methamphetamine treatment admissions exceed alcohol abuse treatment admissions.

"Ice" purity levels ranging from 96-99% are readily available and consumed by the user population throughout the State. Crystal methamphetamine prices for Hawaii vary depending on where it is purchased and are typically proportional to the distance from the mainland. In Hawaii one gram of "Ice" costs $200 - $300. One ounce ranges from $2,200 - $2,800. The wholesale price for one pound of "Ice" ranges from $22,000 to $40,000. When sold at the retail level, the same pound of "Ice" sells for approximately $300,000. In Guam and Saipan, retail and wholesale prices are several times higher than these amounts. The price of crystal methamphetamine in Hawaii and Guam are among the highest in the nation.

In Hawaii, "Ice" abusers have been linked to violent crimes including child abuse, hostage situations, and homicides. Hawaii's violent crime rates, which historically have been among the lowest in the nation, are on the rise. "Ice" abusers are also linked to Hawaii's high property crime rate, which is one of the worst in the nation. Methamphetamine and the violence associated with the drug threaten the well-being of all of Hawaii's citizens and continue to challenge not only the DEA, but all law enforcement, health care, and social services entities within the state. This epidemic is fueled by the ever increasing number of drug trafficking organizations operating in conjunction with larger organizations located in Mexico and on the U.S. West Coast.

"Ice" in Paradise

Historically, "Ice" production and distribution has been associated with Asian drug trafficking organizations. This drug first appeared in Hawaii around 1985 and was considered to be the "poor man's cocaine". During mid 1980s "Ice" was distributed by Asian youth gangs. At that time, the pure "Ice" crystals came primarily from the Philippines, South Korea, Hong Kong, Taiwan and Japan. Asian organizations routinely transported drugs from source countries such as Korea, Thailand, and the Philippines through Canada to Hawaii via California to avoid Hawaii's strict U.S. Customs and Border Protection inspections. In the 1990's, the trend shifted and Mexican organizations became the principal "Ice" suppliers for traffickers in Hawaii.

The DEA has recently emphasized, and had significant success with investigations targeting the flow of precursor chemicals used to produce methamphetamine. Due to the successes of OCDETF investigations Operations Mountain Express III and Northern Star between 2002 and 2003, U.S. importation of bulk pseudoephedrine from Canada dramatically dropped and the U.S. price of bulk pseudoephedrine more than doubled. These enforcement successes at the Northern border have forced traffickers to import pseudoephedrine to Mexico from Hong Kong, increased methamphetamine manufacturing in Mexico, and increased the smuggling of finished methamphetamine from Mexico into the U.S. across the Southwest Border.

Presently, Mexican organizations are producing "Ice" in Mexico, California, and Southwestern states and are using their established transportation networks to distribute the drug throughout the United States, including Hawaii. Clandestine labs located in Mexico and the Southwestern United States are responsible for most of the "Ice" distributed in Hawaii.

While Hawaii has not been inundated with clandestine laboratory operations, the state is intensely concerned and motivated to protect indigenous flora and fauna to avoid the devastating environmental damage suffered throughout the mainland. The DEA uses a precursor control program to identify and target the most significant sources of methamphetamine precursor chemicals. The DEA also works domestically with legitimate handlers of precursor chemicals to ensure that these chemicals are not diverted for illicit use.

Through DEA's State and Local Task Force Program and the HIDTA program, the DEA Honolulu District Office has joined forces with our state and local partners to address methamphetamine-related trends from large Mexican trafficking organizations down to the small-time producers operating out of their homes. For example, in March 2004, in a joint investigation with the Bureau of Customs and Border Protection, the DEA Airport Task Force seized 20 pounds of crystal methamphetamine concealed inside aluminum pipes sent from an individual in Mexico to Honolulu, as well as $200,000 in proceeds. At the bottom end of the chain, in February 2004, the Maui Post of Duty arrested an individual with 15 grams of "Ice". This individual allegedly supplied high school students and was the source for other dealers on Lanai since July 2003.

Significant Investigations and Seizures

The Honolulu District Office has DEA Task Forces in Maui and Hilo and at the Honolulu Airport. These federally deputized state and local officers have the same authority and jurisdiction as DEA Special Agents. This Task Force concept acts as a force multiplier for the DEA and allows participating agencies to participate in major investigations. This team effort has led to significant investigations allowing law enforcement to jointly attack crystal methamphetamine trafficking.

For example, a joint investigation between the DEA and the Honolulu Office of Immigration and Customs Enforcement (ICE), lead to the seizure of five gallons of red phosphorous in the possession of a Canadian citizen in February 2004. The individual was identified as a methamphetamine chemist shipping substantial quantities of "Ice" to distributors in Hawaii and elsewhere. This investigation eliminated a clandestine manufacturing operation based in Canada. The individual was responsible for distribution of approximately 30 to 40 pounds of "Ice" per month from February 2002 through March 2003.

More recently, the DEA Airport Task Force, which included state and local officers deputized with DEA authority, seized 1.8 kilograms of "Ice" shipped from California to Kihei, Maui and 1.44 kilograms of "Ice" from two individuals arriving in Honolulu from Las Vegas, Nevada. Also, our Guam office seized 200 grams of liquid methamphetamine sent from the Philippines to Guam.

Conclusion

The DEA is committed to protecting the American public's health and safety from the serious consequences resulting from the methamphetamine threat. The DEA has had a significant impact on the trafficking of precursor chemicals and continues to target Mexican trafficking organizations controlling the majority of the methamphetamine produced and distributed in our country.

Thank you again for the opportunity to testify before the Subcommittee today. I will be happy to answer any questions at the appropriate time.

Mr. SOUDER. I thank you each for your testimony. Let me say that it's unusual; I've never done this with a lei before, let alone without a tie. I appreciate Congressman Case because he wore a lei, actually, when he testified in front of the committee in Washington. I just want everybody back in Hawaii to know that he's very consistent in making statements for his home State and his concern on this issue and I appreciate it.

There are a number of things in your testimony that are dramatically different than what we've heard elsewhere. I want to make sure that I highlight some of these, both FBI, DEA, and I know from talking to HIDTA that you've said this, too, but I want to highlight this, 90 percent of property crime is believed to be drug related, 90 percent of child abuse, I believe you said Mr. Goodwin, was methamphetamine, crystal methamphetamine related, assaults on police officers increased fivefold over the last 5 years.

So am I taking from that the associated crime and violence from meth, even if meth has been a historic problem, has jumped?

Mr. GOODWIN. I think that's a fair assumption and I think it's pretty well based on both reports from the media and police reports. The incident of violent crimes actually in Hawaii is, we believe, down somewhat. But those assaults, for instance, aggravated assault, assaults on police officers and those personal types of crimes and certainly property crime has continued to be on the rise, and we do believe it's directly attributed to the methamphetamine problem.

Mr. AIONA. As far as the child welfare cases and our collection of the statistics on the State level, I can't say that we have had the best collection system of data available. I think the number that you got is an estimate based on field interviews and response from social workers who are in the field and on the line and reporting back as to what they've encountered most recently. I think that's within the past few years. And I think it's a good assessment. I don't know if it's accurate, but I wouldn't say that's——

Mr. SOUDER. Hard.

Mr. AIONA. Yeah, hard facts.

Mr. SOUDER. Now, when you were in Family Court, what we've heard around the country is anywhere from 60 to 85 percent of all court cases in crime has some nexus with marijuana, alcohol, usually poly users and then to meth, which would include child support enforcement, divorce cases, and spouse abuse.

Is that true here as well? Is it usually poly drug, and here what seems to be more of a relationship with crystal meth is a higher percentage?

Mr. AIONA. Again, I don't have any hard data on that, but from my experience I would agree with that wholeheartedly, poly substance or multi substance abuse, you're correct. In Drug Court that's all I saw. Methamphetamine was usually the drug of choice, it usually was, but they'd mix it with marijuana and alcohol and cocaine and everything else you can imagine, so yes, that's an accurate statement.

Mr. SOUDER. Mr. Burnett, when we talked the other day, one of the things that we were discussing was how the relationship of marijuana to some degree alcohol with crystal methamphetamine and the coming down process.

Could you describe that, somebody maybe high on ice and then come down with marijuana?

Mr. BURNETT. I assume you're speaking of the tweaking process?

Mr. SOUDER. Right.

Mr. BURNETT. When individuals get high on ice, especially smoking in the form that we do here in Hawaii, it's an immediate rush and it's an extremely high high and a prolonged high. It lasts for a long time. But in order to maintain that, there is always the opposite side, like anything else, and it's called tweaking where you start to twitch and go into a deep depression.

And with ice, and that's part of the problem with violence that is associated with it, you go into a real deep depression, emotionally and physically. And what we see here is that they use marijuana and other drugs in order to mitigate that and try and even out that experience and try to take the edge off of the depression.

Mr. SOUDER. Have any of you seen any ice users who didn't use marijuana and/or alcohol.

Mr. BURNETT. I'm sure that there is somewhere. What we normally say with our statistics is that almost everybody that tests positive, and that's 40 percent of the males that are picked up for any crime in the State, that's the highest in the Nation, 40 percent test positive for meth. And when they test positive for meth, they are poly drug users. It's usually accompanied by alcohol and marijuana.

Mr. SOUDER. I want to pursue another round of questions before I go to Mr. Case. I want to pursue the Canada question a little bit. First off, one other thing I want to note for the record is several of you said, and I thought it was very helpful to understand, the historic ties to Asia which is the way we normally think of this, it would have not been self evident that Mexican drug trafficking organizations are taking over the meth in Hawaii. Walking around and talking to people you would not assume that's your major challenge.

Also, for the record, you're saying that there are fewer meth labs because normally in all the other States and we're talking Tennessee, Missouri, Kansas, Arkansas, Indiana which are the five highest, we're talking labs, even though we have these superlabs in California, and here you're basically talking about it coming in and then being turned into crystal methamphetamine. Is that correct?

Could you explain to me as someone who sits both on Border Committee on Homeland Security and has oversight here and we spent a couple years working on border issues, what do you mean by this statement?

And you made this Mr. Goodwin and Mr. Grey made a similar and actually, even more specific statement about how the meth, crystal meth, comes in through Canada sometimes through California and you made the statement to avoid strict custom and border patrol inspections conducted in the Hawaii ports of entry?

And I believe you had a case, Mr. Grey, where you talked about a recent one where a person came in, Canadian citizen came in with five gallons. That wasn't UPS or Fed Ex which most of them are, but could you describe what you mean by they can get in through Canada easier than Hawaii?

Mr. GOODWIN. First of all, we mentioned that we know the large quantities of drugs, first of all, come through Mexico and so they'll move through Mexico to the West Coast and then can be transhipped to Hawaii.

We also see precursors coming out of Asia as well. And in both cases they can ship product to Canada and then move it over land to California or Nevada to move it to Hawaii. And coming from the West Coast to Hawaii, they're not subject to customs inspection.

Mr. SOUDER. Even from Canada.

Mr. GOODWIN. Well, if they tranship it from Canada to Nevada, for instance, or California, and then ship it out, then it doesn't get looked at coming from the West Coast, the United States, to Hawaii. Now, in theory you would look at it between Canada and the United States, but the reality there is it's pretty much an open border.

I'd like to also just mention as we talk about more and more methamphetamine produced in the United States. But also being produced in big quantities in Mexico, moved to the West Coast and transhipped. The other thing we're starting to see is—we've always seen precursors coming from the Far East, but just recently, for instance, the Australian Federal Police brought a case to us. It was a superlab that they had interdicted in Fiji and it looked like a portable cement mixer. It was about three stories high and was capable of producing $1 billion a year worth of methamphetamine.

Now, in that particular case it was destined primarily for Australia and New Zealand and other Pacific Rim countries. But once something like that is established there, moved through Guam and Saipan, it would be pretty easy to ship it to Hawaii as well.

Mr. SOUDER. I'm going to come back for another round on the Asia side, but I want to do one more thing coming from our mainland West Coast this direction. One of the things we documented over and over, we're having a huge problem with hydroponic, we'll talk about marijuana in just a minute, but the cocaine coming up from Columbia and then meth going up California, across the Washington border swapping in British Columbia, then coming down and they get their cocaine, heroin coming north bringing the hydroponic seeds or marijuana or meth precursors down.

And what you're telling me is the route isn't usually Canada to here. What we're seeing is the swapping of the cocaine and heroin we're seeing in California going north is coming down from Canada, sometimes from Asia, sometimes from Belgium, and the Netherlands, which are still the biggest labs. Then they swap them and then they go Las Vegas or western California are the most logical places and then head this way and your meth problems are directly related to marijuana and cocaine problem going on the Coast because they're swapping it out.

Is that a fair statement, accurate? Any comments?

Mr. GREY. Yes, I think that's an accurate assessment. For swapping the drugs in the State of California.

Mr. SOUDER. Or Washington State?

Mr. GREY. Washington State. I think the key is getting it into the United States once it clears the border there, they don't have to go through another critical inspection prior to getting it over to Hawaii. And again, they're not talking bulk shipments. It can be a pound at a time, five pounds, easily able to go on a person's body, Fed Ex shipments are small, air cargo freight shipment, so the detection would be much less than if it was going across the open port.

Mr. SOUDER. It is certainly identified in the Yakima area of Washington State a swapping area in Yakima, the Tri Cities, that's going heavy into the Midwest as well with fighting traffic and going to Georgia and finding swaps that are occurring up in that region going north and south of California.

Mr. BURNETT. That's exactly right, Chairman.

What has happened is a lot of the nations out in the Pacific, both Australia, New Zealand, and Hong Kong when Hong Kong was handed back to the mainland Chinese, they all belonged to the Commonwealth, the British Commonwealth, and as such they can travel amongst the Commonwealth with relative ease.

So you have a mass migration of Chinese into British Columbia and they bring with them their ties from Asia. And there is a criminal group that is attendant with all parts of society, and so not only did you get the business but you also got the criminal group that preyed upon them that also went to British Columbia.

Then you couple that with the northern border, and as you're saying, as you start moving east along the northern border, there is a million and one roads where they move all the brain trucks back and forth.

So it is a pretty porous border. And then when it comes into Washington, the loads get broken down. And why risk 100 pounds of meth going to the Midwest or going to Hawaii or Guam, it's easier to break them down into one to two pound parcels, put them in Fed Ex, U.S. Postal Service, DHL, all of those services, and flood the market. All you have to do is look at our system we have out here. We have both a domestic and international mail branch and they handle millions, millions of pieces every month.

Mr. SOUDER. Congressman Blackburn is on this subcommittee and we're planning to do probably either late fall or early next year, the Fed Ex headquarters in Memphis.

Mr. CASE. Thank you, Mr. Chair. I'm going to come back to one question at the end for each of you, and I'd like to ask the same question of everyone else that is going to testify; and that is, this is your Federal Government. Maybe we don't look like, at least he does, maybe I don't.

This is your U.S. Congress, and if you had one thing to ask, one thing to ask of your U.S. Congress today to deal with meth from the perspective that you take it from, whether it's law enforcement, rehabilitation, preventative education, whatever, what is that one thing?

Let me leave that for you to think about, and let me ask you because I'm back to the front porch of the Lanai police station after a long day with the police officers, County of Maui police officers, by the way, that are on the front lines and dealing with how to go after the manufacturers. And I asked them what's really what you need.

And I'm going to paraphrase the answer, but what it came down to was we don't have the tools, the law enforcement tools to catch them. They're moving too fast on us. They mostly come in from the outside.

They come in by airplane, they come in by ferry, they come in by jet skis to the north shore, at least this is what they think, and they set up operations and they identify pretty fast. The Lanai population is 2,500 to 3,000. Everybody pretty much knows what's happening.

But by the time they can get the legal enforcement mechanisms in place to bust them, these guys have sold it and left the island; or what they told me was the old concept of an ice house is fast disappearing. They're really much more into a mobile operation where the dealers and sellers are one step ahead of the law. And what they have said is that the State law enforcement mechanisms aren't fast enough to give them the ability to bust them.

So therefore, what they are doing is they're basically skipping the State and going to the Feds because of the mechanisms of their rules and their inabilities there to respond a lot faster. Now that strikes me as an action of necessity but not a particular course of action. We clearly want both sides, both Federal and State ability. And it seems to me that stretches even more the Federal law enforcement system.

One of you alluded to Federal guidelines for—so you may get the most immediate, and that lets those 30 people go back on the streets. And it goes back to the point I made earlier which is we either need more Federal law enforcement officials on the ground in Hawaii, and especially in my Second Congressional District, and/or we need somehow to fix the State mechanisms so the State law enforcement can take some of the load off of you, the Feds, who are stretched out with ice, other forms of drugs, not to mention civil law enforcement, not to mention homeland security obligations.

So I guess I want to ask you is that something that is true throughout the State, No. 1; No. 2, what are the solutions because it seems we need to fix the State law enforcement mechanisms and/or No. 2, put Federal law enforcement out there in the communities.

Maybe I can start with you Lieutenant Governor because I think that has been an initiative by the Governor to move these kind of reasonable modifications to State laws.

Mr. AIONA. You call it reasonable, but obviously there are some people who don't feel that it's reasonable and as such we haven't had much success with the legislation that we proposed, especially this past legislative session. What we did propose were a couple of things.

First of all, we wanted to bring back the walk and talk issue; in other words, what we wanted to do was amend the Constitution for the execution of the walk and talk—the tool, if you want to call it, law enforcement has successfully used back in the 1990's on the local level, on the State level.

And then, of course, our electronic surveillance of laws, what they're calling the adversarial process; in other words, how we're going about getting wiretaps, etc. by local law enforcement personnel.

The other thing that we tried was to have a little bit more mandatory sentences in regards to people who had been using or dealing—that's an issue, when it comes to what amounts, to dealer quantities, but we had pushed for more stringent sentences, so to speak, in regards to that. Unfortunately, like I said, there was resistance on that. There were people that felt that it—one, it was too invasive, it was a violation of civil rights, they felt it shouldn't happen here in Hawaii. And of course, it became to a certain extent a policy issue in regards to emphasis being placed maybe more on treatment, as opposed to intervention.

And so what had happened as a result of that is you had the continuation of what we're calling act 161 which basically allows someone who has a previous arrest who now has a current arrest for a drug-related offense to undergo treatment and be placed on probation. And that, again, like I said, was a policy question that we were dealing with. We weren't in favor of that. The administration definitely was not in favor of that. Being a proponent of Drug Court, we felt that Drug Court provided that access to treatment and yet at the same time provided enough of the hammer, so to speak, to deal with that problem.

So your assessment of what you said I agree with it, but I don't agree that we should go more Federal law enforcement. I think if you talk to everyone who is going to come up here this morning, they're going to say we have tremendous collaboration.

Mr. Burnett said and we have to continue it. And I think everything has to shoulder that burden, so to speak, on an equal basis, if not more so the State, as opposed to the Federal Government.

The FBI, for instance, doesn't only deal with drug enforcement, it deals with terrorism and everything else we have going on in this region. So their resources would be better used, I would say better used, but you can see the balance that they need.

Mr. CASE. That's true in an ideal world. In an ideal world we would have a State law enforcement mechanism where you could, in fact, go after people with alacrity and commitment, but there are handicaps. Representative Voight comments on that.

But I guess what I'm trying to get at here is if we can't get there, and this is a policy determination made by the local Governor and State legislature, if we can't get there, which I think we should, I agree with you, I agree with you, then we got to do something. And I don't know where else to go because there is a whole level that's not being caught here under the circumstances.

Mr. AIONA. And I want to make one last comment, if I can, Congressman. Having HIDTA is obviously an advantage for us, but that's also a designation that I would prefer to have in this jurisdiction and I'll leave it at that.

Mr. CASE. We want to get to the next panel. A quick comment by you on what is the one thing you would ask Congress, just a quick comment on the——

Mr. BURNETT. About the State and local?

Mr. CASE. Yes.

Mr. BURNETT. It is a real problem for us, inasmuch as—I made the comment about individuals and it is very common to have individuals out there with 30 arrests and still out loose in the neighborhoods. And these 30 arrests are not like they're simple possession charges. We don't go after those kind. These 30 arrests are assaults. We have burglaries. We have larcenies. They have welfare charges against them from our State child endangerment. It's a critical problem for us and we need the State to be able to step up to the plate and do their job.

By the same token, from our standpoint, a standpoint where we organize strike forces and task forces, it is much easier to commingle and build a task force if we have those Federal resources on the ground, although our Lieutenant Governor might be without a job. I'd probably give that up and get rid of it as an issue here. I'd gladly give it up. I have grandkids and kids that live here and work here.

It is important, I think, to have the Federal resources, at least as a minimal amount, both here on the Big Island and on Kauai where they're totally lacking.

Mr. CASE. One thing from Congress.

Mr. GOODWIN. I can't say anything in just one thing. I want to comment that we've got great cooperation and coordination with the State and Federal authorities here. The reason they really like having the Feds here is because of our ability to do wiretaps and our search and seizure and also the minimum sentencing guidelines. When we send somebody away for 15 years, they're gone.

Mr. CASE. I think the other comment, again from the front porch of Lanai, is that the Federal court system moves a little faster in terms of dealing with it.

Mr. GOODWIN. We do want resources and from our standpoint, from the FBI's standpoint, nearly 600 bodies have been refocused from drugs. And drugs really—here in Hawaii, in particular, I mean it's a nationwide problem, but it really does tear up the fabric of the society. And that's the one thing I wish, I could put two more people in Hilo, in addition to the two in Kona, and put somebody on Kauai and place them where they're needed to further foster the spirit of cooperation and coordination that we enjoy in Honolulu and here in Kona, Hilo, and Maui.

Mr. CASE. What do you want.

Mr. GREY. Similar to that, I would agree resources is a big issue here, but I think more importantly, let's not forget, we're a user State being targeted both by Mexican traffickers and Asian traffickers; and that with the identification in Hawaii as a paradise, we have the same problems here, if not more so, than the rest of the United States.

So we're in this matter with you and take that with you to get the support and resources out here.

Mr. CASE. I want to make sure I get the Lieutenant Governor.

Mr. AIONA. Of course there are many things on the wish list, Congressman, but I would like Congress to really raise the bar, raise the standard, as far as the substance abuse and the effect it has on our family, to raise it not the top 10 percent, within the top 2 percent; and of course, with that it comes from policy statements, but I think some commitment to resources, a lot more than what's been happening now.

And I really believe that Access to Recovery initiative as being proposed by SAMHSA at this point in time is something that I really, really would like is, more money. Thank you.

Mr. GOODWIN. Just what you're doing right now, hold hearings, find out what's effective. In this time of tight budgets, make sure that what we are doing is prioritized and we get the information to your subcommittees as quick as possible.

Mr. SOUDER. I want to make sure we get a couple of additional things in the record. My understanding was Hawaii has the highest prices for meth.

Mr. BURNETT. If you look at prices on the West Coast, the rule of thumb is that Hawaii is about double the West Coast. Guam and Saipan are and some of the territories of the Pacific are about double here.

Mr. SOUDER. And as I recall, you were telling me that one of the reasons you see the Mexican trafficking organizations moving in this direction is they can make more money.

Mr. BURNETT. That's correct.

Mr. SOUDER. I also understood concerning marijuana, that we're not even talking about what we're seeing on the West Coast. My understanding is some of the THC is up to 40 percent, that 20, 30 would be——

Mr. BURNETT. THC, marijuana historically has been fairly low, 5, 6, 7 percent. We've intercepted seeds like you were talking about coming out of Canada, cross-pollination. Our growers here kick back seeds to no one. I can tell you that right now. We seized 200 tons of pot out of the State last year and kept it from going to, basically to the mainland.

We have seen some hydro plants that have done as high, I believe, I'm aware of about 28 percent THC, but that's about the highest. I think Chris Tally was talking to you at a meeting before where something was higher, but I'm not sure exactly the lab report. That's the highest one I've seen come back.

Mr. SOUDER. 28 percent. So that would be marijuana almost five times to—because we're not going to spend tens of millions of dollars here to address one problem because when you get up to 28 percent higher and you're approaching meth's impact.

Mr. BURNETT. It's a problem and I don't know exactly. We haven't seen a lot whole of that here. It is a problem.

Mr. SOUDER. You also mentioned across the board which is something we don't hear about in the mainland, particularly when you're from the West Coast or the islands way out there, the concept of Guam, Saipan, the Mariana Islands, the America Micronesia, all that type of thing is totally an alien concept.

You're saying you've seen the stuff coming from the Mexican traffickers, you're seeing historic patterns from Asia, and I believe that in the superlabs, Mr. Burnett, you expressed some concern that China was going to basically knock out the Europeans.

Could any of you elaborate on that and then, Mr. Goodwin, if you could explain some of the potential how you're going to watch the organizations out of Indonesia and others who recently are getting a hold of that drug trade as a means of financing and Al Qaeda, their sister organizations?

Mr. BURNETT. What Mr. Goodwin and the FBI talked about was this lab that was in the Fiji Islands and it was as big as an asphalt batch plant. The precipitator on it alone was almost two stories high. It was massive. And it wasn't only there, it took off. There are two similar labs in Malaysia and one in Manila, in the Philippines, and so there are at least four there.

And each one of those have the opportunity to make about $1 billion in profit for these organizations. And the individual behind this and the financier was Chinese organized crime so I mean it's coming. If we get a handle on the Colombians and Mexicans, you can almost see where the pressure is going to come from. These guys are organized, and that neck of the woods is not foreign to the people of Hawaii. That is our ohana. A lot of the people that make up this unique blend that we have come from the Philippines, come from Asia, and the Pacific Rim.

Mr. SOUDER. Not to mention, talk about Vancouver and Vietnam getting control.

Mr. BURNETT. We do see that. We see through our international branches customs continually picking off shipments that go from the harvest into the Midwest because there is a huge population there.

Mr. SOUDER. Mr. Goodwin, do you have anything to add.

Mr. GOODWIN. I wanted to mention in the Fiji case the precursors also came from China and so certainly China is really extending its influence through the Pacific Rim as is Korea and a number of the other countries.

The concern for us in terms of narcoterrorism and financing is the southern Philippines, Indonesia, some of the largest groups of Islamic followers, fundamentalists Muslims. And it's probably fair to say that it's potentially the next big recruiting ground for Al Qaeda, the J.I., Abu Sayaf which is already in the southern Philippines and financing drugs and trafficking drugs, using the same routes that you use now to move people or to move weapons of mass destruction, that's a big concern, and it's a big concern for Hawaii, too.

We've recently done a study looking at the Philippines and Indonesia and the crews that come on boats and the lack of oversight. We're really drilling down on that right now with those customs and immigration. So we're identifying through intelligence and it's some of the new things that we're doing. Now we're talking a close look at it.

Apparently, it's a problem. But these same routes that you use to smuggle people and drugs, you could use for smuggling money and terrorist financing of criminal enterprises.

Mr. SOUDER. We're not talking high percents here. We're talking when you have 270 million Muslims in Indonesia, 1 percent is 2.7 million, one-tenth of 1 percent is 270,000. When you're dealing with 23 million in a country like Iraq or Afghanistan, it's a totally different base we're looking at.

Mr. GOODWIN. And if you look at the level of poverty in those counties and the lack of any law enforcement, in terms of recruiting for Al Qaeda and terrorist organizations, it would be a very fertile ground. People really don't have anything much to live for there. You offer them an opportunity to make money through State-sponsored trafficking drugs and the opportunities are endless.

Mr. SOUDER. I appreciate all your efforts and Mr. Aiona, Lieutenant Governor, we appreciate your leadership. One of the things from the Federal level that we're looking really hard at it, and this is what's partly disturbing about some of the State law problems, and that is that we're dealing with. If you look at the narcotics question to the degree we don't get it on the ground in Columbia, say coca or the meth labs themselves, the further we move down into the system, if we fail here and fail here, by the time we get to local enforcement, we're down to smaller and smaller cases. By the time we get them into treatment, that means the system has totally failed them.

They're in treatment, prevention. We're trying to do the best we can, and we need to get more effective at that. But there is only a certain amount of dollars that the Federal Government is going to put in for treatment into the State if the State won't take the initiative and says, unlike the other 49 States, that we're going to use local law enforcement to go after this stuff. We'll have the laws—I understand Hawaii has different traditions and it's a newer State and Alaska has a little bit of the same questions.

But when, in fact, you say we want to have a cost shifting from 49 States in the mainland, each State has to take care of its load, too. We're having this discussion aggressively in California because they can't say, oh, we need more dollars for marijuana treatment, we need more dollars for treating meth but we're not going to take some of the steps with which to address the question.

And I know you've been an advocate of that, and hopefully, this hearing helps highlight the interconnection with this because when we see this is clearly the highest meth use problem we've seen anywhere in the United States, it should be a primary focus. Property crime—I mean tourism is your life blood. Already just coming over here, I'm hearing certain things about how I you should behave in the car, what to do in your hotels, where you go. You don't need to have that spread through the people who are coming to Hawaii.

Mr. AIONA. You're right, you're absolutely right. Thank you for making those comments. You're absolutely right. Thank you.

Mr. SOUDER. Thank you very much for coming.

Mr. CASE. I just want to recognize, for the record, someone that is not represented here which you all would agree deserves recognition and that's our U.S. Attorney's office and Ed Kubo who has been very much a part of the effort and he deserves to be recognized. Thank you.

Mr. SOUDER. If the second panel will come forward; Honorable Harry Kim who is mayor of the county of Hawaii. And I understand that means mayor of the city within; Mr. Keith Kamita, chief of the Narcotics Division, Hawaii Department of Public Safety; Mr. Lawrence Mahuna, police chief of the Hawaii County Police Department; and Mr. Richard Botti, executive director of the Hawaii Food Industry Administration.

[Recess.]

[Witnesses sworn.]

Mr. SOUDER. Let the record show is that each of witnesses respond inside the affirmative. We're going to start with Deputy Mayor William Kenoi, right? Did I get that close?

Mr. KENOI. Close enough. I'll go with that.

STATEMENT OF WILLIAM P. KENOI, EXECUTIVE ASSISTANT TO MAYOR HARRY KIM, COUNTY OF HAWAII

Mr. KENOI. Thank you very much, Mr. Chairman. Chairman Souder, Congressman Case, thank you for traveling to Hawaii Island for your commitment to finding a solution to this terrible problem.

My name is William P. Kenoi, and I am proud and honored to serve Mayor Harry Kim and the people of Hawaii Island as an executive assistant tasked with coordinating the communities response to ice.

Three years ago we collectively embarked on a mission, to stem the tide of ice that threatened the quality of life for our children, our families, and our neighborhoods. We took this important first step because the data, statistics, and more importantly, the personal stories were impossible to ignore.

Children were being abused and neglected at an alarming rate. An increase in amount and severity of domestic violence complaints; horror stories from the emergency rooms; violence that stunned the law enforcement community, and a criminal justice system that was being crushed by ice. It was time to take action.

Ice has been ravaging our community for between 10 and 15 years. We couldn't talk about this problem anymore. We needed immediate execution and implementation. This would only be possible with two key elements; No. 1, broad-based community support; and two, the commitment of resource providers at every level.

To this end the Hawaii Island Methamphetamine Summit was held in August 2002. This summit brought together everyone in the community, business, government, community members, elected officials, unions, churches, cultural groups, nonprofits, law enforcement, treatment specialists, and prevention and education people. This collaboration and focus was unprecedented in Hawaii.

Why did the community rally and the resource providers commit? Because ice affected everyone in community. No one was untouched by the terrible effects of ice. Ice brought everyone in the community to the table to find a solution. The collective effort has resulted in substantial progress in the past 3 years.

We knew there was no simple solution to such a complex problem. However, if we focused on taking small steps hand in hand with the community, we would improve the health and well being of the entire community. So our approach was a simple one; focus on improving our community's capacity in the areas of enforcement, treatment, and prevention.

We needed to ensure that we didn't just talk about, but that we actually improved enforcement capabilities, that we funded increased treatment options, and we provided for prevention and education that focused on our youth.

There is no denying that ice threatens our future and our way of life. We lack adequate treatment programs and alternatives on all islands. We lack treatment options for those incarcerated for drug offenses. We lack a transportation system that allows youth and families to access important programs and services. We lack enough manpower and resources to our law enforcement community to eliminate ice. But Chairman Souder and Congressman Case, we do not lack community awareness, community commitment, and community momentum. And it is at the community level that we will be successful in eliminating ice from our islands.

All of us commit to the community that will stand side by side with them in this effort. There is no alternative. Anything short of a collective, committed, sustained initiative we'll fail to save our babies, our children, and our families from dying and being torn apart. We have no choice in this effort.

We commit to this effort and support our communities or we lose everyone we have.

Thank you very much for the opportunity to testify before the distinguished subcommittee on the U.S. House of Representatives.

Mr. SOUDER. Thank you very much. Mr. Kamita.

STATEMENT OF KEITH KAMITA, ADMINISTRATOR, NARCOTICS ENFORCEMENT DIVISION, HAWAII STATE DEPARTMENT OF PUBLIC SAFETY

Mr. KAMITA. Thank you, Chairman Souder, Congressman Case. My Federal partners that you've heard before us have gone over the State's, I guess, methamphetamine problem quite well. I want to touch on a section that the State is looking at and basically it's the unlawful manufacture of crystal methamphetamine here in Hawaii.

What we are seeing is not the big superlabs, but we are seeing small laboratories, mom-and-pop laboratories, where they are using every day household products such as pseudoephedrine, red phosphorous, iodine to manufacture small batches of methamphetamine which causes just as much danger as a superlab to the neighbors here in Hawaii.

These laboratories that cook up small batches are posing just as much danger as these superlabs by dumping their waste in the ground, by letting and venting their methamphetamine fumes, I would say, to their neighbors.

In Hawaii, we have had a very little amount of small labs, full synthesis laboratories where they're using red phosphorous and iodine, but we have had many conversion labs where they are bringing in the methamphetamine from California and just icing it up here in Hawaii.

In Hawaii we have a problem with monitoring certain precursor chemicals, one of which is pseudoephedrine. Hawaii's law right now is less than that of Federal law. We do not or we do have a full exemption on pseudoephedrine and ephedrine combination products. We are looking toward the Federal Government and utilizing their laws which do put on some restriction which is called Safe Harbor Products, anything which is three grams in a blister pack, such as something like this that is sold here in Hawaii every day. All of Hawaii's pseudoephedrine that we're finding in these laboratories are blister packs.

What we ask of the Federal Government is that you look at your law regarding blister packs, and hopefully, reevaluate that these blister packs that are utilized in laboratories they do not deter the meth user from manufacturing. These blister packs were made, I guess, as an ease to the consumer. However, a person on methamphetamine doesn't mind punching out 300 to 1,000 of these tablets, just sitting there and doing it.

The blister pack law, I think, is outdated and that exemption should be taken away. And to answer your question, that one thing the Federal Government can do for us, is to review that law. We don't want to make this a Schedule V controlled substance. The next best step is to look at some regulation. And we have worked with small retail shops and our Long's Drugs and other stores at educating and we did 98 presentations last year, educating both the public and retailers about the dangers of methamphetamine and how it's manufactured. We are working with, as a partnership, with Mr. Botti and some of the other people who are selling these over-the-counter items.

In ending, that's the one thing you can help us with. Thank you very much. Any questions, I'll answer later.

[The prepared statement of Mr. Kamita follows:]

LINDA LINGLE
GOVERNOR

STATE OF HAWAII
DEPARTMENT OF PUBLIC SAFETY
NARCOTICS ENFORCEMENT DIVISION
3375 Koapaka Street, Suite D-100
Honolulu, Hawaii 96819
(808) 837-8470

JOHN F. PEYTON, JR.
DIRECTOR

CLAIRE Y. NAKAMURA
Deputy Director
Administration

FRANK J. LOPEZ
Deputy Director
Corrections

JAMES L. PROPOTNICK
Deputy Director
Law Enforcement

No. ____________

THE POISONING OF PARADISE: CRYSTAL METHAPHETAMINE IN HAWAII

Written Testimony of Keith Kamita
Administrator, Narcotics Enforcement Division,
Hawaii State Department of Public Safety

Submitted to the U.S. House Government Reform Committee
Subcommittee on Criminal Justice, Drug Policy, and Human Resources

August 2, 2004

Chairman Tom Davis and Ranking Member Henry A. Waxman:

Substance abuse continues to have a profound social and economic impact on Hawaii. The Department of Public Safety sees its devastating effects daily, particularly in our corrections and law enforcement operations.

70% of those entering Hawaii's criminal justice system has a substance abuse problem. 85% of the incarcerated population has a history of drug abuse. 90% of all parole failures are linked to substance abuse.

The statistics are as dismal with the problem of crystal methamphetamine, also known as ice. Ice is considered to be the most significant drug threat in Hawaii. Ice abusers have been linked to violent crimes in Hawaii, including an alarming number of domestic crimes such as child neglect cases, hostage situations and homicides. In 2001, a survey among cities indicated that Honolulu had the highest percentage of male arrestees who tested positive for ice abuse.

As a major crossroads of the Pacific and Asia, the Hawaiian Islands are ideal distribution points for ice. Local, Mexican, Pacific Islander and Asian drug trafficking organizations distribute ice at the wholesale level throughout Hawaii. Approximately 80-90% of ice seized in Hawaii enters the State in mailed packages and on commercial flights by couriers via the Honolulu International Airport, where we have Federal, State and County law enforcement working together in an attempt to interdict drug entering our State. The number of drug cases initiated by the department's Sheriff Airport Unit through routine searches at x-ray machines and checkpoints has increased dramatically. These cases are investigated by the Narcotics Enforcement Division (NED) which has witnessed a 700% increase in the number of controlled substances cases handled by since July 2001. This upward spiral is certain to continue. Additional resources for law enforcement personnel at the Honolulu International Airport and narcotics enforcement investigators statewide are needed in the fight against Hawaii's number one illicit drug problem crystal methamphetamine. Hawaii would also be better equipped to combat ice in the community with a forensic laboratory for standardized drug analysis and forensic testing to support our existing Chemical Diversion Program which tracks and identifies suspect diverting regulated chemicals for the unlawful manufacture of drugs like crystal methamphetamine. The Narcotics Enforcement Division in an attempt to stem the unlawful manufacture of crystal methamphetamine in Hawaii has focused its attention on regulating and tracking the sales of these essential precursor chemicals. Pseudoephedrine has been the primary precursor chemical utilized to manufacture crystal methamphetamine "ice" here in Hawaii and is readily available in over the counter cold products that are diverted to these clandestine laboratories by individuals purchasing multiple boxes of these products or by stealing these items off the shelves of retail stores. Presently across the nation there is a trend toward placing over-the-counter products that contain pseudoephedrine behind the counter or by limiting the quantity that a customer can purchase in a single retail transaction (July 2003 Scheduling/Regulation study done on pseudoephedrine by the National Alliance for Model State Drug Laws). Even here in Hawaii there has been several Bills that propose that proposed limits on the sale of over the counter pseudoephedrine or resolutions that request that the Department of Public Safety to review and consider whether the exception of pseudoephedrine from the reporting, record keeping, and permit requirements generally applicable to list I chemicals should be repealed.

Presently Hawaii's laws on the sale or distribution of over-the-counter cold medications containing pseudoephedrine, norpseudoephedrine, or an ephedrine combination products is less stringent than that of Federal language and is causing a loop hole for individuals hired or tasked by street chemist in obtaining these precursor chemicals to be later sold to individuals manufacturing methamphetamine.

The Hawaii Revised Statutes contains no language that restricts the sale of "safe harbor" products containing ephedrine, pseudoephedrine, norpseudoephedrine, or phenylpropanoline. Only under administrative rules listed in Title 23, Chapter 201-9, does it require that any retail distributor that sells, transfers, or furnishes any products containing ephedrine, pseudoephedrine, norpseudoephedrine, or phenylpropanoline in a single transaction that is not in "safe harbor packaging" and is over 24 grams shall keep records of that transaction. The Federal Methamphetamine Anti-Proliferation Act (MAPA) currently limits the threshold of pseudoephedrine drug products that are not in blister packs ("Safe Harbor" products), to 9 grams in a single transaction and places reporting and registration requirements on distributors of over the counter pseudoephedrine products. The term "safe harbor packaging" means a product that is, if not a liquid, sold in packages of not more than three grams of the base ingredient and is packed in blister packs of not more than two tablets per blister, or if a liquid, sold in package size of not more than three grams of the base ingredient. This exemption given to over the counter pseudoephedrine products packed in "Safe Harbor Product" blister packs do not deter street chemist that utilize this product to manufacture methamphetamine.

During this past legislative session the Department proposed language to better regulates the retail sale of over the counter pseudoephedrine products on the State level but was unsuccessful. House Bill 2499 would have amend existing language in section 329-64(a)(4) that exempt retail distributors who sell, transfer, or furnish any over-the-counter drug product in a single transaction not to exceed three packages or 6 grams to an individual for legitimate medical use that contains pseudoephedrine, norpseudoephedrine, or an ephedrine combination product.

The Department is requesting that Congress also review Federal statutes to plug this "safe Harbor Product" loophole and require wholesale distributors and retail distributors to report all suspicious sales and over threshold sales of all pseudoephedrine and ephedrine combination products.

In July 1994, the Narcotics Enforcement Division to assist the Department took on a secondary mission and developed a new program to assist the Department in the investigation of all felony cases relating to controlled substances imitated by Deputies of the Sheriff, Maritime Law Enforcement, Protective Services Divisions and correctional facilities located on all islands. This program was named the "**FELONY ARREST LOCK-UP INVESTIGATION PROGRAM FOR THE DEPARTMENT OF PUBLIC SAFETY."** In Fiscal Year 2003 NED assigned two Investigators from its Diversion Branch to exclusively handle all cases initiated by the Airport Sheriff Detail and all correctional facilities on all islands.

In Fiscal year 2004 the Narcotics Enforcement Division responded to and investigated 217 cases that originated from the Airport Sheriff's Detail and 335 controlled substance or regulated chemical cases referred by US Customs Service, BICE or US Postal Service relating to the illegal importation of controlled substances or regulated chemicals by passengers or mail.

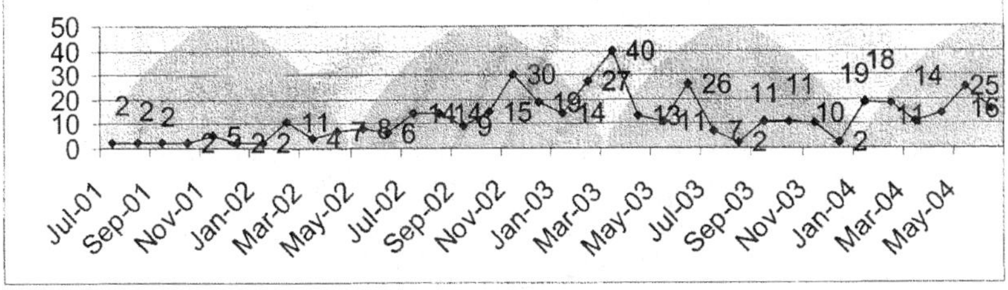

NED Airport Controlled Substance Cases July 2001 through June 2004

The Narcotics Enforcement Division in an effort to do more with less has invested its manpower with several of the Hawaii High Intensity Drug Trafficking Area (HIDTA) taskforces. The Narcotics Enforcement Division is presently a member of the following HIDTA taskforces:

HIGHT INTENSITY DRUG TRAFFICING AREA (STATEWIDE MULTI-AGENCY CLANDESTINE LABRITORY COORDINATION)

NED is the lead agency coordinating HIDTA's Statewide Multi-agency Clandestine Laboratory Coordination initiative which provides oversight, consolidated training, and to coordinate a first response to clandestine laboratories involved in the manufacturing of crystal methamphetamine "ice", gamma Hydroxyl-butyrate (GHB), phencyclidine (PCP), phenyl-2-propanone (P-2-P), methlenedioxtmethaphetamine (MDMA/Ecstasy), and lysergic acid diethylamide (LSD). The primary goal of this initiative is to coordinate and support all other HIDTA initiatives and regional law enforcement agencies as a resource to train, detect, dismantle, disrupt, arrest and prosecute individuals, drug organizations, drug gangs, and organized crime groups involved in clandestine laboratories, the diverting of regulated chemicals and the manufacturing of illicit narcotics. During FY 2004, this initiative initiated 23 clandestine laboratories investigations, 1regulated chemical diversion case, and 36 inspections of controlled substance or regulated chemical registrants. This initiative is headquartered within the Narcotics Enforcement Division and is supported by 1 primary investigator and 9 Clandestine Laboratory certified NED Investigators.

HIGHT INTENSITY DRUG TRAFFICING AREA (AIRPORT INTRADICTION)

The Narcotics Enforcement Division continues to be a member of HIDTA and has dedicating one full time position to the Airport Interdiction Taskforce stationed at the Honolulu International airport. The mission of this taskforce is the interdiction of drugs at all of the commercial airports statewide. A NED Investigator is assigned full time to this taskforce and is based out of the Honolulu International Airport.

HIGHT INTENSITY DRUG TRAFFICING AREA (FOREIGN INTERDICTION TASK FORCE)

The Narcotics Enforcement Division continues to be a member of a Customs HIDTA initiative, which identifies and investigates controlled substances, shipped, mailed or smuggled from a foreign country into Hawaii. During FY 2004, the Narcotics Enforcement Division investigated 335 pharmaceutical controlled substance or regulated chemical cases referred by US Customs Service, BICE or US Postal Service relating to the illegal importation of controlled substances by passengers or mail and issued 278 NED Customs Warnings.

HIGHT INTENSITY DRUG TRAFFICING AREA (MONEY LAUNDERING / ASSET FORFEITURE TASK FORCE)

In February of 2004, the Narcotics Enforcement Division became a full time member of the HIDTA Money Laundering / Asset Forfeiture Task Force, which is a multi agency initiative to detect, disrupt and dismantle drug organizations that use real property and launder proceeds from illegal activities by tracing assets and the flow of drug money proceeds both internationally and domestically into and out of the State of Hawaii. NED contributes one investigator to this initiative.

HIGHT INTENSITY DRUG TRAFFICING AREA (HILO IMPACT)

Ned has one Investigator participating in the HI IMPACT initiative which is HIDTA's primary investigative initiative utilized to dismantle, arrest and prosecute drug trafficking organizations, drug gangs, and organized groups involved in the drug distribution, drug manufacturing, money laundering, and other drug related crimes. NED has assigned its Hilo based Investigator to participate in this initiative.

DRUGS IN PRISON

Random drug testing of Hawaii inmates reveals that the drug of choice for offenders is ice. 70% of all positive urinalysis test results are attributed to ice. The Narcotics Enforcement Division during FY 2004 responded to 49 cases at our correctional facilities statewide, 3 from Hawaii Paroling Authority and initiated

36 prison contraband cases relating to the drugs resulting in arrest and seizures. In the majority of these drug cases crystal methamphetamine was the drug of choice.

NED Investigators respond to all controlled substance cases originating from correctional facilities on the island of Oahu on a 24-hour a day, 7-days a week call out system. NED's one Hilo based Investigator who responds to all controlled substance cases initiated out of HCCC and Kulani Correctional Facility with the assistance of the Hilo Narcotics Vice Office. Presently NED must depend upon the Maui and Kauai Police Departments for assistance in responding to any drug case originating from KCCC or MCCC due to the lack of presence of NED Investigators on both islands. Violations reported on these two islands are investigated by the local police departments and information later referred to NED.

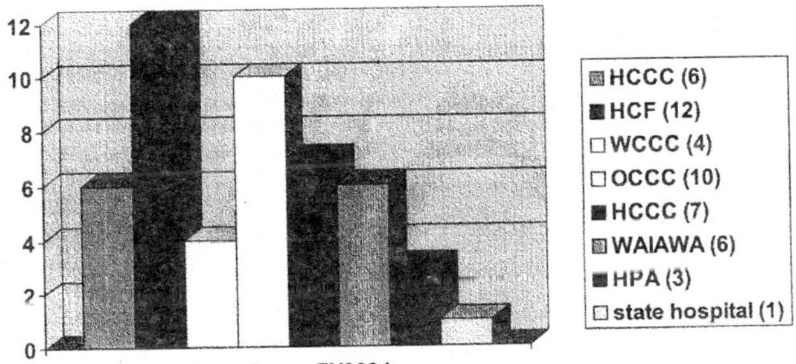

Drug Cases FY2004

Due to the increase in investigative services needed at Hawaii's airports, prison Facilities and other state controlled areas on all islands, the Narcotics Enforcement Division (NED) is in need of additional manpower and resources to be able to adequately investigate felony controlled substances and regulated chemicals investigations in these areas. NED presently lacks investigative personnel on the islands of Maui (to include Molokai, Niihau and Lanai), Kauai and in Kona on the island of Hawaii.

TRAINING AND EDUCATION

During FY 2004, NED took a leadership role in informing the community of Hawaii's methamphetamine problem. During FY 2004, the Narcotics

Enforcement Division put on 98 drug and clandestine laboratory presentations and training sessions to law enforcement, schools, the medical community and the public across the State. These various presentations on were attended by 9150 individuals as well as had media coverage. NED's education programs covers Hawaii's drug trends, drug identification, the physical and psychological effects as well as the damage that drugs can do to the human body. NED has partnered up with Laulima Hawaii and other State, County and Federal Agencies in an attempt to educate the public on the dangers of drugs. During FY 2004, NED participated in the making of two video documentaries, one made by Edgy Lee on Hawaii's Ice problem and another by Catholic Charities called "Try Wait." NED also participated as guest speakers on radio shows and television interviews to try and educate the public on Hawaii's drug trends and problems.

There is also a statewide effort to engage the community in Governor Linda Lingle and Lieutenant Governor Duke Aiona's ongoing efforts to control illegal drug use, particularly with the problem of ice as a major concern. The development of Hawaii's Drug Control Strategy, "A New Beginning," will reduce illegal drug use in Hawaii, intervene in the distribution of illicit drugs, increase access to treatment, and enhance law enforcement efforts.

The Department of Public Safety fully supports the Subcommittee's efforts to reduce drug abuse and address the methamphetamine problem in Hawaii and the rest of the country.

Thank you for the opportunity to testify on this important matter.

Mr. SOUDER. Thank you. Chief Mahuna.

STATEMENT OF LAWRENCE K. MAHUNA, POLICE CHIEF, HAWAII COUNTY POLICE DEPARTMENT

Mr. MAHUNA. Chairman Souder, Congressman Case, it's a pleasure to be here to look at our ice, what I would call, epidemic. We are a paradise. We have long-standing relationships. We have ohanas, which means families, that have been broken apart, families being affected. I've lived in areas that have been affected by ice houses.

Like September 11, it's changed the course in the way we travel, ice has changed the course of the way people live in their own neighborhoods. People no longer can leave their house unlocked, they can't leave their garage with items such as lawn mowers and that type of thing. We're seeing an increase in violence, both domestic violence and violence in nightclubs, violence in general, violence toward police officers.

So we're, basically, looking at trying to cooperate with our Federal partners, trying to cope with the lack of personnel because I think that's one of the ways that the Federal Government could help, is to help and assist us in having more FBI agents, more DEA agents, more ATF agents, customs agents here, because as Mr. Kamita said we don't have these big laboratories, we have small ones.

And yes, they are as insidious as these big giant labs. However, what is more insidious is that this drug is a generation killer. It is not a drug that we can say, well, maybe we can treat these people and the treatment of these individuals is not real successful, No. 1; No. 2, when you talk to child protective people, these people that use ice are one of the few people that don't want their children back. And that's what you always find at an ice house.

You'll find living conditions that you wouldn't have an animal live in, No. 1. You'll find young children. You'll find poly use of drugs. You'll find at least one or two pregnant women. You'll find high rates of domestic violence, and you will have people that are afraid to leave their houses for fear that either their house is going to be entered and their valuable items taken. And when we talk about valuable items, value is based upon what you feel.

I've had a good friend that had poi pounders that are 200 years old that were in the family stolen and sold for $10. These things are irreplaceable things, these things that affect the heart and soul of people on this island.

It has affected people from children 12 years old, 11 years old, as far as selling the drug. We've caught kids on campus that are 13 years old with 10, 12 grams of ice so they can sell, and they've been instructed by the parents to go and sell these drugs because No. 1, if the kid gets caught, he or she does not face the same kind of penalties as, say, an adult would selling it in the school.

So we have to set up two task forces in the police department to strictly look at ice itself, but we have not only looked at the big organization. One of our issues here is to dismantle the large organizations, of course. But the other issue is to take away the social terrorism that our people are actually involved in day-to-day. And when you live that thing day-to-day, that is pure terrorism to me.

And we ask that the Federal Government, hopefully, will step up outside of the main island of Oahu and look at the smaller islands and the bigger islands and provide us with adequate funds, adequate resources. And I think it's a holistic way of looking at it.

The community has to get involved and has been involved. The mayor's office and everybody else, treatment people, the demand reduction people. So I plead with you to help the people that have lived here hundreds of years. You're taking away their source of who they are and what they are and where they're coming from. Thank you very much.

Mr. SOUDER. Thank you.

[The prepared statement of Mr. Mahuna follows:]

July 27, 2004

Mark E. Souder
Chairman
Subcommittee on Criminal Justice
Drug Policy and Human Resources
Congress of the United States
House of Representatives
2157 Rayburn House Office Building
Washington, DC 20515-6143

Dear Chairman Souder:

Mr. Chairman and members of the Subcommittee:

Thank you for your invitation to address this investigative hearing entitled, "The Poisoning of Paradise: Crystal Methamphetamine in Hawaii.

The State of Hawaii and in my personal opinion, particularly the island of Hawaii are indeed a paradise. Because of its size and economic diversity, the 4,000-square-mile Big Island of Hawaii, although incorporated as a single county, finds itself challenged. Much of the western part of the island, with its reputation as both a tourist destination and an area with many upscale residences, enjoys a higher standard of living. The eastern part of the island, lacking major industrial job providers, suffers from a reduced economy. This results in higher unemployment in the East and an abundance of lower paying service jobs in the West to which many people from the East are forced to commute on a daily basis.

The economically distinct sides of the island do share an unfortunate common trait; a large segment of their population addicted to the drug crystal methamphetamine, also commonly known by its street name of "ice." This highly addictive drug has provided suppliers and distributors from both here and abroad with a large and highly profitable market here in Hawaii.

The increased supply and demand for "ice" in the County of Hawaii is a continuous threat to the safety and welfare of the general public and is therefore a primary law enforcement concern. Our local media, elected officials, and members of the public have repeatedly stated the abuse of "ice" on the Big Island has reached epidemic levels. Our Honorable Mayor Harry Kim has publicly declared "war" on "ice."

We have learned through several investigations that much of the crystal methamphetamine distribution on our island can be traced back to California and Mexico, and it includes elements of the so-called Mexican Mafia.

In order to be more proactive, our Department has established two Ice Task Force units, one in East Hawaii and one here in West Hawaii. These Task Forces, comprised entirely of personnel from within our Department are in response to this growing menace to our community. We have also dedicated two telephone lines as "Ice" Hotlines for use by the public for reporting of crystal methamphetamine possession and or distribution. The primary goal of our task forces is to identify, dismantle, disrupt, arrest, and prosecute street, mid-and upper-level drug trafficking organizations and organized crime groups involved in methamphetamine distribution, methamphetamine manufacturing, and money laundering.

Although we may concentrate on the large organizations, even "ice" houses have been targeted although the quantities of "ice" recovered is small at times. Removal of the occupants of the house is primary, as the high rate of domestic violence, parental neglect and property crimes, which occur within these neighborhoods, becomes a form of social terrorism which is unacceptable.

A secondary yet perhaps more crucial goal is to have our task force personnel maintain a drug prevention and educational program in our schools and community. Our department seeks to remain both connected to our community and hopeful for their continuing support in reporting suspected "ice" dealers and sharing a vision that together we can overcome this peril, which seeks to rob our youth of their future and our elderly of their possessions, which are often stolen to support "ice" addicted persons. We firmly believe this is not an effort in futility, but rather a partnership towards an eventual victory.

Our efforts to date have disrupted the activities of several large drug organizations on the Island of Hawaii. In conjunction with Federal agents and attorneys, we have prosecuted the leaders of these organizations in Federal Court. Additionally, in concert with community partners we have participated in roadside sign waving campaigns to bring further attention to the problem and to seek additional community support.

Our seizures of crystal methamphetamine have increased from 2.6 pounds in 2002 to 13.5 pounds in 2003, as well as 6.5 pounds through June of this year. This may not sound like a huge amount in terms of volume, but it is important to know street-level "ice" sales often deal in tenth of a gram quantities.

We understand no recitation of statistical data in terms of seizures, numbers of cases and/or arrests can compare to the agony and pain suffered by relatives and friends of "ice" users. In June of this year we conducted a daytime search warrant raid on a suspected ice dealer. What was found aside from the "ice"-using suspect, and a quantity of "ice", were the suspect's six children ranging in age from 5 to 17 none was at school on that day. When asked by a detective why they were not in school, they indicated they had wanted to go but their mother could not be awakened to take them. There are numerous documented accounts or incidents that have taken place whereby crimes of violence have occurred to infants, and spouses due to the use of "ice".

I am aware the purpose of this hearing is to examine the problem of methamphetamine trafficking and abuse and how we on the local level in partnership with the Federal Government can address this problem.

In terms of methamphetamine trafficking, as an island state we are dependent upon the maritime and aviation industries for all of our imported goods, and based on our intelligence most of our "ice" is imported in the same manner. Our State Supreme Court has interpreted our State Constitution as forbidding local law enforcement from utilizing the "Walk and Talk" method of drug interdiction which is both allowed and used by Federal agents. Our island, about the size of the state of Connecticut, currently has only one fulltime Drug Enforcement Administration agent and two agents from the Bureau of Alcohol, Tobacco and Firearms, all located on the East side of our island but no presence on the West side. We do have two FBI agents on the West side of the island, but none in the East. We believe a larger presence in terms of Federal Law Enforcement Agents on our island working with Hawaii Police Department personnel will help to slow the importation of "ice".

Approximately 82 percent of all cases assigned to our Crime Laboratory are for drug analysis, including analysis for other state and certain Federal Agencies. Because of its age and limited space our Crime Laboratory will never be confused with that of the CSI television show. We have had Federal assistance in the past in terms of funding for new equipment, but a state of the art Crime Laboratory designed in the mid-1970's is hard-pressed to keep up with the 21st Century technology available to those who reap massive profits, estimated at 300 to 400 percent here in Hawaii, from the illicit manufacture and subsequent sales of crystal methamphetamine. We are in need of Federal financial assistance to improve and expand our Crime Lab.

Since February 2000, a number of joint federal, state and local law enforcement operations targeting specific drug trafficking organizations have resulted in significant drug seizures, drug-related arrests and forfeitures in Hawaii County alone. We believe continuing results of these types of investigations can only be achieved through additional manpower and federal law enforcement support with a primary focus on stemming the importation and distribution of crystal methamphetamine in the State of Hawaii.

Thank you for allowing me this opportunity to provide testimony today.

Sincerely,

LAWRENCE K. MAHUNA
POLICE CHIEF

STATEMENT OF RICHARD BOTTI, EXECUTIVE DIRECTOR, HAWAII FOOD INDUSTRY ASSOCIATION

Mr. BOTTI. Thank you, Chairman Souder and Representative Case for the opportunity to testify before your subcommittee. I'm the President of the Hawaii Food Industry, a trade association, representing over 225 of Hawaii retailers, distributors, and suppliers of food and related items.

I'm here to express our concerns about the placement of pseudoephedrine on Schedule V where commonly sold medicine products would be required to be placed behind the pharmacy counter, sold only by a pharmacy and customers would be required to show identification and sign a register when they made the purchases.

Retailers would be forced to eliminate the variety or products and customers would be denied access and availability. Most store do not have a pharmacy, thus Schedule V would mean that most over-the-counter cold and allergy medicines could not be purchased at airports, hotel gift shops, convenience stores, or any other retail outlet that does not have a pharmacist on duty.

Schedule V would also present a public health problem because it would limit the amount of medicine that families can legitimately purchase in 1 month. Because there is no central recording of all pseudoephedrine purchases in the State, this provision will be impossible to implement and law enforcement would have difficulty enforcing the law without going store to store to compare names in the log books.

Schedule V will have no impact on internet sales of pseudoephedrine. FDA and U.S. Customs have testified before Congress that they are able to inspect less than 5 percent of drug packages that go through U.S. Postal facilities from overseas.

Schedule V places an unfair burden on retailers and their employees, most of whom are trying to do the right thing.

We agree that our industry has a responsibility to help in this crisis we face. We are taking action. Without the placement of pseudoephedrine on Schedule V, the Hawaii Food Industry is supporting what we call Meth Watch that started in Kansas 2001 and has a proven track record of success with the reduction and sales of pseudoephedrine for illegal purposes.

It has reduced the number of meth labs in the State. It has also resulted in dramatic reductions in the theft of products used to make meth.

Most important, it addresses a larger problem.

It involves the whole community, law enforcement, retailers, business leaders, and citizens through the education and prevention efforts and it appears to be having an impact on actual meth usage.

There is, however, an important element that law enforcement needs; that is, a list of all retailers that sell targeted products. For this reason we support the registration of all retailers in the State who sell OTC or over-the-counter drugs, medicines, that contain pseudoephedrine. This will provide law enforcement with an accurate list of where the medicines are being sold. Comparing this list with distribution data that is available under Federal law will allow law enforcement to determine whether stores are selling excessive amounts.

HFIA acknowledges that serious action must be taken to prevent the diversion of precursor chemicals to meth labs, and we want to be a part of the solution. There are less restrictive alternatives to Schedule V that include many of the things that I mentioned at the beginning of my testimony. Demand reduction, prevention, education and partnerships with law enforcement will serve the community at large. There is much that we can do to reduce the meth problem in this State without placing unreasonable burdens on consumers to purchase the medicines they need and on the retailers who provide them.

Added to our testimony I would like to include what we will do without a law and the logo for the Meth Watch program that is taken off from the Kansas City one. Thank you.

[The prepared statement of Mr. Botti follows:]

Testimony of

RICHARD C. BOTTI
PRESIDENT
HAWAII FOOD INDUSTRY ASSOCIATION

SUBCOMMITTEE ON CRIMINAL JUSTICE, DRUG POLICY, AND HUMAN RESOUCES
COMMITTEE ON GOVERNMENT REFORM
UNITED STATE HOUSE OF REPRESENTATIVES

Presented on August 2, 2004

Chairman Souder and Members of the Subcommittee:

Good morning, welcome to Hawaii, and thank you for the opportunity to testify before the subcommittee. I am the President of the Hawaii Food Industry Association (HFIA), a trade association representing over 225 of Hawaii's retailers, distributors, and suppliers of food and related items.

HFIA has been working proactively on the methamphetamine issue for many years because our members distribute and sell many of the ingredients, or precursor chemicals, that are diverted to make meth. These products include over-the-counter medicines for colds, allergies, and asthma, lithium batteries, coffee filters, drain cleaner, rock salt, iodine, and several other household products. HFIA members have worked closely with law enforcement officials to prevent the diversion of precursor chemicals from our stores. Many stores around the state have taken voluntary measures to prevent diversion, such as rigorous employee education, limiting sales of certain products, moving meth ingredients close to cash registers and other high traffic areas of the store, and limiting the amount of products on the shelf. Even though we have been informed by law enforcement that the real problem with diversion in Hawaii comes from small, independent neighborhood stores, HFIA members have been working hard to insure that they do not become part of the problem.

This morning, I would like to offer my comments and concerns about the placement of pseudoephedrine on Schedule V of the Controlled Substances Schedule. Oklahoma enacted a law placing pseudoephedrine on Schedule V in April of 2004 and legislation has been introduced in Congress to do the same thing at the national level.

Pseudoephedrine has been approved by the U.S. Food & Drug Administration (FDA) as a decongestant for over-the-counter (OTC) sale in retail outlets in the U.S. Pseudoephedrine is a proven, trusted decongestant, probably the most effective on the market. HFIA stores carry hundreds of OTC medicines that contain pseudoephedrine insuring that consumers have a wide variety of choices between solid dose, liquid-gels, gel-caps, liquids, and several pediatric formulations.

If pseudoephedrine were placed on Schedule V, these products would be required to be placed behind a pharmacy counter, sold only by a pharmacist, and customers would be required to show identification and sign a register when they made a purchase. Because stores don't have the room to place products behind the counter, they will be forced to carry only a small variety of products and customers would be denied access and availability. Because of the fact that most of our stores don't even have a pharmacy, food retailers will not be able to carry the medicines and consumers will not be able to get the medicine they need for themselves or their families. Additionally, families living in rural areas, where pharmacies are limited, will not be able to get the medicines at all. Schedule V means that most OTC cold and allergy medicines could not be purchased at airports, hotel gift shops, convenience stores, or any other retail outlet that does not have a pharmacist on duty.

Schedule V also presents a public health problem because it limits the amount of medicine that families can legitimately purchase in one month. Larger families with children may not be able to purchase enough OTC medicines to treat their colds, allergies, asthma, and coughs as needed. Furthermore, because there is no central recording of all pseudoephedrine purchases in the state, this provision will be impossible for retailers to implement. Law enforcement will also have difficulty enforcing the law without going store-to-store to compare names in the log books.

Schedule V will have no impact on internet sales of pseudoephedrine. FDA and U.S. Customs have testified before Congress that they are able to inspect less than 5 percent of drug packages that go through U.S. Postal facilities from overseas. Scheduling pseudoephedrine will have no impact on internet sales and distribution.

In summary, the placement of pseudoephedrine on Schedule V will limit access and availability, two important factors that help reduce the costs of healthcare in Hawaii and around the U.S. In addition to creating an unnecessary hardship for consumers, Schedule V places an unfair burden on retailers and their employees, most of whom are trying to do the right thing.

There is a better way to address the problem of precursor chemicals being diverted to clandestine meth labs – it's called Meth Watch. Started in Kansas in 2001, Meth Watch is a proven and successful program that has cut sales of pseudoephedrine for illegal purposes and reduced the number of meth labs in the state. Implementation of Meth Watch has also resulted in dramatic reductions in theft of products used to make meth. It also addresses the larger problem: it involves the whole community – law enforcement, retailers, business leaders, and citizens – through education and prevention efforts, and appears to be having an impact on actual meth usage.

Meth Watch is a voluntary program that involves a variety of people at the community and state level, although retail involvement is the cornerstone. Participating retailers place the precursor products where they can be easily monitored, and strategically post Meth Watch signs and tags on their doors and windows, around their cash registers and on the shelves where precursor products are located. They may impose purchase limits to prevent high volume sales. They train their employees to recognize, but not to confront, suspicious customers and to contact law enforcement with as much information as possible. HFIA is a proud supporter of the Meth Watch program and we will be working hard to on implementation throughout the state.

HFIA also supports the registration of all retailers in the state who sell OTC medicines that contain pseudoephedrine. This will provide law enforcement with an accurate list of where the medicines are being sold. Comparing this list with distribution data that is available under federal law will allow law enforcement to determine whether stores are selling excessive amounts.

HFIA acknowledges that serious action must be taken to prevent the diversion of precursor chemicals to meth labs, and we want to be part of the solution. There are less restrictive alternatives to Schedule V that include many of the things that I mentioned at the beginning of my testimony. Demand reduction, prevention, education and partnerships with law enforcement will serve the community at large. There is much that we can do to reduce the meth problem in this state without placing unreasonable burdens on consumers to purchase the medicines they need and on the retailers who provide them.

Again, thank you for the opportunity to testify before the subcommittee.

Mr. SOUDER. Thank you each for your testimony.

I think I'm going to start backward with the Meth Watch program and tying this in with the blister pack question. Then I'll move to Mr. Case and come back to Mr. Kenoi. One of the things the Big Island received—let me start with this.

Did the grant that came in the appropriations process come to the Big Island directly? Was it solely for this island? What amount did you get in the appropriation bill? Was it $5 million?

Mr. KENOI. Last year it was $4 million. It went to the Hawaii Community Foundation to administer.

This year it's $4.5, but it's going to be—last year we received for the Hawaii Island meth initiative, we received $4 million. That moneys went from Department of Justice to the Community Oriented Police and Services Program to the Hawaii Community Foundation for a couple of reasons.

One, they had the grant making capability to administer a broad-based initiative that included enforcement, treatment, and prevention. Two, they had a long-standing commitment of grant making to the community, grass roots level, and for their reputation for honesty and integrity. Hawaii County, unfortunately, didn't have the administrative capability to administer this grant.

We were fortunate enough to secure a second round of funding, but that second round of funding in the amount of $4.5 million will be shared equally amongst Kauai, Maui, Molokai, Lanai, and Hawaii Island. And in the spirit of aloha we are happy to share that with our fellow residents because everybody in Hawaii is suffering from this drug.

Mr. SOUDER. And in this drug plan you gave me, does it have a split out of what you did with the $4.5 million.

Mr. KENOI. There is a breakdown. That was done before we, actually, issued all of the moneys, but I broke it down exactly how we did.

What we did, just general for you, Mr. Chairman, is $1 million went to enforcement. Under that enforcement 525,000 went to HPD. We created an ice task force in east and west Hawaii. We created an anti-smuggling unit here on Hawaii Island based on west Hawaii because of the amount of drugs that are coming in, being targeted to Hawaii with the direct flights from international, as well as source city destinations on the West Coast.

We also used that money under the enforcement arena, gave a couple hundred thousand to the Prosecutor's Office to have a drug prosecutor designated in both east and west Hawaii so that all of the cases that were being generated by HPD could be addressed at the Prosecutor's level.

Another couple hundred thousand went to the Judiciary and the Hawaii Island Drug Court both in east and east Hawaii so that there was an alternative to incarceration for those who wanted and needed treatment. So that was the enforcement component.

Under the treatment component we, actually, put $1.5 million into treatment; $500,000 went equally to every treatment provider around Hawaii Island, $100,000 a piece, not for existing treatment but for each of the programs to expand treatment services on the island.

A million dollars that was in the treatment balance went to the establishment of an adolescent residential treatment program for Hawaii Island. What we found out, Chairman Souder, was that all of our adolescents who need high end treatment were being sent off island to Maui, Kauai. We were sending teenagers as young as 13, pulling them out of their communities, away from their schools, away from everything they knew, and sending them without any support to a residential program off island.

We had been doing this for decades, failing miserably at it. And we didn't want to just take our kids, stick them in a home, give them a drug counselor, and say now you have residential treatment, we did our part. We felt like if our children are our most precious resources, then let us give them the best possible residential program we could. To that end, a million came out of this grant; 900,000 came from SAMHSA.

Mr. SOUDER. That's on top of the $4.5 million.

Mr. KENOI. Yes, on top. And we were able to secure $300,000 from the State legislature last year for a total of $2.2 million and that program just opened a couple weeks ago in Laupahoehoe, 14 acres. It's a community-based, culturally based, and experientially based program so that our kids are active, they're participating in cultural programs, they're using the ocean, the land to help them heal.

So we're really proud of that initiative, taking that step, because people said it's out of your area of jurisdiction, it's out of your area of expertise, and you have no money, you're reaching too far. We said if we fail, we fail, but we've got to try. So we were able to pull that together.

The other 1.5 went into prevention and demand reduction. And what we did was we went around the island and we held grant seminars and grant workshops and we wanted to get the balance of the resources into the community and asked existing programs and service providers to come forward and submit grants as to how they would utilize recreational, cultural, art activities for youth as a way to reduce the demand for crystal meth and ice. And these include island-wide mentoring programs, supplementing the Boys and Girls Club. And we did this island wide because we have a 4,028 square mile island populated by 150,000 people lacking in an adequate transportation system.

So given that we couldn't do one or two programs. We'd have to do programs in all of our communities.

So we set up an independent review panel and we asked people to solicit and provide technical support.

Mr. SOUDER. Did you say $2 million for prevention.

Mr. KENOI. $1.5.

Mr. SOUDER. $1.5 in three categories.

Mr. KENOI. Yeah, and included in the 1.5 for prevention is the administrative costs, the evaluation costs to understand if we're achieving our outcomes, do we have measurable outcomes, are we achieving our goals and objectives.

Mr. SOUDER. And were those 12 month programs, had to be done within 12 months, or——

Mr. KENOI. We got an extension. It was Federal moneys that came down, we got it announced, President Bush post September

11 didn't sign any of the budgets except defense appropriations and so everything went back, it's on the omnibus bill, then it came out, then DOJ, and Department of Justice——

Mr. SOUDER. It's basically 12 months. You didn't ask people for like a 3-year prevention program.

Mr. KENOI. Yeah, we asked people for 1 year with the understanding that we'll probably stretch this money over 2 years because it's a model program. It hasn't been done anywhere else in the country. As you know, DOJ top moneys are enforcement based usually resources and we asked DOJ to help us, work with us and let's make this an across the spectrum program, and they've been very cooperative at the Federal level.

There was hesitancy on their part initially like what is this adolescent residential treatment. This is Department of Justice moneys. What is this island-wide mentoring program so the youth can connect with the career or vocation or opportunity; how does that relate to drug abuse and we had to go and explain using the data that we had that we can't just hire more police officers, we can't just build more prisons. We got to reach our children. We got to reach our families.

Mr. SOUDER. How many people are there on the Big Island.

Mr. KENOI. Approximately, 150,000. I've heard from 148 to 162, somewhere thereabouts.

Mr. SOUDER. One of the reasons we need to have good monitoring is to see some reaction. This grant is the biggest grant that's gone anywhere in the United States for meth. The standard is a million, and those usually cover whole States; that $4.5 million for 150,000 people means it's less than half the size of my hometown. It's less than half the size of some of my rural counties, and it's less than half the size of two other counties I have.

This is incredibly intensive dollars in a problem to address the meth, particularly when you add in 900,000 SAMHSA on top of it and you're trying to do it in 12 months because often this size grant would be over 3 years in an area that may address 3 million people.

And so if you don't see some results that are fairly dramatic, it calls into question whether money is really going to have much of a reaction.

Now, the adolescent youth facility, there the $2.2 million was allotted in the structure, was it?

Mr. KENOI. It was both CIP, as well as operational.

Mr. SOUDER. What would you say was the split of those dollars?

Mr. KENOI. We issued our request for proposal, we're talking 300,000 CIP, the rest operational. Now, the cost for an adolescent for treatment is between 275 and $325 per day, per bed. So just an 8-bed residential facility, it's $100,000 per bed per year to treat one of our children for dramatic substance abuse addiction. So it's $800,000 for 1 year just operational because when you're dealing with adolescents, you're dealing with 24-hour care, 7 days a week, both educational care, healthcare, and substance abuse counseling so it's rather intensive and costly.

And that's the reason we haven't had—if you're on the mainland and you need residential treatment, your parents can drive 2 hours to see you, to support you. Here, you're sent on an airplane that's very expensive, and you might not be seen by your family or friends for another 4 or 5 months.

It was something we needed to do to step up. I mean how can we say we have the highest rate of crystal meth abuse and substance abuse in the entire Nation and we ask our children to step forward and ask for help and when we do so, we pull them away and send them away.

That caused incredible damage and it really makes a farce of any initiative. You cannot say we have the highest rate of substance abuse of our adolescents, ask for money based on that statistic, and then when we get those resources, we say, oooh, it's too expensive, it's a high risk investment.

Mr. SOUDER. For example, in Montana where you have people spread out 1,200 miles, they can't stay in their home area. Now, it is different moving islands and the cultures are difficult, and I understand that, but it's not like in the mountain West we don't have similar things. If somebody from my district needs adolescent care, they may have to go a minimum of 6 hours to the other end of the State, for example, and I'm in a pretty heavily populated area.

I agree it's a little bit more of a mental challenge because I'm trying to get adjusted as I've been here to this concept of ex-pats, people who have left here when you say you don't have job opportunities for young people to stay on the islands and they want to stay on the islands, it's like, well, that's true in every State because less than 40 percent of the people, sometimes as low as 20 percent stay in their home State. We're a highly mobile Nation.

But the difference is you're way out in the middle of the ocean and water between the different islands and there is a much more of a—almost a—particularly among the native Hawaiian population some of the other immigrant groups have fixation to land in the immediate area more like the Native American nations inside the United States. And that presents a different type of a challenge, much like what happened in the Indian schools in the West which were not particularly effective when they moved the kids from the reservation into Phoenix, say, and the impact on the education system.

So I agree it's a different challenge and I'm trying to work that through. On the other hand, it's not unusual that young people have to move long distances away from their families all over the United States and Alaska, for example. Let me yield to.

Mr. CASE. Do you want to make a followup.

Mr KENOI. Yes. I completely agree with you, and there are times when you need to be sent off island when there are too many negative dynamics around them in their home area. I completely agree with you, Chairman Souder, and we understood it from day 1, that we were fortunate we were given an opportunity to be a model program. We knew that we were getting resources that weren't available to other communities across this entire country.

So it wasn't an idea of let's get this money and do our thing with it. It was give us the opportunity with these resources to see how we can create a unique program. And if we're effective, we can replicate this elsewhere in the country. Instead of giving a little bit and guessing what works and what doesn't work, let us be the guinea pig, if you will, let us be a test.

And I think on our island community has done a good job with it. We'll see with the specific data and measurables. But we have a community that the mayor, the police chief, the prosecutor are all on the same page and committed. We're looking at a community that anywhere you go on the island, people come out, they respond, they take the time to be there.

People put aside their political and personal differences, ideological differences, and understand that the only way we're going to succeed is if we collectively and collaboratively work together. So we understand that. This is a unique opportunity and we feel the importance of doing right by it.

Mr. CASE. Just staying with the question because I think you're exactly right, Billy, this was represented to the Congress and Congress approved it and through Senator Inouye's efforts a test, a national test. This is the model. What works and what doesn't?

So with that there is an opportunity, a tremendous opportunity that, frankly, the rest of our State doesn't have but also a tremendous responsibility. And I think there is also a responsibility at the end of the day to recognize and honestly assess what the results were. Because I think what I'm hearing in the Chair's questions are basically we do have to analyze the cost effectiveness at the end of the day.

Are there any results—not results, do you have any sense of what really is working and what is still open for question? Do we know, for example, in your opinion, that the moneys allocated to, for example, we spent the whole first panel talking about law enforcement, trying to give our law enforcement community the tools it needs. And it doesn't have the tools. It doesn't have the tools in the State books, and it doesn't have the tools within the Federal reach or both really, and you have supplemented in that way. You got people out in the community on a law enforcement basis. Rehabilitation, we've always known that was expensive and we have never devoted these kind of resources to it. Preventative education has always been touted as the way to go but at the expense of rehabilitation.

Is it honestly too early to give the committee any indication of what really is a slam dunk or what is out there? Do you have any answers?

Mr. KENOI. Yes, I'll take a stab at that because I'm constantly asking and curious. Nobody is going to stand up and say this is what we know. For example, SAMHSA's directory, I sent a letter to every chemical dependency, substance abuse agency, office, university, department across the country just to see and ask do we know what works.

It's amazing how much billions of dollars we spend every year on substance abuse related issues and a lot of people still shrug, they're still not sure. That's no reason to sit around and—you know, analysis by paralysis.

But to get back to your question what works, I will say this. We contracted with the University of Hawaii Manoa, Center for the Family. They do excellent work in terms of evaluating programs and resources and it's an independent review of resources and programs and services and how effective, what is the effectiveness of that.

But if you ask me, walking around, because people ask every day, you go to a family party, somebody will stop you, how's it going, what's working. Senator Inouye was here a couple weeks ago and we had a briefing from HPD, and they used what indicators they had, whether it's working. Price on the street for crystal meth doubled. That's an indication that things are working. We created an ice hotline.

The community's No. 1 concern, police/law enforcement not effective. Ice house on my street 5 years, 3 years, 6 months, nobody is doing anything. That ice house is a plague on our community and on our children. We started an ice hotline, I think, maybe 50, 60 calls a week, people saying what can we do with this ice house. And what we did with this ice hotline—I want to give Chief Mahuna credit for this, is that we documented every call, so that when a person called in to speak to a sergeant and the next time a patrolman and the next time dispatch.

They documented every call. Now we have one to two complaints a week.

Mr. CASE. Were those efforts funded out of the money; in other words, you had the resources to do that out of the moneys that were provided.

Mr. KENOI. What we were told when we were given Federal moneys is that you guys have to get State moneys and county moneys put forward so that it's not just all of us relaying on the State, and this was part of the county's contribution, to supplement the Federal moneys.

So that's why we were told right off the top by Senator Inouye's office, as well as yourself, Congressman Case, is that when you get congressional money, you can't just ask Congress and the Federal Government to step up and pay for it. The community has to do their part, the county government has to put in something, and the State, you guys have to ask the State legislature, and they stepped for us and supplemented only what little they put. Those are the indicators that are working.

I've had people stop me as recently as last week telling me thank you. I said, it's not me, it's the communities. I'm just trying to do my job to help the communities. They said, you know, 3 years ago we wouldn't go to the beach anymore, Billy. We wouldn't go to the parks, it was scary. It seemed like the drug dealers and the people who were using and dealing owned the public areas. And now it feels safe, we all go out, families use the community parks, they use the beaches, there is no fear. People were terrified a couple years ago, scared. Nobody wanted to even talk to me about the problem and these are anecdotal. It's not documentation.

But I think if you were to ask most people in this community for their fair opinion, I think people will say that it's not magic, there are still bad things going on, but have we progressed. Have these resources made a difference? Absolutely.

The biggest difference is we always ask communities to do it themselves, to step up to the plate because that's true sustainability. These moneys will come and these moneys will go. That's the reality. Grants come and grants go. But the community stays, and they're the key to sustainability. But communities won't participate if they feel they're just being given lip service.

If the media is there and there is a big clap of hands and everybody rah-rah and all these promises made and 6 months, a year down the road, nothing happens, they're not coming back to the meeting. In fact, you're going to have twice a hard time for getting them back the next time, whatever the next issue might be, affordable housing, homelessness, whatever, economic development.

But the reason this works and the reason we're 3 years in and people care and people participate is because the government did step up and there are resources to address communities needs and there is a difference being made, so people are willing to participate.

Mr. CASE. Chief Mahuna, thank you for the true manao. That was very well put. Comments on the first panel's observations on the limitations on your powers and abilities to do what you think you need to do to bust people.

Were the first panel's observations or limitations on State law—and what I heard on Lanai, your officers actually utilizing Federal resources because the State says it doesn't work down on the street, is that your experience here on the Island of Hawaii as well?

Mr. MAHUNA. I think it's a fair assessment to be made. I think every case may require a wiretap, every case may look at large organizations that affect our island because for Federal, simply the fact that the laws are not the same. The adversary hearing when it comes to the wiretap is a hindrance. The unconstitutionality of the "walk and talk" inhibits us from doing our job.

So what we've done and successfully done is use island work in conjunction with our cohorts on the Federal level and I think we've become very successful. We've looked at other intensive ways.

When I look at the terror that people feel, when a parent comes up to me and says thank you very much for arresting my child with tears in their eyes, you don't see that. Usually, you get a pie in the face for arresting my kid.

In small rural areas where we didn't have the type of law enforcement presence, we went down there and we cleaned up a bunch of ice houses. And they said, my God, thank you very much because it makes them breathe better. It makes the fear level decrease and the cooperativeness increase. It gives them a feeling that someone cares about them.

So the task forces were developed. Yes, we are looking at the dismantling of large meth labs and meth organizations, but we're also looking at those ice houses, the ones that plague our people more than anything else because the community cannot take care of their very young and very old. And the very old usually end up being the victims of some sort of crime against persons or some sort of property offense where things of value have been taken from them. And this is not—just trying to get very material with this. I mean things that were passed down from their father's father, things that mean so much to their heart.

For example, the passage of these items and artifacts to their children and to their families are no longer there. And to me that is the measure of how effective we can be, and I think we can be effective given the same type of laws and the same type of criminal justice system Statewide, that we could get the same kind of action and the same type of penalties by Honolulu and probably keep everything on a State level.

But because we can't, the biggest bang for the buck is to go the Federal way. And I think people will think twice, hopefully, that if you deal with large quantities and get 25, 30 years, period, you don't get probation, you don't get anything else, it will make an effect on them. But there are other things that the addiction has not addressed, and I think that is an issue for money. Because we took down an organization, yes, it's slow in coming, but the addiction to money is there, too. So what happens is we have replacement people, people that move up in the tiers of the organization. So when we take an organization down, we have to take the entire organization. That way we get not only the people that run the organization but we get second, third, fourth tier people that move up when we make those arrests of these large leaders of the organization.

Mr. CASE. Thank you very much. Thank you very much.

Mr. SOUDER. Thank you. I'm going to ask to insert two statements from Elaine Wilson, Chief of Alcohol and Drug Abuse Division, Hawaii Department of Health that were given to the Joint House Senate Committee. We met with her Friday, last Friday, and went through a couple of things. And the good thing about having a long-term problem like Hawaii has had, is you have more tracking than anywhere else we have in the United States. We're getting hit.

And one of the things that's really interesting here, not saying the Big Island, per se, but in the State of Hawaii, is that from the tracking data she has which is not perfect because it's voluntary and parents have to give permission for the kids to give the data, in the juveniles it looks like the use of ice has dropped at a fairly steady rate, but adults are going up because the previous high school ice users are hitting the adult market.

And you have a potential tipping point among youth to hammer at home while you're—a lot of times when you're fighting uphill, it takes a lot more dollars if you got a tipping point to close down on this prevention. But the problem you're going to have which has happened with marijuana certainly all over the United States, particularly people think of it as 1960's stuff, a high THC type of variation. And then the adults that have used marijuana and they're not willing to crack down on their kids, say, oh, well, this is OK, I used it back when I was a kid. That group of meth users who are now becoming adults, you don't want to counter-infiltrate the kids in school as they move in and get another wave of meth, even if you accomplish this now.

Because you have a track record in looking at what impact you have is a way we can see to some degree your variables in other States. Because meth is the fastest growing category, we're seeing different parts of the United States doing that which is why Senator Inouye and your delegation was able to get an incredible amount of dollars concentrated in one place, on one island, in a very small State.

So we wanted to see some of that and you have this great track record data to add to what we already have and it's very interesting. On the law enforcement side it's very unusual to have the cops go that way, but I can see why, because it's difficult for you to utilize the dollars if he's hearing, oh, we all hear this a lot.

In my area, crack is a big problem. Oh, there's a crack house over there and the police aren't going for it. There's things like you have to prove it, what size bust is it, you have to go through the court process. Sometimes you're trying to track a bigger case in which stuff is coming in. But if you don't have basic law enforcement tools, it weakens that. If you continue to turn up in your survey that's one of the problems, if you can't get the State legislature to change the laws so you can get more local law enforcement, then you need to figure it out, because we talked to the HIDTA.

There are ways you can get the Federal Government involved in the middle of that because if that undermines your prevention tools, if they think they find something, they work at it, they can't get the bad guys cracked down on, it also sends a bad message to the kids, swift certain punishment.

No matter what treatment program, what prevention program ultimately many of them say but you could go to jail. That's the stick part of the carrot efforts in the Boys and Girls Clubs and everything else.

I want to move to the blister packs. We very much appreciate your testimony, Mr. Kamita, because we're dealing with this legislation at the Federal level. And let me say I have had a drug chairman who is very concerned about the nature of the methamphetamine breaking down after and everything else.

I grew up in the retail business. I'm one of you. There are at least five of us in Congress who aren't attorneys. Actually, there's more than that. There are 5 or 10 of us who are actually retailers, and we actually had a very small grocery store and not a pharmacy. And I know exactly what you're saying. Just driving around on the island here, you can see the concept, not to mention ABC stores everywhere, but the little grocery stores as well present a challenge.

Do you see that if there was a size cutoff, let me deal with the basic thing, that could it be handled like cigarettes; in other words, behind the counter but not up front?

Mr. BOTTI. It could, but it's going to be very inconvenient for the consumer, unlike tobacco products, which we definitely do not want the children to have. And if you look at the tax and the costs because in order to produce tobacco, government came in and tax, tax, tax, tax, we wouldn't want that to happen with cold medicines. You want the people to have them and you want people to have them at the least possible price.

The way I'm looking at this after this hearing is the retailers are not the problem, but the retailers are the visibility. Everybody sees the retailer, but they don't see the drug dealer. They don't see what's coming in from behind the scene. So therefore, it's the retailer's responsibility to act and be aggressive on helping the knowledge area.

We can do this without a law. The photo that I passed out was KTA Superstores. I happen to be a resident in Waikoloa Village now, and this is the Village Market. They have a limit of five packages per day. It doesn't really mean anything because if somebody wants it, they're going to be limited to one, but they're going to come in every day to get it.

But what this does is it allows them to put up a sign that creates education for all consumers. They put it in a highly visible area. And this is based on us going to the Keith Kamita, School of Manufacturing Methamphetamine, because Keith put on a workshop for KTA managers and it was amazing the attitude change because they didn't know how to make it. Now that they know how to make it, they know what people are looking for and that changes.

It's highly visible. They limit the number of quantity to seven of any one item on the shelf, so therefore, you don't have the shelf going all the way back. The problem is not the customer buying it, it's the stealing of it. So this is where they're going to get the quantity. They're going to come and sweep the shelf.

So we have stuff going on-line and we just signed on to the Meth Watch Program, and I think we're like the sixth State to sign-off on it. So working with Keith, getting the education out, educating the retailers, having them educate the public through publicity of these items and then we're not going to be a problem.

Now, we would be a problem if we didn't do this because as law enforcement dries up the hard core stuff, then they will start working the shelves at the store. But like with cigarettes, they have a bust, they stop at every store, 10 people get off and they each buy the limit. That was happening with cigarettes until—I think Ed was there when they passed that law, that they put real stiff regulations on the cigarettes. That's what stopped it, and the State gave $20 million in tax revenue. Thank you.

Mr. SOUDER. Mr. Kamita, well, Oklahoma has a restriction. Well, one of the problems there is at a hearing in Arkansas where we had some testimony, I learned that, for example, to get around it in Oklahoma, they happen to come to my home State of Indiana which is 800 miles—actually, they went to Chicago, but the guy was operating out of Indianapolis, Indiana which is about 150 miles from Chicago. Chicago is about 600 to 800 miles, actually, 800 to 1,000 from Oklahoma because Chicago had no limits, they hadn't had small meth labs and would just bring a whole car load of this stuff back to Oklahoma.

That type of pressure is really putting pressure on the Federal Government right now because clearly in at least the mainland contiguous States, it isn't really working very well.

And the question is, are we going to grandfather in States, and at what level? This is going to be a big issue, probably, next year as we work through this and that's why this question is important. I don't want to have a small business problem versus a big business problem, but I'm very familiar with Wal-Mart, having been to the distribution centers, they've got the scanners, they know basically between 9 and 9:15 how many people with slightly gray hair, black, how much toothpaste of this kind and they can get in their computer systems. A small grocer would not have that ability. But I don't think it's as hard to do the tracking when they move store to store as more move to scanners.

Could you discuss a little bit how the smaller stores move as compared to the bigger stores and how you see that working?

Mr. KAMITA. Well, some of our problem is not so much big stores like Long's Drugs or Safeway who are connected among themselves or if they have a pharmacy within themselves. We have in Hawaii what we call a pharmacy alert system where we can put out an alert to every pharmacy in this State as to a suspected person who's, what we call, smurfing pharmaceuticals or smurfing regulated chemicals. It's the little mom-and-pop stores, the ABC stores that don't have pharmacies inside where an individual can come in with a crew and maybe buy small quantities.

Mr. Botti is correct. A lot of the time the biggest problem is them coming in and sweeping the shelf because maybe that facility had too much product on the shelf. With KTA we told them to limit their box count. It will save them money. It also limits the amount of pseudoephedrine they can get on the street.

We've trained a lot of these pharmacies, a lot of these retailers as to what to watch for. But as you can tell Mr. Botti here, there are some pharmacies who give out seven packages, some that will only allow three packages so it's not a consistent message.

We're looking at saying three packages and no more, and that kind of drives it home that any clerk would know three packages of any one item, that's it, versus having to worry about how many milligrams was that and calculate it up.

We know that each blister pack can have no more than 3 grams. That's why we set a 9 gram limit.

Mr. SOUDER. Is Meth Watch voluntary right now by individual store and chain, or is that a Statewide effort, the Kansas variation.

Mr. BOTTI. It's voluntary. We will be promoting it for all stores. And I think on what Keith is talking about if the legislature, say, adopted a resolution stating that they're asking the stores to do it, we can do that without a law. The problem with the law is then you get a clerk that messes up. And if you've been in the grocery store, you get food stamps, you get WIC, you get cigarettes, you get liquor, and now you've got pseudoephedrine.

Mr. SOUDER. Fortunately, you have graduate students who are 40 years old watching that. That was a joke, by the way, for the record.

Mr. BOTTI. So the issue is we don't have to make criminals out of the customers signing in and getting proprietary information also. You're talking about social security number, driver's license number, address, phone number. If we can avoid that and have the visibility, go along with the high visibility, go in and voluntarily limit the program, limit what's on the shelf, come in with a reporting form that would go to Keith Kamita's office, that is something that would be much more preferable than stating that if they don't do it right, it's a misdemeanor, and then go to jail.

Mr. SOUDER. Do you have a problem with the repeal of the Federal Business Act?

Mr. BOTTI. I can't answer that, but I know they are working on a chemical that would go in there that would make it nonusable for making ice. I don't know how far away that is. I think that's something that should be looked at if they're going to change the blister pack which was made in order to help resolve this problem and keep the product on the shelf for those consumers that need it.

If that's going to be a year away, then I would say no sense in tampering with it if the manufacturers are going to go ahead and do that. I would say that would be far preferable than changing the law.

Mr. SOUDER. Yeah, I have a feeling it's 1 year away, but it would be preferable if we could get that in. And I would be interested in getting further input into the committee to see how you're moving on the Meth Watch, how widely it's being accepted, the effectiveness it's having. They're enthusiastic in Kansas, but they're still having more rapid growth of labs so Kansas is struggling with what to do right now, too.

Congressman Jerry Moran represents that a lot of the west has just exploded in spite of the Meth Watch, so we need to continue that. Retailers often are the tax collectors for sales tax because we're that distribution point. And since businesses don't pay taxes, individuals pay taxes, so it's not like you're going to get it out of—your costs go up because of this. It doesn't mean your profits are going to go down. It means consumer prices are going to go up.

At the same time we've had to do this for cigarettes because as a major point of distribution, and bartenders get hit for distributing alcohol to somebody who's drunk, but there is different accountability. We prefer not to do it that way. If we can address it in some of these other kinds of ways of putting things inside the blister pack, changing the blister pack law, trying to do Meth Watch and that type of thing.

But it's really important for the retail industry to understand they need to be cooperative here because government has clearly shown they're not oversympathetic to the problems of the retailers and the challenges. People love to complain how come everybody is going to Wal-Mart and the big stores. Well, this is the type of pressure that's very difficult for smaller stores.

At the same time you can't tolerate a community that's being overrun with meth and we have to figure out how to do deal with it.

Do you have any further comments?

Mr. CASE. My question from the last panel, Keith I think you've answered it. Chief Mahuna, one thing from Congress.

Mr. MAHUNA. Well, the only thing, as far as our department is concerned, it's resources to at least start programs that are—when you look at prior to the ice teams or ice task force; 2002, recovered 2.6 covered pounds versus 13.5 pound, triple the cases, with more people in keeping programs than institutions.

And I think everybody is asking for resources, but when you look at an island like this that is connected by basically one road, we have small pockets of rural people that if they have a problem, they try to take care of it. And it may exacerbate the problem by trying to keep the person there.

You have a police force that quite frankly is one-fifth or one-sixth that of Oahu. Yes, you have the density on Oahu, we have the size. Anything we can put a seed, whether it's through task force type of operations where we can accept at least a year or 2 years of the Federal Government's money and then, of course, we'll pick up as we go along. We start picking up these individuals.

But right now you're looking at the war and the activation of the National Guard, our people are down. I think the last count at least 40 positions so you're looking——

Mr. CASE. Out of.

Mr. MAHUNA. Out of about 400.

Mr. CASE. Down 10 percent.

Mr. MAHUNA. It's about 10 percent and it's not counting people that are not there for whatever reason, long-term, industrial accidents, and that type of thing.

So when you're looking at a police department trying to take in an effective law enforcement strategy working on an island this large with pockets of community that are stretched 60, 90 miles apart, it may seem small comparison to States the size of Montana. But 90 miles in travel—we have areas where basically can't go on patrol because we don't have the individuals to do that. Response times are horrendous. So anything that could give some seed to law enforcement locally, I think would benefit, not only the county, the State, but I think it would also facilitate the Federal collaboration that we have.

Mr. CASE. Thank you. Mr. Kenoi.

Mr. KENOI. I think if we ask for anything, Congressman Case, it would just be continued support and cooperation. No one level of government, whether it's Federal, State, county, no one entity, no one sector within the community is going to make the difference or has the resources or has all the energy and ideas.

But if we can continue working together and cooperating and moving forward and sharing information back and forth, we'll be happy to share any information we have for the last couple years, but as long as we stick together we'll be better for it in the community. The community will see that cooperation. It will give them that feeling that they're not wasting their time and effort in continuing to address this problem, and that's all.

Mr. CASE. I think we're going to be called to account for this island because at some point the jury is going to come in and it's going to be our turn to report back to the rest of the country how we did. I think that's an effort you've been very good at leading.

And I think I do want to recognize, for the record, somebody who is not here physically but is simply here in spirit and that's Mayor Kim.

Lieutenant Governor, and he talked for his wishlist about our Federal Government specifically at the top of the list and Mayor Kim has not just talked it, he's lived it, so he deserves our recognition. Thank you.

Mr. SOUDER. Thank you. In North Dakota at the Canadian border, there in the northwest corner, there is a little crossing home port, and I think the county is 90 miles by 120 miles. They have two policemen, a chief and a deputy chief.

Now, the good thing is that's more than the number of trees, and it's so flat that anybody who tries to get away, you can see them for almost 100 miles. That's the other difference here in Hawaii in trying to move through all the tropicals and mountains.

We appreciate your work, if you can pass that to all the people who work with you, too. I look forward to getting updated. Thank you for taking the time to be with us today. We'll take a brief break if the third panel could come forward.

[Recess.]

Mr. SOUDER. Our third panel is Mr. Grayson Hashida. You're from the Big Island Substance Abuse Council; Mr. Allen Salavea, Office of the Prosecuting Attorney with the Youth Builder's; and Dr. Jamal Wasan, the Lokahi Treatment Program.

Dr. WASAN. Centers.

Mr. SOUDER. And would you each raise your right hands.

[Witnesses sworn.]

Mr. SOUDER. Let the record show that they each responded in the affirmative and we're going to start off with Mr. Hashida.

STATEMENT OF GRAYSON HASHIDA, BIG ISLAND SUBSTANCE ABUSE COUNCIL

Mr. HASHIDA. Thank you, Congressman Souder and Congressman Case, for this opportunity to share. The Big Island Substance Abuse Council has been responding to those who are reaching out for help from addiction and alcoholism for many years. This is evident by the 40 years of service this non-profit organization has been operating here on the island of Hawaii.

Drugs are not a new phenomenon to the island, but much has changed in recent years. What is a phenomenon is the incredible impact that the drug methamphetamine known as ice has created. Few Big Island residents can state that they have not been touched in one way or another by this terrible drug. Addiction, violence, and crime now recognize ice as the motive or reason behind the action.

At the Big Island Substance Abuse Council the impact began in the mid 1990's as the number of consumers presenting themselves with ice as their drug of choice began a steady increase. In the year 2000, ice became the most common addiction being treated at our programs. Today, the number of individuals in the Big Island Substance Abuse Council programs who will report addiction or abuse of methamphetamine is overwhelming. All ages, all cultures, all income levels, no one is ignored by this addiction.

There are many opinions as to why this trend has occurred. These opinions are as diverse as the people who occupy this beautiful island, and the speculation will undoubtedly continue. The Big Island Substance Abuse Council has moved beyond the question why and is now looking to the solution. Local, State, and Federal Government departments began efforts to reach out to the people of Hawaii County and take a lead in developing the strategy and solution to the problem. Partnerships and collaborative efforts have begun a new trend related to ice that is "Healing Our Island."

A combination of law enforcement, prevention, and treatment efforts has resulted in a comprehensive approach to turn the tide. Details related to the Big Island Substance Abuse Council's role in these efforts include the development and implementation of many new programs and opportunities for those impacted by ice addiction. The primary objective is to increase capacity of programs while reducing barriers to accessing services.

Providing services to children and adolescents is one of the primary objectives. The Big Island Substance Abuse Council is now in all of Hawaii County's public high schools. A full-time substance abuse counselor is available in the familiar environment of the school and can be accessed in confidence. Adolescents who present evidence of substance abuse can also be referred directly. The behaviors and patterns that lead to substance abuse are addressed where and when it is appropriate, not after it has progressed to addiction.

For the adolescents who have progressed past early intervention, the Big Island Substance Abuse Council is a partner in developing and implementing a comprehensive Residential Substance Abuse Treatment Program. This experiential program is designed on the Big Island, by Big Island professionals, for Big Island kids.

These adolescent programs are provided in addition to the outpatient treatment services established by Big Island Substance Abuse Council in Kona, Waimea, and Hilo many years ago. These programs work directly with Judiciary and family referrals for adolescents appropriate for an outpatient level of care such as The Big Island Juvenile Drug Court. Treatment services are provided to this target population while the Drug Court monitors progress and provides accountability through incentives and sanctions for the participant. This program has demonstrated excellent outcomes throughout the mainland and expectations are high as the Big Island Drug Court is implemented in Hawaii County.

Families have experienced a significant amount of turmoil and damage due to ice as demonstrated through increased domestic violence, child abuse, and homelessness. The Big Island Substance Abuse Council responded to this community need through the development of therapeutic living programs. These homes accommodate target populations in a homelike setting with the reinforcement of full-time staffing. Programs for new mothers and their infant children and the home for single fathers and their children are examples of how the therapeutic living programs reach out to meet the specific needs of the families.

With 24 programs throughout the island of Hawaii, the Big Island Substance Abuse Council continues to provide effective and efficient services to those in need. Regardless of age, cultural identity, or income level, our programs are developed to provide immediate access and to reduce barriers to appropriate treatment and prevention services.

The Big Island Substance Abuse Council is honored to be a part of the solution in the efforts of Healing Our Island. The responses to our community needs and development of solutions to the ice epidemic were possible only through a collaborative and strategic effort of everyone involved. Support from our government officials such as Senator Daniel Inouye, Governor Linda Lingle, and County of Hawaii Mayor Harry Kim provided leadership and inspiration to stand firm.

While much progress has been made, and the efforts have been rewarded with success, there remains tremendous needs. Support for the individuals, families, and communities throughout the island of Hawaii will be necessary as the work continues. Many rural areas hit hard by economic turmoil and the devastation of ice still have little or no services for their residents.

Longer durations of treatment have been proven effective for methamphetamine addiction, but treatment episodes continue to be limited in length. Specific target populations such as those with co-occurring disorders struggle to find appropriate care.

The island of Hawaii continues to need the support of our Federal agencies to maintain the course and develop all of the resources necessary to overcome this epidemic. Please continue providing the funding opportunities and support that have allowed the progress to occur and will continue to support the efforts toward Healing Our Island. Thank you.

Mr. SOUDER. Thank you. Mr. Salavea.

STATEMENT OF ALLEN SALAVEA, OFFICE OF THE PROSECUTING ATTORNEY WITH THE YOUTH BUILDERS

Mr. SALAVEA. Aloha mai kakou, Chairman Souder, Representative Case. I would like to begin by thanking you for this opportunity to testify on the impact of crystal methamphetamine or ice as it is locally known. Part of my testimony is to quantify the ice problem and its impact on the youth of Hawaii island. And the other part is to give you a preview of the prevention, treatment, law enforcement, and community mobilization initiatives that have taken place in response to the crisis.

My testimony is about the hope we have in our people, as well as the promise we are making to future generations by taking action now to purge the poison of ice out of our communities.

Hawaii island is in a fight for the lives and futures of our children. In 2002 Alcohol, Tobacco, and Other Drug survey for the County of Hawaii stated that 2.3 percent of eighth graders and 6.1 percent of seniors had tried ice at least once in their lives.

The survey goes on to report that 60.9 percent of eighth graders felt that laws and norms in Hawaii island are favorable to drug use.

Statistics on the impact of ice in other domains of a young person's life are also poor. According to Child Welfare Services, children living without the presence of either parent rose from 2,669 in 1997 to 3,326 in 1999. Cases of neglect have also doubled from 91 cases confirmed in 1995 to 203 in 1999. These numbers illustrate the early onset of ice use, as well as the disintegration of the family unit.

In response, Hawaii County has developed a system of prevention programs, effective treatment options, and law enforcement resources to prosecute ice-related crime. Community based drug prevention programs is an important facet of Hawaii Island's strategy. The Pulama project administered by the Bay Clinic and funded through a grant from the Substance Abuse and Mental Health Services Administration extend prevention resources and services island-wide by collaborating with other non-profit and government agencies.

In the area of treatment the role and acceptance of drug treatment and addiction from a public health perspective has gained widespread acceptance in the community. The Third Circuit Court of Hawaii island has initiated Drug Court based on national models as an alternative for convicted drug users. The response by the community has been very positive with citizen groups asking what type of supports are needed.

Another welcome addition to the array of services available to you is an on-island adolescent treatment facility. County, State, and Federal agencies along with community-based organizations have developed a program grounded and tested and effective methods and incorporated experiential and cultural components.

Law enforcement is the next critical piece in controlling ice and reducing the available supply. Hawaii County Police Department in cooperation with the Drug Enforcement Agency, the U.S. Attorney's Office, and the County of Hawaii Prosecutor's office have formed an ice task force to identify, arrest, and prosecute ice dealers.

The last piece in this effort is community empowerment. Over the last 2 years we have seen mobilization of citizen groups on an unprecedented scale from neighborhood watch groups to coordinating island-wide anti-ice sign waving events to community coalitions engaging in community planning. The citizens of Hawaii island understand their stake in this effort and have risen to the challenge.

The Federal Government's support of community-based prevention and treatment programs along with the continued presence of Federal law enforcement are an integral supports of Hawaii island's ice strategy. In addition, Federal assistance to communities and neighborhoods to complete assessments and action plans help to empower citizens.

In closing, the ice epidemic has caused a wide array of social problems for children and families of Hawaii island. The aforementioned statistics pull at our sense of responsibility and motivate us to act. I have given you an abbreviated glimpse of the four aspects of Hawaii County's response to the ice problem to illustrate the cohesiveness of our community. We hope for continued support from the Federal Government to purge our island paradise of ice.

[The prepared statement of Mr. Salavea follows:]

Testimony of Allen A. Salavea
Youth Builders Coordinator, Office of the Prosecuting Attorney County of Hawaii

Before the
Subcommittee on Criminal Justice, Drug Policy, and Human Resources
of the Committee on Government Reform
U.S. House of Representatives

The Poisoning of Paradise: Crystal Methamphetamine in Hawaii

Monday, August 2, 2004

Introduction

Aloha mai kakou, Chairman Souder, distinguished committee members. I would like to begin by thanking you for this opportunity to testify on the topic crystal methamphetamine and its impact on the people, communities and society of Hawaii Island. As you may already know, Crystal Methamphetamine or "Ice" as it is commonly referred to has made its way to paradise and has destroyed many lives and families on this Island.

A part of what I want to share with you today is to quantify the Ice problem and its impact on youth on Hawaii Island. In addition, I also want to tell you about the prevention, treatment, law enforcement, and community mobilization initiatives that have taken place in response to this crisis. My testimony is about the hope we have in our people as well as the promise we are making to future generations by taking action now to purge the poison of ice out of our communities.

Impact on Children and the Family

Hawaii Island is in a fight for the lives and futures of our children. The State of Hawaii's Department of Health reported in the 2002 Alcohol, Tobacco, and Other Drug (ATOD) survey for the County of Hawaii County (COH) that .4% of sixth graders, 2.3% of eighth graders, 5.2% of high school sophomores, and 6.1% of seniors had tried Ice at least once. The 2002 ATOD survey goes on to report that 60.9% of eighth graders felt that laws and norms in Hawaii Island are favorable to drug use and 59.3% of eighth graders acknowledge that they have been exposed to family ATOD use (the COH led or exceeded the state average in these categories for each of mentioned grade levels). These statistics illustrate statistically the extent of the "drug culture" prevalent on Hawaii Island and reveal that children as young as eleven or twelve are experimenting with Ice. This is not acceptable in paradise.

Statistics on the impact of Ice in other domains of a young person's life are also poor. According to the Child Welfare Services, children living without the presence of either parent rose from 2,669 in 1997 to 3,326 in 1999. Cases of neglect have also doubled from 91cases confirmed in 1995 to 203 confirmed in 1999. Finally the number of runaways rose from 579 reports in 1998 to 649 in 2000. Although the correlation between these statistics and Ice use varies, these numbers serve as a statistical representation of the disintegration of the family unit and the need for support from other aspects of the community.

In the face of such daunting statistics, it would be simple to crawl into a hole a hide from the impending doom. However one important characteristic of the Hawaii Island community is resiliency. The health and well being of children are priority and the result of the Ice crisis has been the mobilization of business, government, private citizens, and youth. The development of a system of prevention resources and programs, effective treatment options, and a commitment by law enforcement to police and expeditiously prosecute Ice related crime is a direct product of this mobilization.

Prevention

The youth of Hawaii Island were instrumental in identifying the Ice problem and have taken a proactive approach to creating opportunities for children, teenagers, and families. To date Hawaii Island youth have formed a civic action group called Na Leo O Na Opio and have coordinated more than 20 events over the past two years and reached out to thousands of parents and youth. Their goal is to increase the number of positive activities utilizing the abundant natural, cultural, and existing programs to promote the positive aspects of living a drug free lifestyle. Partners have included Prince Kuhio Mall, Rotary Club of Hilo, Family Support Service of West Hawaii, Department of Education, Workforce Investment Board, and Ku Haaheo.

Community based drug prevention programs are an important facet in fighting the Ice problem locally. The Hawaii Island community understands that parents and the family are important influences in raising a drug free child. However in today's society, parents need help to prevent substance abuse. The Pulama project administered by the Bay Clinic Inc. and funded through a grant from the Substance Abuse and Mental Health Services Administration extends prevention resources and services island-wide by collaborating with other non-profit and government agencies. The result has been a dramatic increase in drug prevention services through the pooling of resources and the creation of a team environment where agencies work together to provide an array of preventions services that range from mentoring to monitoring school performance to drug counseling. Program partners include the Bay Clinic, Department of Education, Office of the Mayor (COH), Office of the Prosecuting Attorney (COH), Family Court, Ku Haaheo, Big Island Substance Abuse Counsel, Neighborhood Place of Kona, and the Catalyst Group.

Drug Treatment

The role and acceptance of drug treatment and addiction from a public health perspective has gained wide spread acceptance. In response to Ice use by many criminal offenders, the third circuit court of Hawaii Island have initiated a drug court based on national models as an alternative for convicted drug users. The response by the community in support of the project has been very positive. This past May, the drug court was featured at a local Neighborhood Watch conference and participants were eager to learn how the program works and what type of community supports are needed.

Another welcome addition to the array of services available to youth is an on island adolescent treatment facility. County, State and Federal agencies along with community based organizations have developed a program grounded in tested and effective adolescent treatment methods and incorporated experiential and cultural components. The program treats the clinical aspects of drug addiction and builds confidence and self esteem of the individual through the use of culturally appropriate activities. This newfound confidence serves as protective factors to help the youth to stay drug free. Again we see unique partnerships between government and community entities that build on existing resources and multiply the effort by the individual parts through effective collaboration.

Enforcement

Law enforcement is the next critical piece in controlling Ice and reducing the available supply. Hawaii County Police Department in cooperation with the Drug Enforcement Agency, the U.S. Attorney's Office, and the COH Prosecutor's office have formed a Ice task force to identify, arrest, and prosecute individuals and groups engaged in the trafficking and distribution of Ice. By expediting and making Ice distribution activity a priority, a clear message is being sent to criminal elements in the community that Ice trafficking is not tolerated and will be dealt with swiftly. We have taken what was once the primary method of dealing with drug abuse and incorporated it into a comprehensive and multi-faceted approach to purging Ice from our community.

Mobilizing Citizen Groups

The last piece in this effort is community empowerment. Over the last two years, we have seen the mobilization of the citizen groups and the business sector on an unprecedented scale. From neighborhood watch groups coordinating island-wide anti-ice sign waving events to community coalitions engaging in community planning, the citizens of Hawaii Island understand their stake in this effort and have risen to the challenge. Groups like the North Hawaii Drug Free Coalition and Hui Laulima exemplify the concept of working within a team environment and set the example for other groups to follow suit. The significance of this movement is the common belief in the destructive nature of Ice at all levels of the community. From children to parents, community and government, everyone shares in the vision of a healthy community.

Conclusion

The Federal government's support of community based prevention and treatment programs along with the continued presence of Federal law enforcement are an integral part of Hawaii Island's Ice strategy. In addition Federal assistance to communities and neighborhoods to complete assessments and action plans will empower citizens.

In closing, the Ice epidemic has caused a wide array of social problems for children and families of Hawaii Island. Statistics regarding the early onset of Ice use by children and their exposure to drugs pull at our sense of responsibility and motivate us to act. I have given you an abbreviated glimpse of the four aspects of the County's response to the Ice problem to illustrate the cohesiveness of our community. This is the foundation of the effort and is an important factor in sustaining it into the future.

Children are the cornerstones of our future. Youth is a time of transition to adulthood and self-empowerment. Parents are our first teachers in life and are there to catch us when we fall. Family is the sacred bond we share with relatives and friends. These are essential components of a community. Which when nurtured, form a strong barrier against the social problems caused by Ice addiction and abuse.

Mr. SOUDER. Thank you.
Dr. Wasan.

STATEMENT OF JAMAL WASAN, LOKAHI TREATMENT PROGRAM

Dr. WASAN. A very famous philosopher once said: "Once you label me, you negate me." And I think a lot of it comes with dealing with rehabilitation for those who are suffering from ice. I think at times we forget where they come from and who they really are.

I am, personally, myself, in recovery, a recovering addict. I was wounded twice in Vietnam, was hospitalized, ended up becoming addicted to Demerol and when I got out of the hospital, stayed on Darvocet and used marijuana for quite a long time. I read a book back in 1970 called Man Searches for Meaning by a person named Victor Franco. In that book it talked about having had a reason, a why to change one's life. And once you have that, you'll find how.

I came to this island in 1993 after successfully completing my own recovery and going back into the military where I retired as colonel for the United States Air Force. I came to this island and I began to work for a place called BISAC, Big Island Substance Abuse Council, and they were dealing at that time—the big issue was not methamphetamine. It was crack cocaine. This was 1993.

And at that time we were told this drug is the most intensive, most addictive drug we've ever run across. Now, unfortunately, we're involved with methamphetamine. I'm here to tell you when methamphetamine goes, there will be another drug that will come along because that's how it works. The question was asked before about cannabis or marijuana, THC, marijuana is a multiphasic drug which is why you will find that people who use methamphetamines will also use THC because it takes of edge off of the effect of ice itself.

It also helps to stimulate their appetite which is something that—in the 1980's and 1990's we had the diet pill which were methamphetamine based which were used to prevent or block appetites. So therefore, THC helps those who are involved with methamphetamines to get an appetite.

I think another issue I really want to address and I put it in here is that having lived on this island in 1993 and understanding the population and working with some very, I should say, renowned people who have been working very hard to deal with this problem, talking about Kanaka Maoles and others, churches, we need to really—the question was asked if I could ask Congress what they could do that could help; I think managed care needs a push in the butt.

If there's two-in-a-lifetime treatment for substance abuse, is there something wrong with that? If I have cancer and I get cured from cancer, if I get it again, I'm going to be treated. If I go in remission, and I get it again, I'll be treated.

We talk about methamphetamines or addiction as being something that is a disease and it is. It's biologically based. It does have signs and symptoms and it does have predictable outcomes, and we know that is the definition of a disease. Yet, when it comes down to treating our addiction process, we often forget that and not treat it the same way it should be.

There are rehabilitation programs. I personally believe that this drug did not come about because it just happened. A vacuum was created on these islands. There was at one time a very dynamic culture here that involved the sugar plantation, pineapple production on other islands. People had a sense and source of identity just like Victor Franco talks about his in book. They knew who they were. The plantation who carried so many things, medical, churches, schools, recreational. A lot of things happened.

When that began to demise—and by the way, pakalolo was here for a long time or marijuana was here a long time and was taken as a nonabusive drug. People just used it. It, actually, was creating an island of addicts. I mean it is a drug. If you take someone off from marijuana, they will go through withdrawal symptoms. It was already there.

But you had this plantation environment which was containing families. Families had a place to go to church, they had community projects they could participate in. Then hotels came and thus we have the tourist industry. That caused a vacuum because that is not the dominant culture for these islands. We're agriculture.

So all of a sudden you're working down in tourism, you're working with the high end, but you're given minimum wage salaries. That required people had to work double wage shifts, double jobs, longer hours. Guess what, methamphetamine is a methamphetamine, it will allow me to work 12 hours, 24 hours, 36 hours, it will keep me up.

It was a natural consequence that occurred and we take it away and create a vacuum. You take away the marijuana which was done under new harvest which was a major drug and you do this for the hotels, you got a problem. Then we go around and we try to say people are not going in for treatment or they need treatment and we place the facilities on this island where they can't even get treatment. There is no transportation on this island. Something needs to be done about that.

Voc rehab is a significant part of treatment. We talked about having a reason for recovery and that is the fundamentally why. The how has to include voc rehabilitation. When I finish treatment, what am I supposed to do then? Or when I get out of residential—residential doesn't work. The stats show that residential and outpatient programs are about the same, unless you add something different.

And that's what Billy Kenoi is trying to do here. You have to add another piece that goes back to identity and also establish some type of after program where the child is then able to then step back in the community and find that he's not only accepted in the community, but he has a place. And that often comes from jobs, my self-esteem, my self-identity.

There's a lot that needs to be done. I think Mayor Harry Kim has done tremendously by stepping up to the plate, talking to Senator Daniel Inouye to bring down here, bring you all down here and bring the money in. But as we very well know, you can't just throw money at something and expect that to cure it.

I mean I'm a Vietnam veteran. They threw a bunch of money in Vietnam and it didn't do anything, right. It didn't cure anything. You can't do that with this problem either.

This is a war. BISAC, Kevin Kunz is not here, but there are different services and we're joining together around this island to try and do what we can to stop it. This is a simple old soldier, but I know the enemy is in front of me. I know how to deal with it. The enemy in front of us right now is methamphetamine. We know how to deal with it.

The county needs to be given more direct funding to be able to do that. I'm not a big State supporter when it comes to that. I believe that at times you need to go to the people who know what the problem is and how to deal with it, and that's the people we elect in our county and that's our mayor and that's our council. They need to be given more grants and aid. They're the ones who call us together. They're they ones that go around the island, Billy Kenoi, Mayor Kim, go to high schools, go to the churches and talk. That's where the funding needs to be hitting more and more of and less to the State where it gets tied up.

If you put it like an old grunt that I was in Vietnam, I know what I'm dealing with and give us the resources, we'll do something about it. And I hope that my testimony will prompt you all to do something about managed care and get them to stop playing these silly games and provide treatment for people and also provide more funding directly to the community which is to the county. Thank you.

[The prepared statement of Dr. Wasan follows:]

The Poisoning of Paradise: Crystal Methamphetamine in Hawaii

AUGUST 2, 2004

TESTIMONY

DR. JAMAL F. WASAN
LOKAHI TREATMENT CENTERS

THE DEMISE OF AGRICULTURE ON THE ISLANDS AND THE RISE OF DISILLUSIONMENT

1835
Sugar was first grown commercially in Hawaii at Koloa Plantation on Kauai in 1835. At one time there were 32 plantations in the State of Hawaii. Collectively, they imported the 385,000 workers from Asia, Europe and North America who created Hawaii's unique multi-cultural society.

1975
Kohala Sugar Co. closes.

1994
Hamakua Sugar Co. closes.

1995
Hilo Sugar closes.

1996
Ka'u Sugar closes.

The Sugar Mill and other plantation closures have affected the rhythm of island life and devastated communities. Displaced workers were now being forced to leave their communities to find employment in other industries that generally provided only minimal pay. Whereas the sugar plantations had provided for families from birth to death with; schools, churches, community centers, sporting events and job security. The new tourism industry was for the wealthy and those coming for a taste of "paradise". In essence, the sugar plantation closures created a huge vacuum that left the population with despair, frustration, and loss of identity. In their frustration, many turned to drug abuse and alcoholism, which led to family violence and depression. While marijuana was previously the "drug of choice" for many drug users, when the Green Harvest Program cracked down on growers, the picture changed dramatically. As marijuana became more difficult to buy, active addicts began using "Ice" (methamphetamine) in epidemic proportion. With Ice use, the Big Island began to experience an increase in acts of violence. This was inevitable as this drug is an amphetamine and when used in large quantities over long periods, it produces neurological damage manifested as paranoia, distorted cognitive processing and organic brain damage. This drug has the potential to devastate centuries of cultural practices, beliefs and essentially destroy an entire generation.

A wave of construction began along the coastal highway, the growth of luxury hotels and resorts along the Kohala coast, and a growing interest and developments of eco-tourism have started to revive the community economically. Agriculture had been replaced by tourism as the prime workforce employer. Presently, West Hawaii is primarily employed in the hotel and visitor industries, which attracted former plantation workers. This includes residents of both East and West Hawaii. However, there is a dark side to this, as many are required to work extra long shifts to earn the income necessary in an attempt to restore what the plantations had provided (Housing, medical . . .). For those working double shifts "Ice" (methamphetamine) is often seen as a way to maintain alertness during extended work hours and long distance traveling. Initially this appears be a viable solution and the word is spread around to other workers. However, what starts off as a way to stay awake becomes an addiction and the worker(s) finds themselves using methamphetamines to "feel normal."

Although the Kohala coast has experienced a growth in tourism, it continues to experience a sense of existential isolation; income, but no cultural identity to who they are as island peoples. The Kohala community is also geographically cut off from the mainstream, as is the southern part of the island, Kau District. There is no viable public transportation connecting Kohala and Kau with other communities on the Big Island, nor is there any viable public transportation within the districts itself. Transportation has often been the cause for those who are unemployed or under-employed (casual/part-time workers), which prolongs the cycle of despair and frustration that leads to increased family violence, drug abuse, alcoholism and depression.

Surviving economically is a struggle in Hawaii, which has one of the highest costs of living in the United States, and resulted in many locally born residents moving to the mainland. Additionally, a significant number of single parents are working two jobs to make ends meet, leaving the children at home unsupervised. For many, opportunities for "family time" much less after school programs and special lessons for their children are out of reach. Our children are missing opportunities for growth and achievement. Their formerly secure futures are now one of doubt, and frustration as they watch their parents struggle to make ends meet but fall further and further behind.

Perhaps it is these circumstances that catalyze the exponential growth rate of drug use on our island today. Anecdotally, we know that a growing number of parents believe that it is okay to drink excessively and use drugs with their kids or in front of their kids. It's how to take the edge and escape the reality of their circumstances. In this way, the drug use is handed down from parent to child and has become an unfortunate part of the Hawaiian culture.

Here's a few suggestions for possible solutions:

- **Support and continue to develop existing programs that provide recreational activities for youths and adults, such as Parks and Recreation, the Boys and Girls Club, YWCA, YMCA . . . .**
- **Support Vocational Rehabilitation Programs. LTC feels that, in addition to counseling, an equally important element to a full recovery is the support and skills gathered through Vocational Educational services.**
- **Support and continue to develop the Parent Community Network that already exists in all of Hawaii's public schools through their Parent Community Network Coordinator. At this time, these are only part-time positions.**
- **Support and continue to develop agricultural cooperatives and eco-tourism.**

LOKAHI TREATMENT CENTERS

When the crystal methamphetamine epidemic escalated on the Big Island of Hawaii in the late 1990's, Dr. Jamal Wasan, PhD responded to the community's concerns by founding The Waikoloa Community-Based Substance Abuse Rehabilitation and Recovery Program a nonprofit community program, now known as LOKAHI TREATMENT CENTERS (LTC). The community quickly learned that drug abuse was not an isolated problem and LTC expanded its services to create an integrated model to address related mental health and anger issues, as well. The mission of LTC is to provide community-based Substance Abuse and Mental health services that are culturally appropriate to Big Island adults, adolescents, and children suffering from chemical dependency and acts of violence.

LTC Invest in the Career Development of Clients

Job training programs are a missing link in substance abuse treatment services. LTC would like to provide a means for helping its' clients by providing them with job training opportunities as part of their treatment plan. LTC will encourage its' clients to make choices and take responsibility for their own employment and self-development. LTC will help clients make informed employment/career choices, to which they become committed. These choices motivate them to take full advantage of the educational programs and services to become better prepared for work. As a result, their attendance in other programs dramatically increases.

As the flow chart below indicates, a quality career choice up front helps clients and staff organize the client's program logically. Clients attend regularly, complete training, get and retain their jobs because of the increased motivation and satisfaction.

LTC Career Development Organizational Model

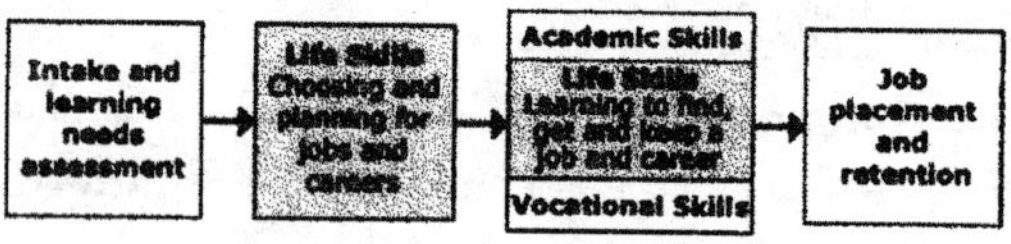

LTC Strengthens Client Motivation

We invest in client training to ensure that our clients are making informed occupational choices that are right for them-choices that they can stick with.

Research shows that clients who have made informed career choices, based on good self and occupational knowledge are more highly motivated and more successful in completing training, getting jobs and staying employed. They are also more satisfied than those who have not given systematic thought to their future options.

LTC Reduces Fragmentation of Services

One goal of LTC is reducing the fragmentation of services to its clients.

Clients who have career plans and who are goal-directed can take full advantage of the multiple opportunities for learning and services that will be available through LTC's treatment plans. There is a tendency on the part of some agencies to help make choices for people instead of helping them to make their own choices. Research shows that people are motivated to pursue choices they themselves make far more than choices made for them.

LTC will address the needs of those:

1. who are job/career ready and self-directed;
2. who need some help with motivational, choice and planning issues; and
3. who need the most help to become job/career ready.

LTC Makes Up for Missed Learning about Life Tasks

LTC Substance abuse programs provides the kind of developmental learning that many persons using drugs or alcohol have missed. This kind of positive learning goes beyond jobs and careers to the essential psychological skills and values of self-direction and self-development that were delayed or impaired during the years of substance abuse.

LTC is the ideal complement to traditional treatment methods that focus on the elimination of negative, self-defeating behaviors.

The program enhances the true rehabilitation of the chemical abuser by focusing on the acquisition of essential coping skills, based on new concepts, new knowledge, different values, and new behaviors which have not yet become part of the individual's repertoire.

LTC Stresses The Positive

LTC requires that the clients become actively involved in conducting inquiries, gaining new experiences, internalizing new learning and practicing new behaviors until they can competently perform the new coping skills.

It is our conviction that the learning of necessary new values, attitudes, strategies, and the making of life-affirming choices requires a different kind of learning process, one that stresses the positive. The process must help the individuals think differently, help them decode emotion, learn new concepts and practice new behaviors to mastery. What the program does is help a person substitute new effective life-sustaining attitudes and behaviors for old ineffective life-draining attitudes and behaviors.

Mr. SOUDER. Thank you for your testimony. Let me ask Dr. Wasan, but the others as well, you're not arguing that drug abuse is predominantly concentrated among the poor.

Dr. WASAN. No, I'm not. If you look at Beverly Hills and L.A., cocaine was the drug of choice. Freud created the cocaine epidemic in Europe. No, I'm not saying that. What I'm trying to say is that when you take away something that is very meaningful to whatever people, that creates a vacuum. Nature abhors a vacuum. Something else is going to rush in and take its place.

In this case what has happened is we've had a whole economy that came in place, that economy also wanted to have results, profit. In order to do that, at times I have to make my people work extra hard, double shifts. And when I do that and they're driving halfway across this island because there is no transportation system, people offer me something. I went to college, what did we use, stay awake to study longer, caffeine.

Mr. SOUDER. I understand that point, but what my question is that—this is a huge debate. I can understand that part of the economy, but are you saying that the middle class doesn't abuse meth here and the upper class doesn't abuse meth here, it's only in that group that's highly stressed.

Dr. WASAN. Well, if you look at who's coming into treatment, that's what you're seeing.

Mr. SOUDER. Well, that's what I want to know because it's not true in other parts of the country.

Dr. WASAN. If you look at who's coming into treatment on this island, you're going to find those that are underserved and under privileged. That's who you find coming into treatment. Now, I do know——

Mr. SOUDER. Are you talking about government funded-based treatment or private facilities? Do the wealthier groups send their family members who are having treatment in the private facilities that may or may not be here or be in Honolulu?

Dr. WASAN. Right. I do know people who have sent their family members back to facilities on the mainland, in California for $35,000 a month so yeah.

Mr. SOUDER. In the schools where you could do the tracking of this, do you find that kids from middle and upper income families have less of a meth problem than those from lower income families?

Dr. WASAN. I do know that the kids that I'm aware of who go to HPA or Parker School, $12,000 a year to go to HPA, there is a marijuana problem and that's there. There is a problem there. But as far as methamphetamine, I have not seen a rush on that among the adolescent. I've seen marijuana. But remember what I just said, though, once you get addicted to marijuana, you've already created an addict. It's simple, you give me another drug and I'll try it.

Mr. SOUDER. Any of the others jump in on any of these questions. Let me followup with that. One of the big debates we're having is how to concentrate on drugs. There is no question that marijuana is overwhelmingly the No. 1 drug of choice. 60 percent of people in treatment in the United States are with marijuana. As THC goes up, it's becoming a greater problem, greater violence problem, greater problem on the road.

One of the arguments is, only 8 percent of the Nation has a meth problem. It's certainly higher here. But one of the arguments we've heard in the hearings is that meth grips you differently. In other words, when you hit ice, it's like all you think about is your next hit, it's tough to work, it's tough to do other things, and it's a little like ecstasy in the sense that addiction may be even greater.

Is that true? Do you agree with that?

Dr. WASAN. I would agree that the addiction to methamphetamine like crack cocaine happens more rapidly. It's because of the effect that your memory is pushing out the normetanephrine which allows you to be stronger, more alert. It's like taking a 75 watt light bulb and making it a 150 watt light bulb so you can see everything and you can do more. And that's a very strong draw, especially if I'm working in a position that I need to be hyperalert. It's a very strong draw.

Mr. SOUDER. We haven't heard this. In fact, we've heard the reverse, that ice doesn't enable you to work. It may be like No Doze, super caffeine keeping you awake at a certain level, but at what point does it debilitate you? In other words, you're starting to make errors at work that are substantial. Pretty soon the impact on your brain cells is like marijuana because it has a lazy effect in many cases.

Dr. WASAN. Right, right, the motivational reference. What you're saying is true, but not initially. The more you use methamphetamine, it creates a neurotoxin that causes brain damage, memory loss, and paranoia, amphetamine psychosis kind of thing. They repetitive in what they're doing so that's nonproductive, but initially, no, like any other amphetamine, it's going to boost me and I think I can do more.

Mr. SOUDER. It's like the rock stars taking a hit before the concert.

Dr. WASAN. Right, right. It's a long-term what you're talking about when reverse effect occurs, because remember the body can only sustain this for so long. This endorphin which is blocked from the brain and keeps me agitated and moving around and moving and moving. The body can only take so much of that and begins to shut down; my ability to concentrate.

Mr. SOUDER. And then in the treatment, how do you treat a drug like ice? We've heard that it's much harder in treatment organizations to get a treatment for ice like crack, as opposed to many of the other drugs. Your points about fallback is true and depends whether the family is abusing and whether they have a job, I understand that portion, but the actual physical addiction, is it substantially harder to treat than other drugs.

Dr. WASAN. It takes a longer period of time, I would say, to treat and that's because of the neurological deficits that also occur, whereas in marijuana it tends to be faster; crack cocaine—you know, cocaine is not a neurotoxin. So yeah, you can be able to—your brain and body compensates quicker than it would from a methamphetamine. Treatment does need to be longer.

I think the thing we have to understand is that because addiction is a process, it's going to go through precontemplation, I don't got a problem; contemplation, I think maybe I need to work on this; and action, I really am working on it and I'm in treatment. The final stage is maintenance, and that's going to be for a lifetime.

So if the drug is still out there, I need to have a strong barrier between me and that drug. You know what, I can say the same thing about marijuana and crack cocaine, so the treatment may be longer. And I also need to have an integrated treatment approach. I need to have medical, I need to have psychiatric when I'm treating methamphetamines? Not necessarily so if I'm treating marijuana or alcoholism, but if I'm treating methamphetamines, yes, I do which is why the expense for treating methamphetamine may be more because I need a more stronger, specialized integrative staff than to treat, say, alcohol, for example.

Mr. SOUDER. Now, in California which is the only other place I've heard this particular thing, meth addicts are the one group that they don't want their children. If you take them into child custody, often they don't want them back particularly if they're a cooker. And I would be interested in the prosecutor's office's comments about that, too.

That suggests there is something also very different going on in this drug than other drugs, if they don't have the normal family attachment for their kids.

Dr. WASAN. Again, if you're talking about the disease and biologically based organism neurotoxin, it does cause deficits within the brain. In other words, tissue begins to die. Methamphetamine, the chemical that's produced in it, causes a neurotoxin effect that does tend to cause organic damage to the brain.

This is why you have certain behavior changes because of the loss of impulse control, damage to the neocortex, damage to the temporal lobe. It does deduce that. The only way you're going to find that is if you have them in treatment for a longer period of time and you have these specialists looking at that. Then you can design a real legitimate program around that to help them overcome these deficits—or I should say not overcome them necessarily, but to compensate for these deficits.

And this is one of the things that has not been happening, and although a number of us have said this for a period of time, it's only just now that I found the first opportunity to be able to sit and talk with you. And if Dr. Kevin Kunz, he's is a physician, were here, he would share some of the things I talked about because it is a neurologically based problem, but it's being addressed more as a behavioral problem than it is being addressed as an organic problem or physical problem because it is.

Mr. SOUDER. Congressman Case.

Mr. CASE. Let me back up and then we'll come back to rehabilitation and talk about prevention.

We've got law enforcement, we've heard about that. We're talking about rehabilitation, but let me focus on prevention just for a second with you, Mr. Salavea, because I think your testimony goes to prevention.

There was a comment by the Chair earlier that the national stats show that ice use may be declining. I think this is a fair statement of what you said, ice use may be declining among youth, but we're seeing it accelerated among young adults and that's simply a [inaudible] going through.

Mr. SOUDER. In Hawaii.

Mr. CASE. In Hawaii, which implies that since we're not having the same type of demographics going through, that we're doing something right. What is it? First of all, are we doing something right and what is it we're doing right in terms of prevention? What is keeping more kids—if that's true, what's keeping more kids off ice and stable through high school.

Mr. SALAVEA. That's an interesting question and we notice through analyzing the statistics from the surveys, that was a trend that, like you mentioned, Chairman, a tipping point for us to take advantage of. And as far as what—if we are doing things right, I think we are.

My testimony really went to the heart or speaking of the cohesiveness of the community, and we have these terrific leaders and motivators like Billy Kenoi to get the community work done and to buy into the problem of ice and methamphetamine abuse here. And from that the community has taken the—taken the initiative and in some instances formed their own community coalitions.

The North Hawaii Drug-Free Coalition is a terrific example of how citizen empowerment really—investment in that movement really has a multiplier effect. You bring in the businesses, you bring in the volunteer help, you bring in the moms, the dads, the civic organizations located in this particular area. And you're able to take advantage of that human resource and use your dollars for direct—to get directly out to the community, as opposed to paying a full-time position with benefits, so I think that's one huge component.

The second thing is probably the—because we come from an island that may not have the same amount of resources as, say, like Honolulu, we've learned over the past 20, 25, 30 years to do more with less and that just has been a tradition.

When I got into the prosecutor's office and we started doing community assessments and surveys to find out what some of the issues were, the other agencies came to the table readily and they put out their resources for everyone to use and to see how we can work together to more effectively do our jobs and that continues to today.

So you don't have this rift between or competition between agencies and that's what we really like to work on or utilize when you bring together projects. It's not about who's going to get the big piece of the pie, rather it's who can provide the best services to the most amount of people for the lowest cost and effectively do that as a team.

Mr. CASE. Do you do it mostly through the schools? Is that the most effective way to get to the kids?

Mr. SALAVEA. The school is definitely a rally point. We're fortunate to have a lot of DOE personnel. Their primary objective is with the education of a child, but it's being hindered by drug use and in this case methamphetamine. So they understand and they come to the table with the hope that if we help them get kids off of drugs, then they can do their jobs better of educating the kids, so definitely the DOE is a big partner.

Mr. CASE. I'm focusing more on kids not getting on drugs to start with. We're trying to take care of what's working. You can track the smoking thing, for example. In Australia they show the brain autopsy to—and we're getting close to that here. I know that something like that is happening in the schools.

Is that where that preventive education effort is going? I guess I'm trying to get a sense of what works in preventive education. What exactly works, or is there just no standard way of doing it? Do you do it differently with a community that has more churches, you go through the churches versus some others?

Dr. WASAN. There was a book that I'm trying to think of the author's name. I think it was Dale Matthews, and they did a study with the public health system down in Texas. And they found that prevention and preventing relapse, they're looking at a real spiritual basis. The churches—as a matter of fact, I think one study was done in 1985 or 1992 or 1996 and it said that the prevention for youth turning to drugs or alcohol was the father's spiritual belief, his value system.

The public health did a study with heroin addicts, for example, and they found those that got involved with spiritual-based or church-based beliefs after 1 year were in a 90 percent not relapse, but 90 percent recovery.

So we need to be able to support those people that are involved with the churches and faith-based group organizations. We need to be able to provide more support for prevention for those that are involved in culturally based programs, and that will serve prevention.

Remember, like I said before, if I have an identity of who I am, I'm less likely to go off that side because it brings shame on me and my ancestors.

I need to know that.

Mr. CASE. Comment. I would love to see an empirical study drug and ice abuse among children in Native Hawaiians because I'll bet you anything that you would see some amazing things going on there which is exactly the point you're making.

Mr. SALAVEA. In regards to your question to the DOE, we do things here in each individual community differently based on what resources are available. Sometimes the staff or logistically it may not be feasible to do the education and prevention in the schools, and therefore, be partnered with a community base. But the key is identifying what is the strength and then working off of that.

And the model is, what we try to do, is once you come up with a successful method and this is the area of community planning, you use that method or you match up a community with similar demographics, similar resources to a previous model that's worked. And then that way you can show them that, OK, with what you have, you're able to take on a prevention program and develop an action plan based on your strengths, not looking at your weaknesses but understanding your strengths and then working from there.

The big part that we've begun to do better I think in Hawaii County, and this goes back to your first question, Representative, is we're getting outreach. We're publicizing what we're doing and making sure that the community at the lowest levels, local neighborhoods, understand that, one, there is an ice problem; and two, from the clinical standpoint it's not all about persons having a personal weakness for a particular substance, it's a disease; and three, there are things you can do as a citizen and get involved.

And it's replicating that message over and over and telling people to get involved because look at what north Hawaii did, look at what Ka'u is doing, look at what Kohala is doing. It's the representation of the message over and over to the other communities that may not be as geared up or effective, that's helping a lot.

Mr. CASE. Mr. Hashida, let me ask you about rehabilitation. Does rehabilitation of crystal methamphetamine, specifically ice, does it have to be so expensive to be effective? Is there any proven, medically proven, because I do agree with you it's a medical condition—does it have to cost $325 a day?

Mr. HASHIDA. That's a good question. Our agency every year collects outcome data on all of our programs, and we can kind of take a look at everything. We are finding that there are extensive services that need to be put in place for treatment—what we call, treatment outcomes and goals to be met, and unfortunately, it does cost money.

Like, for example, one of the programs that we can do, a client can come in and we have a program therapeutic living services, a house, 24/7 type of coverage, and then 30 days they go into what's called outpatient treatment which again costs more money.

The other side of that is they also attend what's called silver support networks which are 12-step groups which are also very effective.

Mr. CASE. What's the success rate of one of those programs? What is the fall off the wagon, if that's the right way to put it? Are there any stats on how many people are addicted, medically addicted to ice and go through a recognized, supervised treatment program and stay off.

Mr. HASHIDA. I can take a look and send some information over to your office about exact stats with specific programs.

Mr. CASE. Just off the top of your head.

Mr. HASHIDA. 30, 40 percent, but that sounds really low. But in actuality, when you compare that to other programs, that's pretty decent.

Mr. CASE. That puts a little bit more emphasis on prevention.

Mr. HASHIDA. Yeah, yeah. I think at the schools and also in the community levels the programs are making an impact. They're creating a sense of urgency so a school teacher or counselor or somebody can identify a potential kid, if there is an ice problem.

There is an urgency there. We get calls, things roll, things happen to prevent that kid from going into further trouble with ice. Even when you talk to the kids, they understand that it's a dangerous drug. They don't minimize it, it's just like cigarettes or pakalolo. They know it's a lot more serious. Some of the programs they've talked about definitely has made an impact on them, but prevention is the way.

Mr. CASE. Thank you.

Mr. SOUDER. It's interesting because one of the things I've heard was that part of the reason behind the drop here is that all of a sudden every elected official and television station and the news stories, say that meth is terrible. The concentrated effort of the community over time seems to have had an impact, at least in the youth thing which is interesting because one of the greatest myths in America is "Just Say No" didn't work. In fact, "Just Say No" dropped drug use in the United States 8 straight years.

It wasn't "Just Say No," that was the starter. Say no, and then you do all the other stuff to help the addicts, to reinforce that through prevention, you still arrest people on the roads. Nobody ever did "Just Say No," but if you don't start with "Just Say No" it is very difficult to move through. And you made an interesting case of that because you've had bipartisan, cross party, cross—when Congressman Case first came to the committee, I know that we really weren't focused on the meth problems and drug problems in Hawaii.

Senators have a lot easier chance to write things into a bill than we do on the House side. We start low in the budget and then they get to add the add-ons and then we scramble to get part of the credit is about the way the system works. But often we'll lay the groundwork for which they can then put the things in and there was a bipartisan effort coming in on meth.

The same thing is happening with tobacco, that when we grab it as a community, we can start to get that. My understanding that I hadn't heard in other places, and this is an interesting cultural question and I don't know where the subgroup would be and where in the community, that some people here in Hawaii have seen family clusters doing drugs together. And we see that in a few parts of the United States with a couple types of drugs, but could you describe that here and do you see that in meth?

Mr. SALAVEA. Are you referring to—when you say family, is that——

Mr. SOUDER. Mother and dad and the kids at the same time.

Mr. SALAVEA. If you talk about marijuana or pakalolo, it's almost at the level of—its use is almost as casual as drinking alcohol. When you go to family parties, that's one of the—used to be one of the old initiations into adulthood for a young boy, when you get to sit down and drink beer with your dad. When you did that, you were a man.

Marijuana in my opinion, and from what I know of from my personal experience, my family, and my friends, approaches that level of use or has that type of community norm associated with it. When you're able to smoke in front of your parents, smoke marijuana in front of your parents, you've crossed into adulthood and now it's OK for you.

One characteristic of ice that makes it extremely attractive to local people is the fact that it's smokeable. If you asked—if meth users or addicts had to inject meth, I don't think we would have the same problem here today. It's a cultural thing that, yeah, it's being done in family groups, in pods. I know a lot of parties where you go to a party and you can pick out every relative who smokes pakalolo. And as soon as they disappear, you go out the door with them because they're going to light up.

Mr. SOUDER. Give me the challenge for treatment here because what we hear in treatment hearings is—the common thing is enablers. In other words, alcohol you hear it, wife doesn't want to crack down, doesn't want to get in an argument, kind of lets it go, kids tend to get out of the way. We're not talking enablers here. How in the world do you treat somebody if they go right back into the family and everybody is smoking pot and maybe doing meth, too?

Do you have a family drug treatment? In other words, if somebody checks themself into drug treatment, if that's the type of culture you're dealing with, taking individuals is almost irrelevant, and you don't bring the family in for 1 day to say, hey, or 3 days, this guy is going to be coming out of drug treatment, how are you going to help him. Well, one thing would be go into drug treatment yourself.

Are there programs that are oriented if you get somebody like—somebody comes in at 18 and says my parents are doing the drug as well, my brothers and sisters, do you approach the whole family, try to get them in together? How do you deal with this? This is a little bit different.

Dr. WASAN. You hit a very natural track there, too. They will not do ice with their kids. You'll hear them say I'd rather have my child do marijuana or pakalolo at home, or smoking cigarettes, at least I know what he's doing, so you'll see that happening.

But I have yet to meet anybody in my treatment program that will sit and smoke ice with their children. They'll say the opposite. I'll smoke in the bathroom, I'll smoke it outside because they do understand there is a difference here.

Now, the other piece, though, and because this is the hard concept to sell on the islands because it's transgenerational. Marijuana has been considered to be OK because it doesn't lead to violent crimes.

It's antimotivational. Who wants to fight me doped up on marijuana, right, so it's more of a hard sell.

You have to bring families into treatment with, as we call it in mental health, the identified patient. It may be the child, it may be the parent, you have to bring a family in. Most treatment when you look at the research will say that, that you have to have the family component added as part of treatment.

Now, has that happened a lot, probably not, but it should. And why hasn't it happened a lot. Well, managed care isn't going to pay for that straight out. Managed care will only pay for the identified patient for treatment. It will not pay for the family treatment like that, they don't believe in it, right. So that's a problem.

So in order to be able to do that, you have to get grants or funding that goes specifically for groups like Parenting Net Inc. or people who are certified in parenting and even getting involved in getting faith based who does family treatment a lot.

It needs to be targeted that way.

Right now it is not targeted that way. The purpose of bringing an adolescent residential program on this island, and Billy is definitely correct with that, 70 percent, I heard the number as high as 70 percent, of the people involved in adolescent treatment off island were from this island. To bring the treatment on this island, allows the families to be involved in treatment and it should be a required component. I imagine it actually is. I can't say for sure or not. But that is a natural draw, you have to have the family.

Now, what that will do at least will make it an awareness. I don't think most people who smoke marijuana on this island really think it's a drug.

They haven't had to sit down and really go through the process of addiction. They could if they were put into a treatment.

Mr. SOUDER. Is there a way in any of your data to check when a person comes out? 30 to 40 percent is probably a 1-year tracking not a multiyear tracking and also if you can get any data in from any of your organizations to see if any of them kept multiyear tracking. It might be actually a little bit easier for multiyear here because you're not as mobile. In the end I'm going to go to Ohio and Michigan and Illinois, and then the differences between, say, one relapse, three lapses, and serious falling back to being an addict, because there are substantial differences.

But in that 30 to 40 percent, what are the differences if no one else in the family is a drug abuser? In other words, if you kick somebody out—somebody graduates from the drug treatment, they're clean, if they're family is using marijuana or ice, I would assume their chances of fallback are much greater than if they're the loan user in that family. And if so, that's the type of statistic that would be helpful in making the argument that the problem is beyond the individual.

Otherwise, we're just spending money. Nobody has ever worked this issue. You can go anywhere and guys will tell you I've been to seven drug treatment programs, I've been to 10 drug treatment programs. I know how to hustle, I know how to pass the drug test. I know what they want to hear, I can say the words they want to say, once they learn to beat the system.

And the question is this: How do we figure out some of the—and one of them is if you put them back in the conditions that were there beforehand, and if the family is the condition, this is huge because if it's the job, you can move them here, you got a locational thing that's more problematic than other areas. But, if it's the family, then you're in the position of the only way to rehab a drug addict is get them away from the family which is a pretty nasty concept.

Mr. SALAVEA. I just wanted to mention we do see that, family dynamic going on, and some of the families are huge. There are huge families. Every corner you turn there are family members.

Mr. SOUDER. Extended family problems, we should make sure we note that in the record because that will be different than any other—when you say that, elaborate on that a little bit.

Mr. SALAVEA. Yeah, the family extensions can go quite a bit in terms of a small town. That's another factor to think about. The way we approach this is I'll tell a client, for example, you've done the treatment successfully, you want to continue to be successful, some of your family members—you just can't go back and live in that same house. You can still have family members and they may or may not seek treatment. They may not be in recovery, but you're not going to be living in that kind of environment and that's how we try to deal with them.

Just to add a little bit more answer to that question, I was discussing with one of the members in the audience previously, when you're part of the scene and you're in it, it seems like everyone is doing it. And when you get out of it, it seems like it's a minority, but you're on the other side of the glass, so to speak, and you don't really see the depth or the extent of it, the true extent.

And in getting back to your question about how do you deal with someone who in the family environment is the enabler or that trigger that will make that person relapse, another part of the adolescent treatment is the cultural component where many of these youth or teenagers have grown up in a cultural family of drug abuse, alcohol abuse, addiction where it's become—not their second nature, it's what life is and that's all they know.

An important aspect is to make them aware that you are not bound by what your family has exposed you to, and therefore, you can set your own sights on where you want to go and use cultural activities, cultural education, history to show that person that you don't come from a long line of addicts and that's your destiny, that's the only way you're going to go. That addiction began one, maybe two generations ago and it's not that deep and it's not far-fetched for you as an individual to make a total, clean break from it.

And in that process, that education process, the person begins to understand, you empower that person and they believe that I am the master of my own destiny and even though my family may choose to do that, I choose not to. And therefore, like counselors from BISAC, you don't have to spend as much time monitoring the individual because that person will for themselves be making the decision. No, that's not my choice, I choose to live a different lifestyle.

Dr. WASAN. I want to add one more piece. Just so you know, the communities on this island were stepping forth long before the funds were given. The Lokahi Treatment Center began in the back room of a church with a counsel one, by myself, but they gave me a building to start it with, they gave me support. I received no funding at that point from the State or from the feds or anyone else. I did receive some funding from the Dr. Earl Bakken Foundation to help me.

We were then given a free location in Kohala because the community said we need help up here. We were then given a location in Hilo for 3 months free to come in. The community is stepping forward. And they couldn't give any money, but what they could give was I'll give you space, I'll give you the time. The people who were coming for treatment were not even able to pay for the treatment, they had yet not been on QUEST or been able to afford the treatment so we treated them for free based on what we were getting from Dr. Earl Bakken. And then the community supplied other means of support.

So this project or this program or this treatment was going on before the Feds and the State stepped in and helped, and will continue. What you all have done is provided us a way to up the ante a little bit. Now we have agencies that are accredited. We're an integrated we're the only integrated programs on these islands that's accredited. We have Dr. Kevin Kunz who's accredited. You've allowed us now to step up to the bar, raise the level, bring in the people to work on this problem and that has helped a large, large amount.

I do see the numbers dropping of those in my program from relapsing and coming back. Something is happening. I see the faith-based communities stepping in and filling the gaps. So I truly thank you for the support you have given us to allow us to raise the bar on treatment and that's what we're trying to do.

You're absolutely correct, prevention is the key and getting—as I said before, getting families involved, supporting the churches more, supporting the cultural programs more. That's the true preventive key. Once I know who I am, I have a less chance of going that direction. I don't want to bring shame.

I'll say it over and over again, this culture is based on that. You do not want to bring shame on our ancestors, those who are of a Polynesian or Japanese or Asian ancestry. You do not want to do that. And one of the ways you're helping them not to do that is allowing the cultural and faith-based programs to be strengthened to give them a place to go and learn who they are.

Mr. CASE. I don't have any more questions, other than to say thank you and to the people who came before you and to the audience who has stayed with us throughout. Trying to be an observer in the hearing, I think you've seen the best of Congress, a good person who cares, down here trying to make a difference, so we want to thank him very much, Chairman Souder, for joining us this afternoon.

We have a tremendous need across our country. We have tremendous resources and the resources are stretched. There are many things Congress needs to attend to. This is one of the opportunities, to come down in our community and have the community so eloquently state to Congress for the record that is being taken what we are, what we need, and what we want, and what we are doing is truly a great opportunity.

I think we have seen here today the similarities that we share with many parts of our country in terms of the drug war such as this epidemic of ice. We've also seen the differences that we have here. Differences in not only needs and challenges but also in opportunities and solutions. I think, in fact, we have been given a rare opportunity to provide really an [inaudible] for our country, an opportunity that no one in the entire country has had.

Unfortunately, we got that opportunity because we have a problem, but we also have the opportunity to demonstrate a solution that's going to work for our entire country. And I think we should all feel a sense of responsibility especially for the people that are responsible—I certainly feel a responsibility to assist you, the people that are on the ground, actually dealing with this on an every day basis and whether you're dealing with law enforcement and prevention, or whether you're dealing with it with rehabilitation. That's a very tough job you're doing. We appreciate very much what you're doing.

I guess I just want to close by telling you a little bit of a story. This is another one of those police station stories. I get a lot of information from communities from dropping into the local police stations and finding the lowest ranking police officer and asking him or her what's happened. In the hierarchy sometimes you'll lose something in the translation.

This was in Hana and it was at the very beginning of my term and I wandered into that community. Now, many of us would not think especially, if we're in Oahu central, that Hana would have an ice problem. It does have an ice problem. A community incredibly deep-knitted culturally, remote, you would think that perhaps there wouldn't be as much of a challenge there, but it is.

And I walked in and I asked the police officer what is your No. 1 challenge in Hana, and he said "ice." I said, "What's happening?" He said, "Well, we don't have enough of any of the three things, prevention, rehabilitation, or law enforcement." The community is like many of this island, remote, far away, supply land, if you put it that way, are stretched. The assets are tending to be focused on the highly centralized population areas.

And I said, "Many bright spots." He said, "You know, something amazing has happened in the last couple of months." He said, "For many, many it is very hard for us in law enforcement to do anything about 'ice' because, essentially, we stood against the entire community."

Ice users were being sheltered by their families, they were being sheltered by their friends. We would find out after the fact that the drug deal was going down. We knew who was having a problem, but we could never really get in on it.

What has happened in the last couple months is we've seen more family members, more community members just saying no, and not saying no because they didn't like their family or friends that were using but because they cared about their family and friends.

They cared to turn people in that they knew, that they had grown up with, that had gone back generations and within that very small, deep-knitted cultural community. And they were just saying for the good of us all, we need to put a stop to this.

And I think what you have on the Big Island is a much better realization of that because this island amazingly has really led the way, in terms of the entire island, many different cultures, many different people, many different socioeconomics, saying that they care about this problem collectively, we're going to do something about it.

And I think if we can keep that spirit going, if we can continue to maintain an attitude that this is all of our problem, every single one of us, whether we have friends or family or know somebody that is using, dealing, manufacturing, and whatever literally they might do, and help in whatever way we can, any one of these three categories, enforcement, prevention, or rehabilitation, I have absolutely no doubt we can eliminate this problem.

Your Federal Government is here to help you, help all of us with our challenges. Again, I thank you for the effort that you have put in on the ground in assisting all of us and I thank your elected officials who have cared about this and for bringing these committee hearings to this island. Mahalo.

Mr. SOUDER. I want to thank our treatment and prevention people. By tradition, this committee always starts with its Federal witnesses who are predominantly Federal oversight agencies and we move through. But we always try to include the treatment and prevention people in every hearing because without the grass roots working away with individuals one at a time, you can only do so much in the larger picture too. Tell your staff, too, and all the organizations they work with, we appreciate their work.

There are a couple of general things I wanted to mention, too, in addition to thanking Congressman Case, again, and the others who have been so hospitable here. Our committee has broad jurisdiction and we probably spend 60 percent of our time on narcotics. We spent a lot of time in this past year because we also oversee the office of faith-based initiatives, so we've been doing a number of regional hearings with that.

And one of the things that is real interesting in narcotics abuse is that everyone, regardless of their approach or feeling about that issue, realizes that unless an individual makes a commitment to change somewhere along the way, aren't probably going to get off, and certainly they aren't going to stay off. And one of the key elements of that is a faith experience, and we've seen some pretty amazing stories that can do it for far less than $325 a day, if, indeed, they make a personal commitment to change their life.

Now, if they don't make that personal commitment, even then you need to have monitoring and support groups, but a major philosophical change often anchored in religion that says I am going to hell, I am going to change my life, I am destroying my family, I am going to change. Then if you don't have that, then the drug testing, the job training, the other types of support become even more critical because internally, they haven't made that change. You have to use more and more external factors. It's amazing when somebody has made a dynamic change. All of a sudden their attitude toward education changes, their attitude toward how they're going to show up for work changes, there are other mental things that come out of that. So that certainly should be an element that goes in the mix and we've been trying to work with that around the country. And by the way, it isn't just for drug treatment, it's in a lot of different areas.

I appreciate you bringing that point out because it's a critical part because much of this is mental. Yes, it's physical, but it's also mental, and particularly the recovery has to be mental, at least after the first stages of addiction as you get over the physical part.

We also—as we work through this, I strongly believe we have to look at more family approaches.

It's also very interesting to see where you can have things that will apply in the other States where you have things that are unique to Hawaii. We need to always respect that from the Federal Government. We try to push things as much as possible down to the State side, you made a good point pushing it to the local community, with minimal pass-through, minimal control should be, obviously, the goal.

When I got elected, I came from a little town of 700 outside of Ft. Wayne. My theme was more Grable, less Washington, but I didn't mean to move it from Grable to Indianapolis either any more than you want to move it to Honolulu. The point should be that you agree to move it down with the monitoring.

When you're spending other peoples' tax dollars from other States, there are going to be more strings, there is going to be more taken out as it moves down in monitoring, it's not just a pure block grant. He who pays the piper picks the tune is the old expression and that will be there. Nevertheless, we want to maximize the dollars on the ground.

I very much appreciate the seeming progress that you're making in a community-wide thing, but it's very important that we also make the end roads on marijuana and the other drugs as you're doing this or it will be self defeating. We don't want a Cheech & Chong or a modern day Ozzie Osbourne family situation.

This committee almost had a very unique hearing.

I say almost because the window was such that I couldn't get in in time, but we actually talked to Ozzie Osbourne and he was going to come to our hearing with his full family before a couple more of them went into drug rehab, Sharon with her own album and all this kind of stuff. But he is one of the most eloquent, in between his ineloquent periods, which are pretty frequent, of saying, look, I got messed up and have blown out part of my brain, I've only blown out part of the brain of my kids because of my behavior.

Unless we kind of understand this is interrelated together, which is the other thing that's been real challenging because the plantation mentality—or the changing limited opportunities in some of the areas of this island isn't that much different than we feel in the rust belt where you can grow up and not even have to graduate from high school, get a steel making job of $55,000, now all of a sudden that's in China. If it's not in Mexico, it's in China.

And the question is now they're working two jobs, have similar kinds of pressures that even the middle and upper classes aren't certainly aware of their next job or how stable that's going to be, it just adds uncertainty. And if you're a temperament that thrives on that, that's fine. But if you're a temperament that likes security, it's a whole different challenge here.

But one of the great things about America, and David Brooks has a new book about this, is that we have outlets beyond just the job in which to identify themselves which is why we don't have some of the class warfare that you have in other nations. It may be you're the greatest ukulele player in a band in Hilo. It may be that you're the bowling champion on a given island or you've written an article or I like to collect miniature lighthouses. I've been to lighthouses and I can pretty much up just about anybody for the number of lighthouses I've been to, and so I'm kind of a lighthouse expert.

And as you teach kids of how self-esteem can come to supplement other than just this daily routine of a job, it's one of challenges and why the Boys and Girls Clubs have increasingly gotten more dollars in the system and why we have to look at creative ways to communicate that jobs are important, I'm the workaholic, this job, other than when you're being attacked which is often, is a great job, but I've also had all kinds of other jobs and so has my family and you can't get your total satisfaction out of your work and that has to be something that you can communicate through to.

Thanks, again, for your efforts. Thanks for this hearing. If you have additional information that you want to come in—and tracking information is very helpful because the problem with meth and ice, in particular, you have more of a track record and have dealt with the variations that when we talk to treatment people in other parts of the United States, we don't have anything. We're dealing with things that are 24 months max, some areas 6 months. It's a whole different ball game.

With that, the subcommittee stands adjourned.

[Whereupon, at 1:15 p.m., the subcommittee was adjourned.]

[Additional information submitted for the hearing record follows:]

BIG ISLAND SUBSTANCE ABUSE COUNCIL

HILO
Corporate Office
234 Waianuenue Avenue
Suite 104
Hilo, Hawaii 96720
(808) 969-9994
(808) 969-7570 Fax
Website: www.bisac.com

Adult & Adolescent Outpatient Treatment
297 Waianuenue Avenue
(808) 935-4927
(808) 969-1861 Fax

Baby S.A.F.E. Program
(808) 961-5022

Ka Wahi Ola Hou - Men Therapeutic Living Program
Hilo, Hawaii 96720

Keola Hou - Men Therapeutic Living Program
Hilo, Hawaii 96720

Ka Wahi Ola Hou - Women Therapeutic Living Program
Hilo, Hawaii 96720

Hale Ho'opulapula O Na Wahine Therapeutic Living Program
Hilo, Hawaii 96720

Hale O'hana Mana Moms & Babies Therapeutic Living Program
Hilo, Hawaii 96720

KONA
Outpatient Treatment and Baby S.A.F.E. Program
P.O. Box 208
Kealakekua, Hawaii 96750
(808) 334-0266
(808) 322-3001 Fax

WAIMEA
Outpatient Treatment
Suite C-12
65-1230 Mamalahoa Highway
Kamuela, Hawaii 96743
(808) 887-2175
(808) 887-0805 Fax

The Big Island Substance Abuse Council has been responding to those who are reaching out for help from addiction and alcoholism for many years. This is evident by the forty (40) years of service this non-profit organization has been operating here on the Island of Hawaii. Drugs are not a new phenomenon to the island, but much has changed in recent years. What is a phenomenon is the incredible impact that the drug methamphetamine known as "Ice" has created. Few Big Island residents can state that they have not been touched in one way or another by this terrible drug. Addiction, violence, and crime now recognize "Ice" as the motive or reason behind the action.

At the Big Island Substance Abuse Council the impact began in the mid 1990's, as the number of consumers presenting themselves with "Ice" as their "drug of choice" began a steady increase. In the year 2000, "Ice" became the most common addiction being treated at our programs. Today, the number of individuals in Big Island Substance Abuse Council programs who will report addiction or abuse of methamphetamine is overwhelming. All ages, all cultures, all income levels, no one is ignored by this addiction.

There are many opinions as to why this trend has occurred. These opinions are as diverse as the people who occupy this beautiful island, and the speculation will undoubtedly continue. The Big Island Substance Abuse Council has moved beyond the question why and is now looking to the solution. Local, State and Federal Government Departments began efforts to reach out to the people of Hawaii County and take a lead in developing the strategy and solution to the problem. Partnerships and collaborative efforts have begun a new trend related to "Ice" that is "Healing Our Island". A combination of law enforcement, prevention and treatment efforts has resulted in a comprehensive approach to turn the tide. Details related to the Big Island Substance Abuse Council's role in these efforts include the development and implementation of many new programs and opportunities for those impacted by "Ice" addiction. The primary objective is to increase capacity of programs while reducing barriers to accessing services.

Providing services to children and adolescents is one of the primary objectives. The Big Island Substance Abuse Council is now in all of Hawaii County's Public High Schools. A full time substance abuse counselor is available in the familiar environment of the school and can be accessed in confidence. Adolescents who present evidence of substance use can also be referred directly. The behaviors and patterns that lead to substance abuse are addressed where and when it is appropriate, not after it has progressed to addiction.

For the adolescents who have progressed past early intervention, the Big Island Substance Abuse Council is a partner in developing and implementing a comprehensive Residential Substance Abuse Treatment Program. This experiential program is designed on the Big Island, by Big Island Professionals, for Big Island kids.

These adolescent programs are provided in addition to the Outpatient Treatment services established by Big Island Substance Abuse Council in Kona, Waimea and Hilo many years ago. These programs work directly with Judiciary and family referrals for adolescents appropriate for an outpatient level of care such as, The Big Island Juvenile Drug Court. Treatment services are provided to this target population while the Drug Court monitors progress and provides accountability through incentives and sanctions for the participant. This program has demonstrated excellent outcomes throughout the mainland and expectations are high as the Big Island Drug Court is implemented in Hawaii County.

Families have experiences a significant amount of turmoil and damage due to "Ice" as demonstrated through increased domestic violence, child abuse, and homelessness. The Big Island Substance Abuse Council responded to this community need through the development of Therapeutic Living Programs. These homes accommodate target populations in a homelike setting with the reinforcement of full time staffing. Programs for new mothers and their infant children and the home for single fathers and their kids are examples of how the Therapeutic Living Programs reach out to meet the specific needs of the families.

With twenty-four (24) programs throughout the Island of Hawaii, the Big Island Substance Abuse Council continues to provide effective and efficient services to those in need. Regardless of age, cultural identity of income level our programs are developed to provide immediate access and to reduce barriers to appropriate treatment and prevention services.

The Big Island Substance Abuse Council is honored to be a part of the solution in the efforts of "Healing Our Island". The responses to community needs and development of solutions to the "Ice" epidemic were possible only through a collaborative and strategic effort of everyone involved. Support from our government officials such as Senator Daniel Inouye, Governor Linda Lingle, and County of Hawaii Mayor Harry Kim provided leadership and inspiration to stand firm battle for freedom from this drug.

While much progress has been made, and the efforts have been rewarded with success there remains tremendous needs. Support for the individuals, families, and communities throughout the Island of Hawaii will be necessary as the work continues. Many rural areas hit hard by economic turmoil and the devastation of "Ice" still have little or no services for their residents. Longer durations of treatment have been proven effective for methamphetamine addiction, but treatment episodes continue to be limited in length. Specific target populations such as those with co-occurring disorders struggle to find appropriate care. The island of Hawaii continues to need the support of our Federal agencies to maintain the course and develop all of the resources necessary to overcome this epidemic. Please continue providing the funding opportunities and support that have allowed the progress to occur and will continue to support the efforts towards "Healing Our Island".

Respectfully Submitted,

Wesley Margheim, CSAC
Director of Business and Community Development

BIG ISLAND SUBSTANCE ABUSE COUNCILS

OVERVIEW OF SERVICES

- Outpatient Substance Abuse Treatment for Adults, and Adolescent (Hilo, Kealakehe and Waimea).
- Eight (8) Therapeutic Living Programs – Gender Specific (24 hour adult supervision and support services), which includes intensive case management. Eight programs which include three men TLP, a women's TLP, a moms and babies TLP, a fathers and children TLP, and a Public Safety women's TLP in Hilo and a men's TLP in North Kohala.
- Mom's and Babies Therapeutic Living Treatment Program substance abuse treatment services for mother and her children under the age of five living together as a family.
- Fathers and children Therapeutic Living Treatment Program substance abuse treatment services for the father and his children from the ages of five to twelve years of age living together as a family.
- Public Safety TLP treatment transition program for adult female sentenced offenders who are concurrently serving their sentence and pretrial defendants on supervised release.
- Specialized Services including mental health care/dual diagnosis and gender specific treatment.
- Employment Core Program-rehabilitation, job preparation, training, and retention.
- Training, Education, and Consulting Services for the community.
- Non-residential services including relapse prevention, continuing care, aftercare and the Alumni Association.
- Transportation services for all consumers (within a 50 mile area of each facility).
- Baby S.A.F.E. (Substance Abuse Free Environment) provides outreach, intervention and pre-treatment services to pregnant and early postpartum women in Hilo and Kealakekua.
- School Based outpatient treatment located in ten (10) high schools across the Big Island of Hawaii.

Big Island Substance Abuse Council
Overview of Services continued

- Supervised Drug Testing-Monitoring individuals and families in order to support and demonstrate a clean and sober life style.

- Community Reintegration-Transitional support for consumers in Aftercare.

- Work Skills Development-Improvement of employment skills to support self-sufficiency.

- Tutoring/Evaluation and basic Educational skill development.

- Children's Milieu Program-Therapeutic nursery services for persons needing childcare to access treatment services.

- Family Program Education-for family education and counseling that supports long-term recovery goals.

BIG ISLAND SUBSTANCE ABUSE COUNCIL'S

DESCRIPTION OF SERVICES

The Big Island Substance Abuse Council has successfully been in operation since May of 1964. For forty (40) years BISAC, through difficult times and economic challenges, has kept our focus on our mission which is to provide "substance abuse treatment to all those in need". The extent and degree of substance abuse on the Big Island is reflective by the need to expand the Big Island Substance Abuse Council's substance abuse treatment services and sites on the Big Island, from two (2) sites in 1997 to twenty three (23) sites in 2004.

BISAC'S Programs include

Three (3) free standing outpatient locations – Hilo, Waimea & Kealakekua

Seven (7) Therapeutic Programs in Hilo and North Kohala

One (1) Safe/Clean and Sober Housing Home in Hilo.

Two (2) Baby S.A.F.E. Programs in East and West Hawaii

Ten (10) School Based programs in High Schools Island wide

BISAC's Mission

The Big Island Substance Abuse Council strives to enhance the quality of care and innovative services in the areas of Substance Abuse Education, Intervention, and Treatment. We are dedicated to the healing of mind, body and spirits of individuals, families and others who suffer as a result of alcohol and other substance use, abuse and addiction.

PROGRAM SERVICES

Ka Wahi Ola Hou "The Healing Place" Mens Therapeutic Living Programs
Located in Hilo

This program was developed to assist the recovering addict in reducing the risk of relapse while obtaining the necessary social and recovery skills to develop safe and substance-free housing. Often these services are offered in conjunction with outpatient treatment to enhance the support offered to the consumer and increase stability in the Therapeutic Living residence. Services are provided as a means of developing, restoring or maintaining community living skills, and remediating deficits in communication, interpersonal skills and medication management. Consumers in this level of care require considerable daily intervention, structure and assistance learning daily living skills through support, education and a comprehensive approach to meet the consumer's needs. These therapeutic living programs promote a safe, drug free lifestyle as the consumer begins his/her transition to more independent housing. The program has gender specific training to educate men in anger and stress management and relapse prevention.

Ka Wahi Ola Hou "The Healing Place" Womens Therapeutic Living Programs
Located in Hilo

This program was developed to assist the recovering addict in reducing the risk of relapse while obtaining the necessary social and recovery skills to develop safe and substance-free housing. Often these services are offered in conjunction with outpatient treatment to enhance the support offered to the consumer and increase stability in the Therapeutic Living residence. Services are provided as a means of developing, restoring or maintaining community living skills, and remediating deficits in communication, interpersonal skills and medication management. Consumers in this level of care require considerable daily intervention, structure and assistance learning daily living skills through support, education and a comprehensive approach to meet the consumer's needs. These therapeutic living programs promote a safe, drug free lifestyle as the consumer begins her transition to more independent housing. The program has gender specific training to educate women in life skills, women's issues and domestic violence.

Keola Hou "The Healing" - Men Therapeutic Living Program
Located in Hilo.

This program was developed to assist the recovering addict in reducing the risk of relapse while obtaining the necessary social and recovery skills to develop safe and substance-free housing. Often these services are offered in conjunction with outpatient treatment to enhance the support offered to the consumer and increase stability in the Therapeutic Living residence. Services are provided as a means of developing, restoring or maintaining community living skills, and remediating deficits in communication, interpersonal skills and medication management. Consumers in this level of care require considerable daily intervention, structure and assistance learning daily living skills through support, education and a comprehensive approach to meet the consumer's needs. These therapeutic living programs promote a safe, drug free lifestyle as the consumer begins his transition to more independent housing. The program has gender specific training to educate men in anger, stress management and relapse prevention.

Ho'omaka Ana Ae Ola Hou "Let the Healing Begin" - Men Therapeutic Living Program
Located in North Kohala

This program was developed to assist the recovering addict in reducing the risk of relapse while obtaining the necessary social and recovery skills to develop safe and substance-free housing. Often these services are offered in conjunction with outpatient treatment to enhance the support offered to the consumer and increase stability in the Therapeutic Living residence. Services are provided as a means of developing, restoring or maintaining community living skills, and remediating deficits in communication, interpersonal skills and medication management. Consumers in this level of care require considerable daily intervention, structure and assistance learning daily living skills through support, education and a comprehensive approach to meet the consumer's needs. These therapeutic living programs promote a safe, drug free lifestyle as the consumer begins his transition to more independent housing. The program has gender specific training to educate men in anger, stress management and relapse prevention.

Department of Public Safety Hale Ho'opulapula "House of Rehabilitation for Women" Therapeutic Living Program
Located in Hilo.

This Therapeutic Living Program is specifically designed for women inmates and addresses the barriers that incarcerated women face in their efforts to engage in professional treatment services and transition back into the community. This program is a long term, 24-hour staff supervised program, providing services to women who committed an offense while they were under the influence of alcohol and/or drugs and who are diagnosed as substance abusers or have other issues that need treatment. Counselors facilitate services such as problem solving, case management, skill building, education, process groups and relapse prevention in addition to individual counseling.

Hale O'hana Mana "House of Working Miracles" Moms and babies Therapeutic Living Program
Located in Hilo.

This is a Therapeutic Living Program for moms and their children ages 0-5 which supports family unification. This program has been recognized as a "model program" for the State of Hawaii. Moms and babies live together while they are in treatment and learn important parenting skills to help the family unit emerge into a "happy and balanced family". This therapeutic living program assists moms in gaining basic life skills needed to be a positive role model to her children.

Fathers and Children Therapeutic Living Program
Located in Hilo.

This is a Therapeutic Living Program for fathers and their children ages 5-12. Fathers and children live together while they are in treatment and learn important parenting skills to help the family unit emerge into a "happy and balanced family." This therapeutic living program assists fathers in gaining basic life skills needed to be a positive role model to his children.

Mauna Loa Clean and Sober Supportive Housing for men
Located in Hilo.

This is a clean and sober supportive affordable housing home available to men who have completed treatment with BISAC or are in recovery. Men are required to be employed or job seeking.

Baby S.A.F.E. (Substance Abuse Free Environment) Program (2 Free standing facilities)
Located in Hilo and Kealakekua.

Baby S.A.F.E. works in conjunction with the Big Island Substance Abuse Council's treatment program and provides an array of outreach and pre-treatment services to Big Island pregnant and postpartum, substance using women and their families. Baby S.A.F.E. uses a variety of outreach methods to assist in early identification providing a greater margin of safety for a healthy birth outcome.

Children's Milieu Program
Located in Hilo and Kona.

BISAC's Children Milieu Program was established in 1998 through the Hawaii Children's Trust Fund and addresses the needs of infants and toddlers identified as "at risk" for drug exposure. Services for children ages 0-5 include comprehensive case management, health and developmental assessments, play therapy and childcare for infants and toddlers of individuals participating in BISAC's substance abuse outpatient treatment program.

Adolescent Services
The Big Island Substance Abuse Council operates three (3) free standing Outpatient Programs for adolescents in Hawaii County. The locations are Kealakekua, Hilo, and Waimea. Each location provides screening/assessment, Intensive Outpatient, Outpatient, individual counseling, and After-Care services. BISAC also provides case-management services to a specific number of adolescent consumers who have been referred to receive treatment through the Pulama/Family Court project.

BISAC's School-Based Programs [Ten (10) Schools Ka'u, Kohala, Konawaena, Kealakehe, Keaau, Honokaa, Laupahoehoe, Hilo, Waiakea, and Pahoa.]

In addition to outpatient services, BISAC also provides School-Based Treatment services at eight Public High Schools in Hawaii County. School-Based Treatment includes screening/assessment, group therapy, individual counseling, after-care, teacher in-service trainings and school education services. School Based programs meet the adolescent consumer needs in an environment that is less intensive then outpatient and provides services immediately after an individual is suspected of having difficulty with substances. Each school has designated office and counseling space for BISAC's program, reducing barriers to care and enhancing greater accessibility to substance abuse treatment. BISAC's School-Based substance abuse treatment programs also provide spring and summer break treatment services.

BISAC's Employment Core Services Program
Located in Hilo program office.

The goal is to promote economic self-sufficiency and self-reliance. The program is available to BISAC's consumers and the public who meet the criteria for recruitment. The training program includes goal setting, personal accountability and other life management skills. Consumers are taught skills such as how to fill out a job application, resume writing, interview skills and job retention. Consumers are taught workplace functioning skills such as gaining more responsibility in the workplace to eventually obtain a promotion. Case management services are given to the consumer in the beginning of the training to determine barriers to employment through interest, skills, values and occupational surveys. Consumers obtain computer experience in our computer lab with the use of the ten (10) computers.

Program Philosophy

The Big Island Substance Abuse Council's Primary goal is reflected in our organizations mission statement. Our goal is to promote public awareness that alcoholism and drug addiction are treatable illnesses and to provide leadership throughout the County and State in the development and establishment of education and treatment of substance abuse.

Mission Statement

The Big Island Substance Abuse Council strives to enhance the quality of care and innovative services in the areas of Substance Abuse Education, Intervention and Treatment. We are dedicated to the healing of mind, body and spirit of individuals, families and others who suffer as a result of alcohol and other substance use, abuse and addiction.

BISAC continues to provide an array of rehabilitation services designed to promote positive attitudes, values and skills. BISAC strives to advance socially positive changes to sustain employment and reduce dependence, crime and anti-social behavior while supporting increased self-reliance, personal productivity, and civic responsibility.

Goals of the Organization

To provide a range of coordinated, comprehensive treatment services that addresses the multiple health and human service needs of adult and adolescent substance abuser in the community.

To decrease the incidence, severity and debilitating consequences of alcohol and drug among Hawaii Island residents through education, psych-educational and individualized treatment modalities.

To effect significant change in the consumers with substance abuse disorders, resulting in an improved quality of life for both the individual and family, to include successful integration into the community.

BISAC's multi-faceted, trans-disciplinary approach is derived from a fundamental philosophical belief that services should be focused on the whole person and as such the organization strives to instill dignity, respect, hope and compassion to all of our consumers.

DIRECTORY

HILO

CORPORATE OFFICES
234 Waianuenue Avenue, Suite 104
Hilo, Hawaii 96720

ADULT & ADOLESCENT
OUTPATIENT TREATMENT
297 Waianuenue Avenue
Hilo, Hawaii 96720

BABY S.A.F.E. (SUBSTANCE ABUSE
FREE ENVIRONMENT) PROGRAM
333 Kauila Street
Hilo, Hawaii 96720

KA WAHI OLA HOU – MEN
THERAPEUTIC LIVING PROGRAM
146 Puueo Street
Hilo, Hawaii 96720

KEOLA HOU – MEN THERAPEUTIC
LIVING PROGRAM
152 Puueo Street
Hilo, Hawaii 96720

KA WAI OLA HOU – WOMEN
THERAPEUTIC LIVING
323 Kauila Street
Hilo, Hawaii 96720

HALE HO'OPULAPULA O NA
WAIHINE THERAPEUTIC LIVING
PROGRAM – Public Safety
160 Puueo Street
Hilo, Hawaii 96720

HALE O'HANA MANA MOM'S AND
BABIES THERAPEUTIC LIVING
PROGRAM
15 Kanoa Street
Hilo, Hawaii 96720

FATHERS AND CHILDREN
THERAPEUTIC LIVING PROGRAM
140 Puueo Street
Hilo, Hawaii 96720

MAUNA LOA THERAPEUTIC
LIVING PROGRAM
69 Mauna Loa Street
Hilo, Hawaii 96720

KONA

ADULT & ADOLESCENT
OUTPATIENT TREATMENT
81-947 Halekii Street
Kealakekua, Hawaii 96750

BABY S.A.F.E. (SUBSTANCE ABUSE
FREE ENVIRONMENT) PROGRAM
81-947 Halekii Street
Kealakekua, Hawaii 96750

WAIMEA

ADULT & ADOLESCENT
OUTPATIENT TREATMENT
65-1158 Mamalahoa Highway, Suite 16
Kamuela, Hawaii 96743

SCHOOL BASED

WAIAKEA HIGH SCHOOL
ADOLESCENT OUTPATIENT
TREATMENT
155 W. Kawili Street
Hilo, Hawaii 96720

PAHOA HIGH SCHOOL
ADOLESCENT OUTPATIENT
TREATMENT
15-3038 Puna Road
Pahoa, Hawaii 96778

KONAWAENA HIGH SCHOOL
ADOLESCENT OUTPATIENT
TREATMENT
81-1043 Konawaena School Road
Kealakekua, Hawaii 96750

KAU HIGH SCHOOL ADOLESCENT
OUTPATIENT TREAMENT
P. O. Box 100
Pahala, Hawaii 96777

Big Island Substance Abuse Council
Directory continued

HILO HIGH SCHOOL ADOLESCENT
OUTPATIENT TREATMENT
556 Waianuenue Avenue
Hilo, Hawaii 96720

KEALAKEHE HIGH SCHOOL
ADOLESCENT OUTPATIENT
TREATMENT
74-500 Puohulihuli Street
Kailua-Kona, Hawaii 96740

HONOKAA HIGH SCHOOL
ADOLESCENT OUTPATIENT
TREATMENT
45-527 Pakalana Street
Honokaa, Hawaii 96727

LAUPAHOEHOE HIGH SCHOOL
ADOLESCENT OUTPATIENT
TREATMENT
35-2065 Old Mamalahoa Highway
Laupahoehoe, Hawaii 96764

KEAAU HIGH SCHOOL
ADOLESCENT OUTPATIENT
TREATMENT
16-725 Keaau-Pahoa Road
Keaau, Hawaii 96749

KOHALA HIGH SCHOOL
ADOLESCENT OUTPATIENT
TREATMENT
P. O. Box 279
Kapaau, Hawaii 96755

MAJOR CONTRIBUTORS

On behalf of the Big Island Substance Abuse Council, grateful acknowledgement is recognized for the generous contributions by the following:

- State of Hawaii, Alcohol and Drug Abuse Division, East and West Hawaii Adult Treatment and Therapeutic Living Programs
- State of Hawaii, Alcohol and Drug Abuse Division, Men's Therapeutic Living Program
- State of Hawaii, Alcohol and Drug Abuse Division, East and West Hawaii School Based Substance Abuse Treatment Services
- State of Hawaii, Department of Public Safety, Women's Therapeutic Living Program
- State of Hawaii, Alcohol and Drug Abuse Division, North Kohala Men's Therapeutic Living Program
- Hawaii Island United Way, Adolescent Substance Abuse Services
- County of Hawaii, East and West Hawaii Substance Abuse Services
- State of Hawaii, Maternal and Child Health Branch, Baby S.A.F.E. Outreach Services for women, East and West Hawaii
- State of Hawaii, Department of Labor and industrial Relations, Employment Core Services
- Hina Mauka, DHS Urinalysis Testing
- Hawaii Community Foundation, Organizational Effectiveness Program
- State of Hawaii, Department of Human Services, Mom's and Babies and Father's and Children Therapeutic Living Programs
- Probation and Parole
- Pulama Contract with Bay Clinic, SAMHSA
- U.S. Drug Courts
- Private trust and foundations
- Hawaii Hotel Industry – Charitable Contribution, East and West Hawaii Treatment Services
- Wal-Mart – Charitable Contribution, Therapeutic Living Program

The Hawaii Island Meth Initiative

I. Mission Statement

The mission of the Hawaii Island Meth Initiative is to have everyone working together to heal our island from the harmful effects of ICE. The goal is to ensure that Hawaii Island is a healthy and safe place for our children and our families.

II. Introduction

In early 2001, Mayor Harry Kim declared a war on the drug crystal methamphetamine or ICE. "It scares me…this is going to take all of us collectively to literally declare war on this drug". Mayor Kim noted that "war" is an ugly word, "I've got to use an ugly word because this is an ugly situation".

In August of 2001, Mayor Kim met with U.S. Senator Daniel K. Inouye, Family Court Judge Ben Gaddis, Police Chief James Correa, Prosecuting Attorney Jay Kimura, Child Welfare Services Supervisor Stewart Maeda and Child Protection Services Supervisor Peggy Hilton. At this meeting, Senator Inouye challenged Mayor Kim to come up with a strategy to address this problem that threatened Hawaii's future. Senator Inouye stated that he needed data and statistics to take back to Washington D.C. along with a strategic plan so that he could convince his colleagues to support a program for Hawaii Island. Senator Inouye made it clear that the briefing was informative and alarming and that something needed to be done about it.

In October of 2001, Mayor Kim assigned this initiative to his new executive assistant, Billy Kenoi. As a former deputy public defender on Oahu for four years and being born and raised on Hawaii Island, Billy was familiar with the issues surrounding crystal methamphetamine and its devastating impact on Hawaii Island. Aware of the complexities of substance abuse, the idea was to create a simple and coherent strategy that would result in positive changes for our Island community. However, this was an effort that would have to do without any initial funding from the County or the State of Hawaii.

Hawaii in the fall of 2001 was just emerging from years of little or no economic growth. Then, September 11, 2001 saw the worst terrorist attack on US soil in our country's history. A tough financial and economic situation became even tougher. Hawaii County in the fall of 2001 was staring at a projected deficit of $7.4 million dollars after nearly 5 years of budget cuts and status quo funding. The State of Hawaii was anticipating a shortfall of $315 million dollars and the dire financial situation of the State required the calling of a special legislative session. Established and worthy programs were being cut while we were moving ahead with a new program requiring millions of dollars. Fortunately, U.S. Senator Daniel K. Inouye had already gone back to Washington D.C. and had made contact with the relevant federal agencies and indicated to them that in spite of the crisis our country was in, Hawaii Island needed help with ICE.

In October of 2001, a few simple principles were established as we planned to create a new model to address ICE. This was to be a three-pronged approach involving public safety (enforcement), public health (treatment), and public education and community awareness (prevention and education). We needed to secure financial commitments prior to planning so that we did not end up going through a year long exercise only to find ourselves back at square one, looking for financial support for established priorities. And finally, we needed to mobilize the entire Island. This could not be a Hilo thing or a Kona thing. This could not be about North or South or East or West Hawaii. This disease called ICE affected everybody and everybody needed to be involved in finding a solution.

Community groups had already begun to meet and to discuss solutions to the problems associated with ICE. North Kohala, Kona, Waimea, and Waikoloa were early pioneers in community mobilization. North Hawaii served as the model for other communities to begin organizing and planning. However, in 2001, although ICE had been around for 10-15 years, many residents still did not know much about the drug and its effects upon the community. This meant that informational sessions and briefings had to be held in every single community and with every single sector in each community.

The Mayor's Office (Billy Kenoi), the Prosecutor's Office (Mitch Roth), the Hawaii County Police Department (Det. Marshall Kanehailua), and the Hawaii National Guard (Sgt. Ha Chi) went to High, Middle, and Elementary schools, businesses, rotary meetings, union meetings, community meetings, churches and faith organizations, chamber of commerce organizations, and any one who was interested in the ICE problem or just needed a speaker for their meeting or luncheon. In addition, Gary Shimabukuro, from Laulima Hawaii, also made multiple visits to Hawaii Island businesses, schools, and community organizations to talk about ICE. These meetings were well attended and a lot of information was shared, including disheartening statistics that showed Hawaii Island with the highest rates of crystal meth abuse in the State.

How did we know that we had the highest rates of substance abuse in the state? In providing the federal government with justification for a Hawaii Island Meth Initiative, we had to have the data and statistics to support it. So we asked the Hawaii County Police Department for their arrest and seizure data for the past four years. We used the Department of Health Needs Assessment Handbook. We asked the Big Island Substance Abuse Council for a graph on drug use trends among those seeking treatment. Finally, the most compelling statistics came from the youth themselves in the 2000 Hawaii Student Alcohol, Tobacco, and Other Drug use study. This data was critical in calling attention to this crisis.

The first two priorities that were identified as being critical to addressing drugs and substance abuse on Hawaii Island were the lack of an updated drug lab and the lack of youth activities and programs. Senator Inouye stepped up and immediately addressed both of those concerns. In December of 2001, Senator Inouye submitted requests for funding for $350,000 for a drug lab and technical assistance through the Department of Labor, Rural Development Assistance Fund. Also, a request for $1.25 Million was earmarked for a Hawaii Island Youth Anti-Drug program. This earmark would later evolve into the Pulama Project, a collaborative effort that would address youth prevention issues Islandwide. Lacking resources to implement a planning process, we were fortunate to have been selected as one of the first sites in the United States to host a Methamphetamine Summit that was sponsored by the Drug Enforcement Administration and the National Crime Prevention Council. Again, Senator Inouye and his staff were instrumental in coordinating this planning process and securing the appearance of DEA Administrator Asa Hutchinson and NCPC CEO Jim Copple to come to Hawaii Island. This was the beginning of Meth Summit I.

Originally planned for 150-200 participants, we realized that we had that many at one ICE meeting. We requested and received permission for 350 participants. Unfortunately, to maintain that number we had to make it an invitation only event. This meant that we had to be diligent in determining who to invite. The planning group numbered 40. In this group were representatives from federal, state, and county government as well as from business, education, faith, treatment, enforcement, cultural groups and community representatives. Each member of the planning group was in turn asked to submit names from their sector or from their community. We aimed to be as balanced and as inclusive as possible.

This comprehensive strategic planning process would involve identifying the problem, identifying solutions to the problem, identifying barriers to implementing the solution, and finally, identifying resources to implement the solutions. The process involved a day long conference where we randomly placed members from different sectors at the same table to generate creative ideas and discussions. This process resulted in over 145 recommendations being generated. Participants were then asked to rank the recommendations according to both importance and feasibility. In December of 2002, a representative from the National Crime Prevention Council returned to Hawaii Island with the survey results. The two areas that generated the most recommendations were Youth and Treatment.

In January of 2003, Hawaii County submitted two pieces of legislation, HB 1603 and HB 1604, relating to establishing an adolescent treatment program and to establishing a community anti-drug fund. These two bills traveled a long and bumpy road through the legislative process, finally ending up as grants-in-aid in the final budget bill. We are eternally grateful for the leadership of Senator Russell Kokubun and Representative Dwight Takamine and our entire Hawaii

Island delegation for making these appropriation requests possible. In addition, we are also appreciative to Governor Linda Lingle for signing off on this legislation and releasing the monies to Hawaii County.

Realizing Federal and State support for this effort, it was important that Hawaii County also contribute to the Hawaii Island Meth Initiative. This contribution came in the allocation of bodies from the police cellblock to a new ICE Task Force established in both East and West Hawaii. In addition, HPD also established and ICE Hotline to ensure that calls from the community were tracked and followed up on in a timely manner. This focus on ICE by our enforcement community led to an unprecedented raid on 37 ICE houses and 49 vehicles island wide, making 123 arrests and seizing over 11.2 lbs. of ICE, over a million dollars worth of crystal methamphetamines. All of this in the first six months of 2003 and before the ICE Task Force was actually up and running.

In July of 2003, Hawaii Island was the first community to engage in an Island wide sign waving event protesting ICE and its impact upon our children and our families. Over 20 locations were involved with an estimated 1,500 people participating. Kohala, Waikoloa, Kona, South Kona, Milolii, HOVE, Naalehu, Pahala, Volcano, Mt. View, Keaau, Pahoa, Lower Puna, Hilo, Papaikou, Pepeekeo, Laupahoehoe, Honoka'a, Waimea – everybody was involved. Some might say that it was only standing on the side of the road and waving, that it was merely a show and nothing more. However, everyone who was involved talked about the power of caring, of meeting new people who were there for different reasons but with one purpose, to rid Hawaii Island of crystal methamphetamine.

In August of 2003, the Hawaii Island Meth Summit II was held. It was only the second site in the USA to have a follow up summit. This summit involved over 300 participants who sat with their own sector – so enforcement, treatment, prevention, community, non-profits, education, faith, etc… all sat together and came up with an action plan that we will hopefully fulfill in the next year. We were fortunate to hear US Senator Inouye and US Attorney Ed Kubo commit to Hawaii Island's success in their Meth Initiative. Congressman Case was also present to share his commitment to this effort. Police Chief Lawrence Mahuna and Mayor Harry Kim continued their commitment to see this through. Dr. Kevin Kunz inspired everyone with his informational and inspirational luncheon address. Finally, the children of Kanu O Ka Aina charter school closed the summit with a chicken skin chant that left everyone realizing why it is we do what we do – because our children deserve no less.

We have come far in two short years, but we have far to go. Our children are still sent off Island, away from family and friends, for treatment. We still are not able to offer treatment to everyone who needs it. Child Protective Services is still seeing abused and neglected children on our Island. Our criminal justice system is still seeing domestic violence related to ICE. Our youth are still without positive drug-free activities. But, because we care, we will make the difference.

III. Goals & Objectives

There are a couple of critical elements that we have to achieve if we are going to be successful in this effort. The following goals and objectives are necessary for Hawaii Island to realize its mission of having a healthy and safe Island for our children and our families.

- Federal, State, and County Government Commitment.
- Community Support – Every single community on Island active and participating in activities to strengthen our children and our families.
- Increase Support for Federal Law Enforcement – Increase DEA, ATF, FBI, HIDTA support for Hawaii Island.
- Increase State Enforcement Support – Increase National Guard Counter-Drug Personnel, Increase Narcotics Enforcement in the Department of Public Safety, Increase Attorney General's commitment to Hawaii Island.
- Increase Local Law Enforcement Capabilities – Dedicate personnel strictly for ICE enforcement, create system for coordinated communication between residents and HPD, improve lab testing capacity.
- Add dedicated senior prosecutors who are assigned strictly to drug cases in both East and West Hawaii.
- Create a Drug Court in both East Hawaii and West Hawaii for both Adults and Juveniles.
- Establish an Adolescent Treatment Program on Island.
- Create more Treatment alternatives for Men, Women, and Children in every community on the Island.
- Establish more School-based Treatment Programs.
- Strengthen Domestic Violence, Native Hawaiian Healing, Mentoring, and Youth Programs – Improve Our Infrastructure Island wide.
- Establish a Community Fund for community-based initiatives.
- Improve our Transportation Infrastructure.
- Create a Healthy, Diversified, and Vibrant Economy.

IV. HAWAII ISLAND METH FUNDING – '02, '03, '04

- Federal Funds in '02
- Priority Items = Drug Lab & Youth Prevention Activities
- SAMHSA - $1.25 Million + 250,000 = $1.5 M for Youth
- Dept. of Labor / Rural D. Fund = $350,000 Drug Lab
- ICE Legislation – Adolescent Residential Treatment + Community Anti-Drug Fund ($300,000 + $100,000) – State of Hawaii
- ICE Task Force – HPD – Hawaii County
- ICE Website – HealingOurIsland.Com – Fairmont Resorts
- Meth Summit I & II – DEA, NCPC, HCF, & PHN
- '03 Appropriation of $4 Million Dollars– D.O.J. to C.O.P.S. to H.C.F. for Hawaii Island Meth Initiative – Enforcement, Treatment, & Prevention.
- SAMHSA - $900,000 – Adolescent Residential Program.
- Dr. Earl Bakken - $900,000 ICE Prevention & Education.
- Communities That Care – State Incentive Grant, North Hawaii $300,000+.
- OJJDP Grant – Five Mountains Hawaii - $100,000 for Community Response to ICE (CRI) groups in North Hawaii.
- Island wide Transportation System upgrade - $3 Million passed Senate appropriations committee for '04.
- Follow Up Funding for Hawaii Island Meth Initiative – Senate appropriations committee passed $4.6 million for '04.
- Legislative Session 2004 – Coordinate priorities with communities, work with Island delegation and Chairman Takamine at House Finance and Vice-Chairman Kokubun at Senate Ways and Means Committees.
- Establish a Hawaii Island Meth Initiative Advisory Task Force to evaluate and monitor effort and assist in coordinating Hawaii Island initiatives.

V. HAWAII ISLAND METH - 25 SIMPLE STEPS

1. Partner with US Senator Daniel K. Inouye's Office

2. Utilize Federal Monies and Federal Agencies For Initial Planning

3. Access Immediate Federal Dollars For Hawaii Island

4. Priorities = Drug Lab & Youth Programs and Activities

5. Mobilize Communities / Increase Community Awareness & Education

6. Commit Federal, State, and County Officials & Agencies To Effort

7. Incremental Implementation Of Priority Items:

    - Federal Resources = '02, '03, '04, '05,...
    - State Resources = '03,'04,'05,...
    - County Resources = '03, '04, '05,...
    - Private Trusts/Foundations – Private $$$ Support
    - Businesses / Local Community – Manpower, Time, Resources

8. Establish Priorities Thru Community Planning & Community Meetings

9. Implement Priorities through Incremental Funding

10. Utilize Community Groups For Sustainability – Maintain Effort

11. Focus On Youth – Demand Reduction – Alternative Activities – Model Programs - Prevention & Education Is the Key!

12. Establishment of An Adolescent Treatment / Rehabilitation Facility

13. Increased Federal Law Enforcement

14. Create New Partnerships (Fed + State + County + Community)

15. Mentoring Program – County / Island wide – Positive Role Models

16. Increased Recreational Activities – Gyms, Pools, Parks, Transportation

17. Increase Social Infrastructure – Programs & Services Focused on ICE

18. Increase Public Information & Resource Directory (211, Website, TV)

19. Utilize Faith Based Organizations, Cultural Organizations, Service Organizations, Business and Educational Partnerships

20. Mobilize Youth Groups, Youth Ministries, Youth Sports Organizations

21. Reverse Cultural Acceptance Of Drugs & Abuse – ICE is NOT cool!

22. Create A Healthy, Positive, Safe Environment For Families

23. Reduce Negativity-Fear, Increase Opportunity-Hope

24. Ensure Continued Resource Commitment – Partner w/ Providers

25. No Simple Answers, No Easy Solutions, No False or Empty Promises

BUT We Can Reduce The Threat Of ICE To Our Community

IF Everyone Works Together To Be Part Of The Solution.

V. HAWAII ISLAND METH DATA & STATISTICS

- HPD reports that arrests for ICE distribution increased 431% from '97-00
- Hawaii County CPS reports that 85-90% of caseload is ICE/Drug related.
- The Big Island Substance Abuse Council (BISAC) reported that Hawaii County had a 50% increase in people meeting the criteria for needing treatment for methamphetamine use (from 690 to 1200).
- Hawaii County had twice the statewide average of 6th graders who reported using ICE (1.0% v. 4%).
- Hawaii County had one third more 8th graders using ICE than the rest of the State (3.0% v. 2.3%).
- Hawaii County had one third more 10th graders using ICE that the rest of the State (6.0% v. 4.5%).
- 22% of Hawaii County high school seniors indicated that ICE was "fairly easy to get".
- In every grade, Hawaii County exceeded the rest of the State in treatment needs for adolescents – 6th (3.5% v. 1.4%), 8th (13.8% v. 7.6%), 10th (27.0% v. 18.4%), and 12th (40.5% v. 27.0%)

VI. HAWAII ISLAND METH CHALLENGES

- Maintaining community momentum and community involvement.
- Maintaining Federal, State, and County funding commitments.
- Increasing Funding For Treatment Programs for Island Residents.
- Establishing a Program for Inmates returning to the community.
- Establishing Multiple Treatment Programs and Options.
- Maintaining Legislative funding and support.
- Establishing Evaluation component for Hawaii Island Meth Initiative.
- Expanding Hawaii Island Transportation System.
- Expanding Employment Opportunities on Hawaii Island.
- Establishing a Mentorship Program for Island Youth.
- Expanding Domestic Violence services for children and families.
- Improving Media and Information dissemination on ICE related issues.
- Expanding Cultural Healing Practices for ICE Treatment (Ho'oponopono).
- Expanding Faith Based programs for ICE impacted families.
- Supporting Non-Profits Organizations who deal with the impact of ICE.
- Increasing Recreational Activities for Youth.
- Expanding Community based initiatives.
- Building Community Capacity to address ICE related problems.
- Minimize Political, Ideological, Geographical and Personal differences.
- Ensure that Infrastructure Improvements occur every year.
- Maintain Network of Providers Committed to Addressing ICE.
- **Support Our Island's Children, Families, and Communities.**

HAWAII DRUG CONTROL STRATEGY: A NEW BEGINNING

(Working Document)

The aim of the *Hawaii Drug Control Strategy: A New Beginning* is to cultivate community capacity and improve the quality of life in the State of Hawaii by reducing illicit drug use and underage drinking. The Strategy provides a prospectus for developing and enhancing prevention, treatment, and drug interdiction programs. This document serves as a framework for the State of Hawaii and will assist policymakers, community leaders, and residents in designing and implementing community-focused, anti-substance abuse approaches based on exemplary, research-based 'best-practices' and evidence-based outcomes.

MISSION

Our mission is to reduce harm to our community by responding to the unique prevention, treatment, criminal justice, and law enforcement needs associated with drug distribution, illicit drug use and underage drinking. Drawing upon government-community partnerships, the Strategy will reduce the factors that put residents at risk for substance abuse and increase protective factors to safeguard the people of Hawaii from the negative consequences associated with illicit drug use and underage drinking.

GOAL

The primary goal of the Hawaii Drug Control Strategy corresponds with the National Drug Control Policy to provide a comprehensive and integrated approach that will:

- stop illicit drug use and underage drinking before they start
- treat drug and alcohol abusers
- intervene in the distribution of illicit drugs

BENCHMARKS

The Hawaii Drug Control Strategy seeks to reduce use of illegal drugs by 10% over three years. This benchmark applies to illicit drug use among youth (ages 12 – 17) and adults. Concurrently, the Strategy proposes a reduction in offender recidivism (for adults) by 10%.

PRIORITIES

Prevention will be the Administration's first line of defense against illegal drug use and underage drinking. This priority seeks to increase prevention services that teach individuals how to avoid illegal drugs while informing them about the ensuing damage to their health and future. Research clearly documents that parental use and/or parental attitudes toward the use of alcohol, tobacco, and illicit drugs correlate with adolescent substance use. Special emphasis will be placed on improving parenting skills and family relationships to reduce adolescent substance abuse.

In addition, community mobilization is central to any prevention initiative. Success would not be possible without strengthening community capacity through interagency collaboration, coalition building and networking. Such private and public efforts, bound by unity of purpose, should demonstrate greater integration and coordination and will be supported through training and technical assistance.

The second priority focuses on providing treatment to individuals otherwise unable to obtain services. Greater access to treatment will be made available to initiate the process of recovery.

Thirdly, new law enforcement policies and legislation will be proposed to reduce offender recidivism, prohibit the sales of pre-cursor chemicals, and treat methamphetamine law violators.

ACHIEVING OUR GOAL

The following section provides an overview of the approaches that will be implemented to achieve the State's goal.

A. Stop Illicit Drug Use and Underage Drinking Before They Start: Prevention and Community Mobilization

Effective drug prevention necessarily involves comprehensive community-based efforts. The two aspects of prevention and education and community mobilization are intertwined and yet distinct.

Community mobilization will enhance the ability of the community to more effectively provide services and includes community and volunteer training, systematic planning, advocacy, multi-agency coordination and collaboration, assessing services and funding, and community team building. The starting point will be the Hawaii Drug Control Strategy Summit, which will utilize a community-based process to foster local decision-making through partnerships. Target areas for the Summit will highlight model drug abuse legislation, administrative policy initiatives, funding issues, and recommendations to improve government-community partnerships.

The prevention and education component will concentrate on information dissemination and the provision of educational services and alternatives to illicit drug use and underage drinking. Information dissemination will furnish awareness and knowledge on the nature and extent of substance use, abuse, and addiction, as well as the devastating effects of drugs on individuals, families, and communities. Secondly, the strategy intends to expand educational services and alternative activities that increase critical life and social skills.

Key features of this approach are summarized below.

? ***Hawaii Drug Control Strategy Summit***
The Hawaii Drug Control Strategy Summit will:

- Convene a group of key stakeholders consisting of local and State authorities to implement a Drug Control Strategy for 2003-2006.
- Provide information from local and statewide experts about the scope of illicit drug use, drug user profiles, risk and protective factors, types of treatment modalities, and model community crime prevention strategies.
- Assist groups in forming and sustaining effective community and anti-drug coalitions to combat the use of illegal drugs and underage drinking.

? ***Further Community Mobilization Steps***
In addition, Community Mobilization will:

- Encourage coalitions to work towards reducing substance abuse among youth and strengthen collaboration among organizations and agencies in both private and public sectors.
- Serve as the catalyst for increased citizen participation in strategic planning.
- Advocate the design and implementation of an annual report card on illicit drug use to assess the efforts of the Strategy by measuring changes in illicit drug use indicators, including arrests, seizures, price, purity, treatment admissions, and overdose deaths.
- Support culturally relevant prevention services on Hawaiian Homelands.

? ***Information Dissemination***
Information Dissemination will focus on the following:

- Develop and implement a comprehensive Anti-Drug Media Campaign that will use paid advertising and grassroots public outreach to educate Hawaii's families, parents, and youth about illicit drug use and underage drinking and their consequences.
- Implement targeted, high impact media messages to reduce illicit drug use and underage drinking by changing attitudes towards drugs and alcohol.
- Test anti-drug television marketing for effectiveness prior to airing; modify the media campaign to focus primarily on the prevention of underage drinking and marijuana and crystal methamphetamine use, and develop a hard-hitting, effective ad style.

- Use student and teen publications and public service announcements, including magazines, radio spots, and television commercials to highlight anti-drug advertisements.
- Distribute anti-methamphetamine brochures or flyers to residents and community groups.
- Coordinate with award-winning local filmmaker Edgy Lee and producer Jeffery Mueller on the debut of their new film, which reveals the severity of the crystal methamphetamine or "ice" epidemic in Hawaii.
- Distribute prevention materials including videotapes and workbooks to targeted schools in 'high-risk' neighborhoods.
- Synthesize data from all available sources to better document local drug problems.
- Investigate new strategies to evaluate program effectiveness in order to better distribute federal and state funds for prevention, treatment, and drug interdiction programs, and adhere to the best and most effective practices in service structure and delivery.

? ***Educational Services and Alternatives***

Educational Services and Alternatives will focus on the following:

- Expand and enhance anti-drug curriculum in local schools.
- Enhance mentorship programs and other services that are gender specific, culturally relevant, and developmentally appropriate.
- Increase alternative activities for youth with an emphasis on recreation, arts, music, etc.
- Provide drug testing, assessment, referral, and interventions to targeted schools.
- Train parents to reduce drug abuse and form parent drug prevention groups.
- Design and implement strategies that will enhance family cohesion by encouraging family involvement in prevention services.
- Support the development and implementation of a charter school designed specifically for at-risk youth.
- Support research collaborations with public health organizations and the University of Hawaii to embark on new initiatives to advance treatment and prevention.

B. Treat Hawaii's Drug and Alcohol Abusers

The overall goal of treatment is to reduce or eliminate the use of alcohol and/or other drugs as a contributing factor to physical, psychological, and social dysfunction and to arrest, retard, or reverse progress of associated problems. (Institute of Medicine, *Broadening the Base of Treatment for Alcohol Problems,* 1990)

The treatment approach will:

- Enhance treatment options for methamphetamine users and expand current residential and outpatient treatment capacity for adolescents.

- Work closely with the Hawaii State Judiciary and the Department of Public Safety in designing and implementing a model for the treatment and supervision of addicted offenders.
- Enhance existing drug court programs to include specific services for drug and alcohol abusers with co-existing disorders.
- Partner with local treatment providers to assist with training on a variety of topics, including the dynamics of methamphetamine use, common side effects, and methods for recovery and how they may differ depending on a person's drug of choice.
- Initiate gender-specific, developmentally sensitive, and criminal justice appropriate substance abuse treatment for youthful offenders at the Hawaii Youth Correctional Facility and the Detention Center.
- Expand and enhance adult and adolescent mental health services for drug and alcohol abusers with co-existing disorders.
- Complete a master plan for the development of a Secure Treatment Facility and re-entry services for addicted sentenced felons.
- Develop specific program models for treating methamphetamine abusers.
- Design evaluation protocols to measure the effectiveness of treatment.

C. Disrupt the Distribution of Illicit Drugs: Law Enforcement

Law enforcement serves as the gatekeeper of the criminal justice processes of arrest, prosecution, incarceration, and court-mandated conditions of probation and parole, used to distinguish users and addicts from dealers and producers. Law enforcement and criminal justice must be linked to community-wide drug prevention efforts, targeting youths and families in rural as well as urban communities. They must be attentive to issues of access to treatment (both community-based and corrections-based), and they must provide the measured criminal justice sanctions that will help drug abusers seek treatment and achieve successful outcomes. (Adapted from *Methamphetamine Interagency Task Force—Final Report: Federal Advisory Committee*, 2000)

The Law Enforcement approach will include the following:

- Evaluate local sales practices and current legislation regarding pre-cursor chemicals.
- Enact legislation or regulations prohibiting the sale of pre-cursor chemicals, including ephedrine and pseudoephedrine.
- Garner support and resources for various law enforcement agencies.
- Work closely with non-law enforcement agencies such as the Department of Health, local hospitals, child and family services, hotel associations, and others who can make a significant impact on identifying, reporting, and addressing methamphetamine problems.
- Enlist the community in the fight against illicit drug use and underage drinking.
- Enhance citizen patrols and Neighborhood Watch programs.
- Draft and implement clear and definitive legislation that mandates decisive consequences for drug offenders and severe consequences for drug dealers.

CONCLUSION

A clear focus is imperative to enable decisions that can be made without compromising the integrity of the effort and that will result in a sound plan that is consistent in form and spirit. This working document is just the first step. Its principles will lay the groundwork to develop a comprehensive and integrated approach to reduce substance abuse and underage drinking throughout the State of Hawaii.

The *Hawaii Drug Control Strategy: A New Beginning* incorporates the most recent research on substance abuse prevention, treatment, and interdiction and outlines a plan of action. Ultimately, the success of the Strategy depends on Hawaii's residents working with government officials and human service agencies to identify and respond to the needs of their communities.

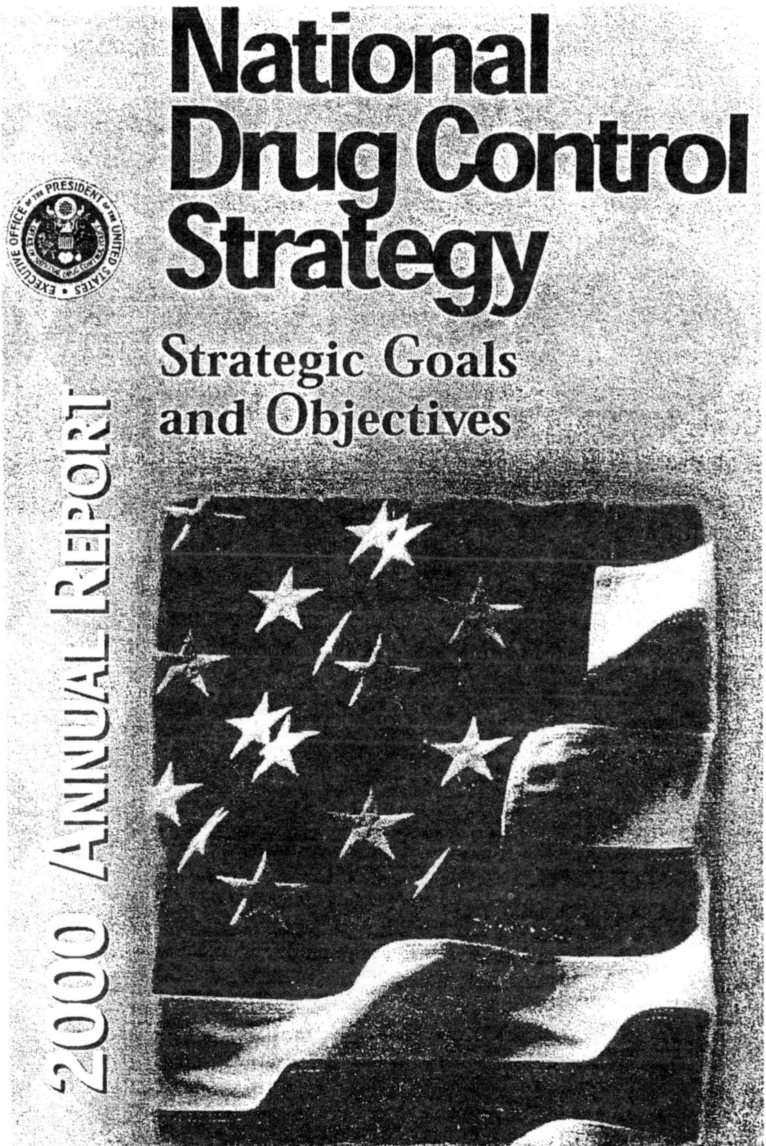
National
Drug Control
Strategy
Strategic Goals
and Objectives
2000 Annual Report

Strategic Goals and Objectives

Goal 1: Educate and enable America's youth to reject illegal drugs as well as alcohol and tobacco.

Objective 1: Educate parents and other care givers, teachers, coaches, clergy, health professionals, and business and community leaders to help youth reject illegal drugs and underage alcohol and tobacco use.

Objective 2: Pursue a vigorous advertising and public communications program dealing with the dangers of illegal drugs, alcohol, and tobacco use by youth.

Objective 3: Promote zero tolerance policies for youth regarding the use of illegal drugs, alcohol, and tobacco within the family, school, workplace, and community.

Objective 4: Provide students in grades K–12 with alcohol, tobacco, and drug prevention programs and policies that are research based.

Objective 5: Support parents and adult mentors in encouraging youth to engage in positive, healthy lifestyles and modeling behavior to be emulated by young people.

Objective 6: Encourage and assist the development of community coalitions and programs in preventing drug abuse and underage alcohol and tobacco use.

Objective 7: Create partnerships with the media, entertainment industry, and professional sports organizations to avoid the glamorization, condoning, or normalization of illegal drugs and the use of alcohol and tobacco by youth.

Objective 8: Develop and implement a set of research-based principles upon which prevention programming can be based.

Objective 9: Support and highlight research, including the development of scientific information, to inform drug, alcohol, and tobacco prevention programs targeting young Americans.

Goal 2: Increase the safety of America's citizens by substantially reducing drug-related crime and violence.

Objective 1: Strengthen law enforcement—including federal, state, and local drug task forces—to combat drug-related violence, disrupt criminal organizations, and arrest and prosecute the leaders of illegal drug syndicates.

Objective 2: Improve the ability of High Intensity Drug Trafficking Areas (HIDTAs) to counter drug trafficking.

Objective 3: Help law enforcement to disrupt money laundering and seize and forfeit criminal assets.

Objective 4: Break the cycle of drug abuse and crime.

Objective 5: Support and highlight research, including the development of scientific information and data, to inform law enforcement, prosecution, incarceration, and treatment of offenders involved with illegal drugs.

National Drug Control Strategy

Goal 3: Reduce health and social costs to the public of illegal drug use.

Objective 1: Support and promote effective, efficient, and accessible drug treatment, ensuring the development of a system that is responsive to emerging trends in drug abuse.

Objective 2: Reduce drug-related health problems, with an emphasis on infectious diseases.

Objective 3: Promote national adoption of drug free workplace programs that emphasize a comprehensive program that includes: drug testing, education, prevention, and intervention.

Objective 4: Support and promote the education, training, and credentialing of professionals who work with substance abusers.

Objective 5: Support research into the development of medications and related protocols to prevent or reduce drug dependence and abuse.

Objective 6: Support and highlight research and technology, including the acquisition and analysis of scientific data, to reduce the health and social costs of illegal drug use.

Objective 7: Support and disseminate scientific research and data on the consequences of legalizing drugs.

Goal 4: Shield America's air, land, and sea frontiers from the drug threat.

Objective 1: Conduct flexible operations to detect, disrupt, deter, and seize illegal drugs in transit to the United States and at U.S. borders.

Objective 2: Improve the coordination and effectiveness of U.S. drug law enforcement programs with particular emphasis on the Southwest Border, Puerto Rico, and the U.S. Virgin Islands.

Objective 3: Improve bilateral and regional cooperation with Mexico as well as other cocaine and heroin transit zone countries in order to reduce the flow of illegal drugs into the United States.

Objective 4: Support and highlight research and technology—including the development of scientific information and data—to detect, disrupt, deter, and seize illegal drugs in transit to the United States and at U.S. borders.

Goal 5: Break foreign and domestic drug sources of supply.

Objective 1: Produce a net reduction in the worldwide cultivation of coca, opium, and marijuana and in the production of other illegal drugs, especially methamphetamine.

Objective 2: Disrupt and dismantle major international drug trafficking organizations and arrest, prosecute, and incarcerate their leaders.

Objective 3: Support and complement source country drug control efforts and strengthen source country political will and drug control capabilities.

Objective 4: Develop and support bilateral, regional, and multilateral initiatives and mobilize international organizational efforts against all aspects of illegal drug production, trafficking, and abuse.

Objective 5: Promote international policies and laws that deter money laundering and facilitate anti-money laundering investigations as well as seizure and forfeiture of associated assets.

Objective 6: Support and highlight research and technology, including the development of scientific data, to reduce the worldwide supply of illegal drugs.

THE NATIONAL DRUG CONTROL STRATEGY

TODAY'S ACTION

Today, ONDCP Director John Walters will unveil the President's new National Drug Control Strategy for 2003 focusing on three core priorities: stopping drug use before it starts, healing America's drug users and disrupting the market.

- The 2003 strategy reports progress toward meeting the President's goals of reducing drug use by 10 percent over two years, and 25 percent over five years, highlighted by reductions in drug use among young people for the first time in nearly a decade.
- The 2003 strategy also highlights a new treatment initiative funded with $600 million over three years to help addicted Americans find needed treatment and support services from the most effective programs, including faith-based and community-based organizations.

Key Points on the National Drug Control Strategy

The strategy proposes a fiscal year 2004 budget of $11.7 billion for drug control serving three core priorities:

- ☑ Stopping drug use before it starts
- ☑ Healing America's drug users
- ☑ Disrupting the market

☑ **Stopping Drug Use Before It Starts:** Continuing the initial reductions in drug use by young people will require action by all Americans through education and community involvement. In homes, schools, places of worship, the workplace, and civic and social organizations, Americans must set standards that reaffirm the values of responsibility and good citizenship while dismissing the image that drug use is consistent with individual freedom. America's children must learn from an early age that avoiding drug use is an expectation and lifelong responsibility.

- The strategy ties national leadership with community-level action to help recreate the formula that has helped America succeed against drugs in the past. The President's budget backs up this goal with a $10 million increase in funding for the expanded Drug-Free Communities Support Program, along with providing $5 million for a new Parents Drug Corps.
- In fiscal year, 2004, the strategy proposes that tools such as student drug testing be available in communities where parents and educators deem them appropriate, and funds them with $8 million.

☑ **Healing America's Drug Users:** Despite substantial drug prevention efforts, some 16 million Americans still use drugs on a monthly basis, and roughly six million meet the clinical criteria for needing drug treatment. Yet the overwhelming majority of users in need of drug treatment fail to recognize their need. The second core priority of the strategy emphasizes the crucial need for family, friends, and former addicts to intercede with and support those fighting to overcome substance abuse. Drug users also need the support of institutions and the people who run them—employers, law enforcement agencies, faith-based and community-based organizations, and health care providers, among others—to help them recognize their drug addiction and to seek treatment.

- Overall, for 2004, the Administration proposes $3.6 billion for drug treatment, an increase of 8.2 percent over 2003.
- The 2004 request includes new funding of $200 million ($600 million over three years) for a new treatment initiative to provide drug treatment to individuals otherwise unable to obtain access to services. People in need of treatment, no matter where they are—emergency rooms, health clinics, the criminal justice system, schools—will receive an evidence-based assessment of their treatment need and will be issued vouchers to obtain help at effective treatment organizations, including faith-based and community-based organizations.

FOR DETAILED DATA TABLES RELATED TO THE NATIONAL DRUG CONTROL STRATEGY, PLEASE VISIT WWW.WHITEHOUSEDRUGPOLICY.GOV

☑ **Disrupting the Market:** The third priority of the strategy seeks to capitalize on the engagement of producer and transit countries like Colombia and Mexico in order to address the drug trade as a business—one that faces numerous and often overlooked obstacles that may be used as pressure points. The drug trade is not an unstoppable force of nature but rather a profit-making enterprise where costs and rewards exist in an equilibrium that can be disrupted. Every action that makes the drug trade more costly and less profitable is a step toward "breaking" the market. Drug traffickers are in business to make money. We intend to deny them that revenue.

- To help secure America's borders, the President's budget includes $2.1 billion for drug interdiction, an increase of 7.3 percent from 2003. Internationally, the Administration will continue to target the supply of illegal drugs in the source countries.
- The Administration is requesting $731 million in dedicated funds in 2004 for the Andean Counterdrug Initiative to be applied in Bolivia, Brazil, Colombia, Ecuador, Panama, Peru, and Venezuela.
- To ensure unity of effort, the strategy advocates the use of a single list (the Consolidated Priority Organization Targeting list) identifying high-level targets among the various agencies involved in domestic drug law enforcement.

☑ **Progress Toward The President's Two- and Five-Year Goals:** Only the first year of the two-year goal period has elapsed, yet already the goal of reducing current drug use by 10 percent among 8th, 10th, and 12th graders, as measured by the *Monitoring the Future* survey, is well on the way to being met (with reductions of 11.1, 8.4, and 1.2 percent respectively). Adjustments to the measuring baseline for the goals have been prompted by discontinuities in the National Household Survey on Drug Abuse (NHSDA). As a result, the goal of reducing drug use among adults will still be measured by the NHSDA, but the baseline has been reset to the 2002 survey, which is not released until mid-year 2003.

FOR DETAILED DATA TABLES RELATED TO THE NATIONAL DRUG CONTROL STRATEGY, PLEASE VISIT WWW.WHITEHOUSEDRUGPOLICY.GOV

National Drug Control Budget Summary

Drug Control Funding: Agency Summary

FY 2002–FY 2004 (Budget Authority in Millions)

	FY 2002 Final	FY 2003 Request	FY 2004 Request
Department of Defense [1]	$852.6	$871.9	$817.4
Department of Education	669.3	634.3	584.3
Dept. of Health & Human Services			
National Institute on Drug Abuse	885.2	960.0	995.6
Substance Abuse and Mental Health Services Administration	2,304.4	2,372.6	2,575.3
Total, HHS	3,189.6	3,332.6	3,570.9
Department of Homeland Security			
Border and Transportation Security [2]	1,183.6	1,271.8	1,372.9
U.S. Coast Guard	609.7	596.1	669.1
Total, DHS	1,793.3	1,867.9	2,041.9
Department of Justice			
Bureau of Prisons	39.4	43.5	45.2
Drug Enforcement Administration	1,562.5	1,659.6	1,677.3
Interagency Crime and Drug Enforcement [3]	446.5	470.3	541.8
Office of Justice Programs	893.2	286.7	301.5
Total, DOJ	2,941.5	2,460.1	2,565.8
ONDCP			
Operations	25.2	25.5	27.3
High Intensity Drug Trafficking Area Program	221.3	206.4	206.4
Counterdrug Technology Assessment Center	42.3	40.0	40.0
Other Federal Drug Control Programs	239.3	251.3	250.0
Total, ONDCP	528.1	523.1	523.6
Department of State			
Bureau of International Narcotics and Law Enforcement Affairs	871.9	877.5	876.9
Department of Veterans Affairs			
Veterans Health Administration	635.7	663.7	690.5
Other Presidential Initiatives [4]	3.0	8.0	8.0
Total, Federal Drug Budget	$11,485.0	$11,239.0	$11,679.3

[1] The FY 2003 funding level for the Department of Defense reflects enacted appropriations.
[2] Drug Control components displayed include the U.S. Customs Service and the Border Patrol.
[3] The FY 2004 Budget proposes the merger of the Treasury ICDE account into Justice's ICDE account. This merger is reflected retrospectively.
[4] This includes $5 million for the Corporation for National Service's Parents Drug Corps beginning in FY 2003 and $3 million for SBA's Drug-Free Workplace programs for all three fiscal years.

FOR DETAILED DATA TABLES RELATED TO THE NATIONAL DRUG CONTROL STRATEGY, PLEASE VISIT WWW.WHITEHOUSEDRUGPOLICY.GOV

Federal Drug Control Spending By Function
FY 2002–FY 2004
(Budget Authority in Millions)

	FY 2002 Final	FY 2003 Request	FY 2004 Request	FY 03–FY 04 Change	
Function:					
Treatment (w/ Research)	$3,151.9	$3,282.2	$3,552.9	270.6	8.2%
Percent	27.4%	29.2%	30.4%		
Prevention (w/ Research)	2,064.5	1,954.9	1,908.1	(46.7)	(2.4%)
Percent	18.0%	17.4%	16.3%		
Domestic Law Enforcement	3,270.3	2,937.9	3,036.1	98.3	3.3%
Percent	28.5%	26.1%	26.0%		
Interdiction	1,913.7	1,960.9	2,103.3	142.3	7.3%
Percent	16.7%	17.4%	18.0%		
International	1,084.5	1,103.1	1,078.9	(24.2)	(2.2%)
Percent	9.4%	9.8%	9.2%		
Total	$11,485.0	$11,239.0	$11,679.3	$440.3	3.9%
Supply / Demand Split:					
Supply	$6,268.6	$6,001.9	$6,218.3	$216.4	3.6%
Percent	54.6%	53.4%	53.2%		
Demand	5,216.4	5,237.1	5,461.0	223.9	4.3%
Percent	45.4%	46.6%	46.8%		
Total	$11,485.0	$11,239.0	$11,679.3	$440.3	3.9%

(Detail may not add to totals due to rounding)

FOR DETAILED DATA TABLES RELATED TO THE NATIONAL DRUG CONTROL STRATEGY, PLEASE VISIT WWW.WHITEHOUSEDRUGPOLICY.GOV

HAWAII ISLAND COMMUNITY ANTI-DRUG FUND

- $100,000 provided by the State of Hawaii for Community Anti-ICE effort
- Community Trainers from the Western Community Policing Center will be on Island later this month to train communities in action planning.
- Grant will be managed by the Hawaii County Resource Center.
- Maximum grant award will be for $2,000.00.
- Evaluation criteria established using point system.
- Application is short, clear, and easy to understand.
- Process is envisioned to take no longer than 30 days to review application and announce award.
- Grants are for non-501(c)(3) community groups.
- Proposals must address drugs and substance abuse in the community.
- Projects will strengthen relationships in the community.
- Preference will be given to projects which show collaboration between two or more community groups.
- Community groups will be accountable for use of monies.
- Evaluation will be conducted to determine effectiveness of effort.
- There should be approximately 50 community anti-drug projects from this fund that will have an impact Island wide.
- This fund should take advantage of the momentum that exists in the community to initiate new projects to address the ICE problem.
- It is hoped that this project will become a success and that continued funding can be obtained to maintain the community anti-drug fund.
- Evaluation committee will probably involve Hawaii County Resource Center, University of Hawaii at Hilo, Department of Health, Office of the Prosecuting Attorney, Office of the Mayor, and Community Representatives.

The Western Community Policing Center (WCPC) is funded by a federal grant awarded to the Department of Public Safety Standards and Training (DPSST) from the COPS Office, US Department of Justice. The purpose of the WCPC is to initiate partnerships and provide resources, information, coordination, and training to law enforcement agencies and community teams in Alaska, Hawaii, Nevada, New Mexico, Oregon, and Utah - increasing their ability to reduce crime and fear of crime in the western region of the United States.

FREE TRAINING
Offered in partnership with the
MAYOR'S OFFICE, DEPARTMENT OF CIVIL DEFENSE, HAWAII COUNTY PROSECUTOR'S OFFICE AND HAWAII COUNTY RESOURCE CENTER

Developing Community-Teams

This two-day course is intended to bring community members and other agencies together to form community action teams. It provides basic information, skills and strategies, and a forum for discussion and planning. The curriculum is built around some basic components of community policing and includes modules on change management, community mobilization, problem solving, and action planning.

Instructors are a mix of police officers and citizen practitioners, who are considered community policing experts in the Western United States. All have personal experience in implementing one or more of the community education components addressed in this curriculum.

Target Audience: Participants register and attend as teams of four to ten people. Ideally, teams are a diverse mix of citizen, government, and law enforcement representatives. Other team members might represent youth, social services, planning, retirees, businesses, parks and recreation, churches, minorities, schools, code enforcement, media, etc.

Dates/Times: October 24-25, 2003
Location: Friday – Saturday, 9:00 a.m. – 5:00 p.m.
U.S. Army National Guard Armory
Kealakekua

October 27-28, 2003
Monday-Tuesday; 12:00 noon – 8:00 p.m.
Pahala Community Center
Pahala

October 30-31, 2003
Thursday-Friday; 9:00 a.m. – 5:00 p.m.
Aupuni Conference Room (old Firestone)
Hawaii County Building, Hilo

Registration: Participants must register and attend as teams. Completed application forms must arrive **at Hawaii County Resource Center Attn: Louise Winn 25 Aupuni St. Rm. 104 Hilo, HI 96720 by October 20, 2003. Or fax to 935-1205**

This training is supported by award 97-CK-WX-0031, awarded by the Office of Community Oriented Policing Services, US Dept of Justice.

Schedule Overview

DAY 1

8:00 - 9:00 Introduction

9:00 – 12:00 Facilitating Change

- This module addresses the effects of change on an individual, an organization, and a community. It discusses some specific changes and suggests strategies for dealing with those changes.
- This module contrasts practices and assumptions of traditional policing with those of community policing. It suggests that everyone in the class has a leadership responsibility, and defines leadership as it relates to facilitating community policing.

1:00 – 3:00 Team Building

- This module endorses team responsibility for transitioning to community action. It discusses group dynamics and the importance of building trust and respect among team members.
- This module discusses the importance of diversity in teams. It teaches that diversity of perception, experience, communication styles, decision making styles, etc. all contribute to sound, comprehensive solutions for community problems.

3:00 – 5:00 Building Community Partnerships

- This module addresses the benefits of building community partnerships and provides strategies for: identifying who should get involved; recruiting involvement; engaging partners; and marketing success.
- It discusses the dynamics of community meetings and some tactics for dealing with them.

DAY 2

8:00 - 10:00 Building Community Partnerships (continued)

10:00 – 5:00 Problem Solving

- This module provides a model for problem solving (SARA) and gives participants practical experience with that model.
- It provides tools and strategies for identifying patterns and to help identify the real problem. It emphasizes the importance of information gathering and analysis prior to thoroughly understand the problem before jumping into solutions.
- This module explains the use of a "partnership agreement" as a means to formalize responsibility for solving a community problem. module emphasizes the importance of looking at the long-term, big picture and discusses strategic planning and action planning processes and who should be involved.
- This module uses an action planning format to guide each team in building a personalized action plan to implement in their own community.
- It also exposes participants to some common terminology and tools of planning

Developing Community Teams

Mail or fax to: *Hawaii County Resource Ctr.* *25 Aupuni St., Hilo 96720* *Phone: (808)961-8035* *Fax: (808)935-1205*

Community name: ______________________________

Total participants on your team: ________

To help our instructors prepare, please list three issues of community concern:

____

____

____

☐ **GOVERNMENT** ☐ **LAW ENFORCEMENT** ☐ **CITIZEN** ☐ **OTHER**

Name: ____________ Title: ____________

Agency/Affiliation: ______________________________

Address: ______________________________

City, State, Zip: ______________________________

Phone: ____________ Fax: ____________

☐ **GOVERNMENT** ☐ **LAW ENFORCEMENT** ☐ **CITIZEN** ☐ **OTHER**

Name: ____________ Title: ____________

Agency/Affiliation: ______________________________

Address: ______________________________

City, State, Zip: ______________________________

Phone: ____________ Fax: ____________

HEALING OUR ISLAND COMMUNITY FUND –Draft#3 this page only

Dear Community Grant Applicant:

Hawaii County Resource Center is administering funds issued by the State Legislature as part of SB1305 as a grant in aid. It is to be used at the neighborhood and community level with a focus on drug use prevention and education, such as community event(s), renovation and beautification, public awareness, mentoring, and youth /family recreation.
Your proposal should reflect the basic goal of drug use prevention and education whether it is a one time event or an ongoing project. It is expected that your project will strengthen relationships within the community.
Preference will be given to projects which promote collaboration of two or more groups.
In preparing your proposal, please be sure it:

√ Does not request more than $2000.00
√ Leads to positive outcomes
√ Is complete, all questions answered
√ Has two signatures on the proposal form
√ Includes County Vendor Form

Make two copies of your proposal. Retain one for your records, and **send one copy to:**

Healing Our Island Community Fund
25 Aupuni St. Room 106
Hilo, HI 96720

Proposals received by the 15th of each month will be reviewed on a monthly basis and notification given within 30 days of decision. We may call you or request a site visit. Grant recipients must have a checking account and shall submit a press release to the local paper announcing the award. Within 30 days of completion of the project a report of the budget, any receipts, and the final evaluation are required. Unspent funds are to be returned at that time.

Mahalo for your commitment to your community!

HEALING OUR ISLAND COMMUNITY FUND Draft #2

Community Grants Proposal Form

Name(s)of your group(s):____

____

____

Contact person: ____________________Phone: ____________________

Address: ____________________City:____________________Zip: __________

E-Mail Address: ____

Amount Requested: $____________________ Expected Completion Date:__________

Program Area: Δ Drug Prevention Education

COMMUNITY DESCRIPTION: Describe your community, including its people and boundaries (physical, social and otherwise).

PROJECT DESCRIPTION: What will you do to meet the need for drug education and prevention in a collaborative way? Who and how many will benefit from this project? What tangible results will this project produce?

Community Grants Proposal Form - page 2

COMMUNITY GROUP DESCRIPTION: Describe your collaborative group. When, why, and how did you get started? Who are the members? (attach a list of their names) Do you have ongoing community projects? What previous projects have you completed, if any? Why do you feel you can work together successfully?

BUDGET: What is the total project cost? How will this grant money be spent? What other funding sources are available to you? **Please use following page or attach a detailed budget.**

EVALUATION: Upon completion of project, a report is required. It shall include a report of expenditures, a statement as to the difference your project made, and the results your project provided. How will you determine if your project has made a difference?

FISCAL RESPONSIBILITY: Who will oversee expenditures? The **two persons** listed below shall accept fiscal responsibility, insuring that any grant monies received will be used for the activities described herein, and that otherwise funds will be **returned** to the Healing our Island Community Fund.

1. ______________________________ Signature ______________
Name (Print or Type)
______________________________ Date ______________
Position in Group

2. ______________________________ Signature ______________
Name (Print or Type)
______________________________ Date ______________
Postion in Group

Community Grants Proposal Form – Page 3

Organization Name: ______________________________

Project costs or expenses:

Type of Cost	Amount
1. ______________________	$__________
2. ______________________	$__________
3. ______________________	$__________
4. ______________________	$__________
5. ______________________	$__________
6. ______________________	$__________

Total project cost: $__________

Healing Our Island Community Grant Proposal Evaluation

Date:____________________ Amount Requested:______________________________
Name of Group Requesting:____
Evaluator:_____________________

EVALUATION CRITERIA	POSSIBLE POINTS	SCORE
Application Information		
Name of Group and Contact Person completed	1	
Total amount of funds requested stated	1	
Expected completion date stated	1	
Program Area is defined	2	
Community Description		
Area to be served clearly defined	3	
Population demographic provided	3	
Project Description		
Clearly states the community need	4	
Collaborative effort clearly defined	4	
Populations and numbers who will benefit clearly define	3	
Clearly states expected outcomes	4	
Timeline is included and is realistic	3	
Community Group Description		
Background of the group clearly defined	3	
List of members/collaborators attached	2	
On-going or previous projects provided	2	
Ability to be successful is explained	4	
How program will be implemented explained	4	
Budget		
Detailed budget submitted	3	
Budget Total equals detailed budget	3	
How money will be spent is clearly defined	4	
Other funding sources are shown if applicable	2	

Evaluation	
Means by which project will be evaluated are clear	4
Desired outcomes appear to be measurable	4
Group appears to have capacity to be successful	4

COMMUNITY GRANT FINAL REPORT FORM

Submit this form with your final receipts and/or any unspent funds within 30 days of completion of your project.
Please answer each question and feel free to add comments of your own. We want to know how it went!

Why was this project important?______________________________

What key actions, resources and people were required?

What barriers or resistance, if any, were encountered?

What changes in the community have occurred due to this project?

What are some overall lessons learned from this project?

What does the future hold for this project?

Send to: HCRC
25 Aupuni St.
Hilo

HB1603

Report Title:
Crystal Methamphetamine Use; Appropriation

Description:
Makes an appropriation to address crystal methamphetamine use and abuse by establishing an Adolescent Substance Abuse Treatment Center on the Island of Hawaii.

HB HMS 2003-3558

03-01-27 17:13 From-HOUSE FINANCE 8085866201 T-720 P.02/11 F-361

HOUSE OF REPRESENTATIVES
TWENTY-SECOND LEGISLATURE, 2003
STATE OF HAWAII

H.B. NO. 1603

A BILL FOR AN ACT

MAKING AN APPROPRIATION TO ESTABLISH AN ADOLESCENT TREATMENT CENTER ON THE ISLAND OF HAWAII.

BE IT ENACTED BY THE LEGISLATURE OF THE STATE OF HAWAII:

SECTION 1. The legislature finds that crystal methamphetamine (ice) is the greatest health and public safety threat to communities on the island of Hawaii. In August of 2001, the Hawaii Island Methamphetamine Summit was held, one of the first four held throughout the country. United States Senator Daniel K. Inouye, Drug Enforcement Administration administrator Asa Hutchinson, National Crime Prevention Council vice president Jim Copple, and Dr. Wesley Clark, director of the Center for Substance Abuse Treatment in Washington, D.C. traveled to the island of Hawaii to address the devastating impact that ice has had on communities across the country.

The purpose of the summit was to focus attention and resources upon the problem of ice and the crisis and epidemic that it has become on the island of Hawaii. Child protective services reported that over one thousand five hundred children on the island of Hawaii have been placed under the jurisdiction of the courts, with over ninety per cent being involved in ice or drugs.

The Hawaii county police department reported that ice arrests between 1997 and 2001 have increased four hundred thirty-one per cent. Ice seizures in Hawaii county increased from almost twenty-seven ounces in 1993 to two hundred nineteen ounces in 2001. The Big Island Substance Abuse Council, the largest substance abuse treatment provider in Hawaii county, reports that ice has become the drug of choice for Big Island residents by a two-to-one margin over any other drug. In 2001-2002, forty-five per cent of those seeking treatment admitted that ice was their first drug of choice, far outpacing cocaine (seven per cent), heroin (three per cent), marijuana (twenty per cent), and alcohol (twenty-five per cent). The U.S. Attorney's Office has also recognized that Hawaii county has been hard hit by ice, reporting that Hawaii's greatest threat is ice and its devastating impact upon families, children, and the safety of the entire community.

In 2001, Hawaii county conducted a comprehensive survey and research into the problem of drugs and substance abuse by adolescents. The juvenile justice comprehensive strategic plan, conducted as a result of a federal grant from the Office of

Juvenile Justice and Drug Prevention, through the Hawaii county office of the prosecuting attorney, revealed that adolescents from Hawaii county were at the highest risk for drug use and abuse in the State of Hawaii. Data from the department of health's report, "The 2000 Hawaii Student Alcohol and Drug Abuse Study (1987-2000)," shows that a greater percentage of students in Hawaii county, in grades six, eight, ten, and twelve have used drugs and engaged in risky behavior or committed crimes more than the rest of the State. This disturbing data was an impetus for Hawaii county to seek federal assistance through the office of Senator Daniel K. Inouye.

However, federal assistance alone will not solve the crisis and epidemic currently affecting children, families, and communities. The only hope to eliminate this threat is for every level of government to do its part and for each community to actively participate in the issues affecting them. Because of the unique challenges posed by a population of approximately one hundred forty thousand spread out over four thousand twenty-eight square miles, with entirely distinct communities with distinct characteristics, the legislature finds that it is important for each community to participate in its own healing and its own initiatives. Through community effort,

03-01-27 17:13 From-HOUSE FINANCE 8085866201 T-720 P 05/11 F-361

neighborhoods must be saved from the devastation of drug use and abuse, or run the risk of losing our most precious resource, our children. The legislature further finds that Hawaii county, the county with the highest rate of substance abuse among youth, should have its own treatment facility, rather than forcing residents to send their children to Oahu or Maui for treatment.

The purpose of this Act is to make an appropriation for the establishment of an adolescent substance abuse treatment facility to address the use of crystal methamphetamine.

SECTION 2. There is appropriated out of the general revenues of the State of Hawaii the sum of $ or so much thereof as may be necessary for fiscal year 2003-2004 for the establishment of an adolescent treatment center aimed at addressing crystal methamphetamine use on the island of Hawaii.

The sum appropriated shall be expended by the department of health, alcohol and drug abuse division, for the purposes of this Act.

SECTION 3. This Act shall take effect on July 1, 2003.

INTRODUCED BY: ____________________

JAN 24 2003

HB1604

Report Title:
Crystal Methamphetamine Use; drug prevention; appropriation

Description:
Makes an appropriation to address crystal methamphetamine use and abuse on the Island of Hawaii.

HB HMS 2003-3559

HOUSE OF REPRESENTATIVES
TWENTY-SECOND LEGISLATURE, 2003
STATE OF HAWAII

H.B. NO. 1604

A BILL FOR AN ACT

MAKING AN APPROPRIATION TO PREVENT CRYSTAL METHAMPHETAMINE USE.

BE IT ENACTED BY THE LEGISLATURE OF THE STATE OF HAWAII:

SECTION 1. The legislature finds that crystal methamphetamine ("ice") is the greatest threat to a community's health and public safety on the Island of Hawaii. In August of 2001, the Hawaii Island Methamphetamine Summit was held, on the island of Hawaii. This was one of the first four held throughout the country. In attendance to address the devastating impact that "ice" has had on communities throughout the country were United States Senator Daniel K. Inouye, Drug Enforcement Administration administrator Asa Hutchinson, National Crime Prevention Council vice president Jim Copple, and Dr. Wesley Clark, director of the Center for Substance Abuse Treatment in Washington, D.C.

The purpose of the summit was to focus attention and resources upon the problem of "ice" use on the island of Hawaii, a problem which has reached epidemic proportions. Indeed, child protective services reports that over one thousand five hundred children on the island of Hawaii have been put under the jurisdiction of the courts, with over ninety per cent being ice or drug related.

The Hawaii county police department has reported that "ice" arrests between 1997 and 2001 have increased by four hundred thirty-one per cent and that "ice" seizures in Hawaii county increased from approximately twenty-seven ounces in 1998 to two hundred nineteen ounces in 2001. Moreover, a report compiled by the Big Island Substance Abuse Council, the largest substance abuse treatment provider in Hawaii county, has indicated that "ice" has become the drug of choice for Big Island residents by a two-to-one margin over any other drug. In 2001-2002, fully forty-five per cent of those seeking treatment admitted that "ice" was their first drug of choice, far outpacing cocaine (seven per cent), heroin (three per cent), marijuana (twenty per cent), and alcohol (twenty five per cent). The U.S. Attorney's Office has also recognized that Hawaii county has been hard hit by "ice," reporting that Hawaii's greatest threat is "ice" and its devastating impact upon families, children, and the community's safety.

Hawaii county in 2001 conducted a comprehensive survey and researched the problem of drug and substance abuse by adolescents. The juvenile justice comprehensive strategic plan, conducted by a federal grant from the Office of Juvenile Justice and Drug Prevention, through the Office of the Prosecuting Attorney, Hawaii county, revealed that adolescents from Hawaii county were at the highest risk for drug use and abuse among all adolescents in the State of Hawaii. Using data from the department of health's report, "The 2000 Hawaii Student Alcohol and Drug Abuse Study (1987-2000)," their research found that a greater percentage of students in grades six, eight, ten, and twelve in Hawaii county have used drugs and engaged in risky behavior or committed crimes as compared to the rest of the State. This disturbing data was an impetus for Hawaii county to seek federal assistance, through the office of Senator Daniel K. Inouye, to combat the problem of drug use and abuse among adolescents.

However, federal assistance alone will not solve the crisis and epidemic currently affecting the children, families, and communities of Hawaii county. The only hope to eliminate this threat is for every level of government to do its part, and for each community to actively participate in the issues affecting them. Because of the unique challenges posed by a population of approximately one hundred forty thousand spread out over four thousand twenty-eight square miles, composed of entirely distinct communities with distinct characteristics, the legislature finds that it is important for each community to participate in its own healing and its own initiatives. In this way, we must take back our neighborhoods from the devastation of drug use and abuse. Too often, untailored programs and services are offered to outlying or rural communities that are neither welcomed nor effective.

The purpose of this Act is to make an appropriation for more effective community based anti-drug programs to prevent the use of crystal methamphetamine.

SECTION 2. There is appropriated out of the general revenues of the State of Hawaii the sum of $250,000 or so much thereof as may be necessary for fiscal year 2003-2004 for community anti-drug efforts aimed at preventing crystal methamphetamine use on the island of Hawaii.

SECTION 3. The sum appropriated shall be expended by the department of health, alcohol drug abuse division, for the purposes of this Act.

SECTION 4. This Act shall take effect on July 1, 2003.

INTRODUCED BY: ______________________

HB HMS 2003-3559

JAN 24 2003

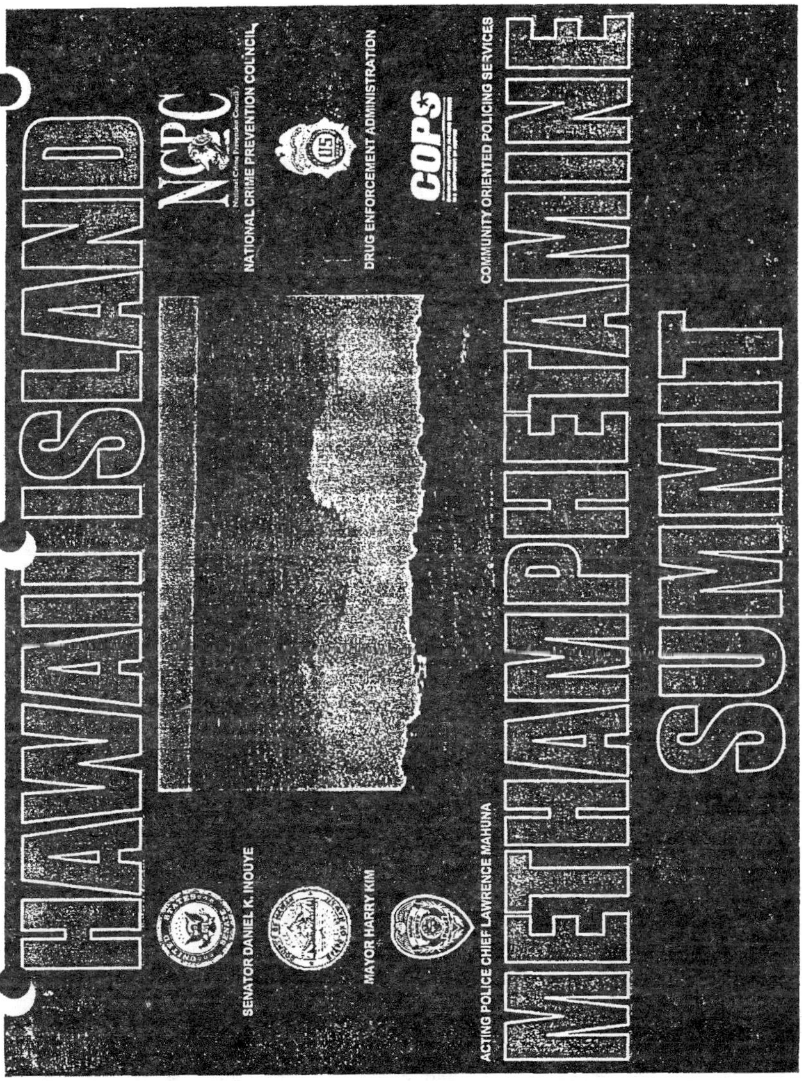
HAWAII ISLAND
NCPC
National Crime Prevention Council
NATIONAL CRIME PREVENTION COUNCIL
DRUG ENFORCEMENT ADMINISTRATION
COPS
COMMUNITY ORIENTED POLICING SERVICES
SENATOR DANIEL K. INOUYE
MAYOR HARRY KIM
ACTING POLICE CHIEF LAWRENCE MAHUNA
METHAMPHETAMINE
SUMMIT

36% of Hawaii high school students and **25%** of middle school students were offered, sold, or given an illegal drug on school property in the past year.

The Hawaii Youth Risk Behavior Survey 1999

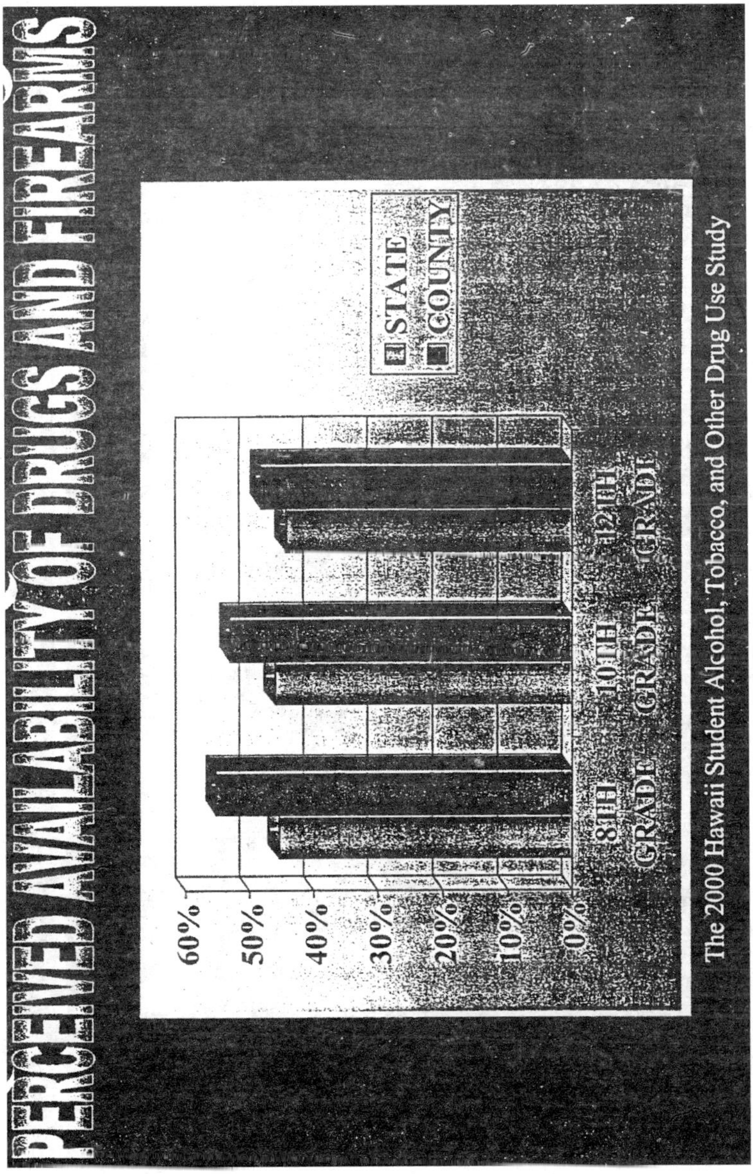
PERCEIVED AVAILABILITY OF DRUGS AND FIREARMS
60%
50%
40%
30%
20%
10%
0%
8TH GRADE
10TH GRADE
12TH GRADE
STATE
COUNTY
The 2000 Hawaii Student Alcohol, Tobacco, and Other Drug Use Study

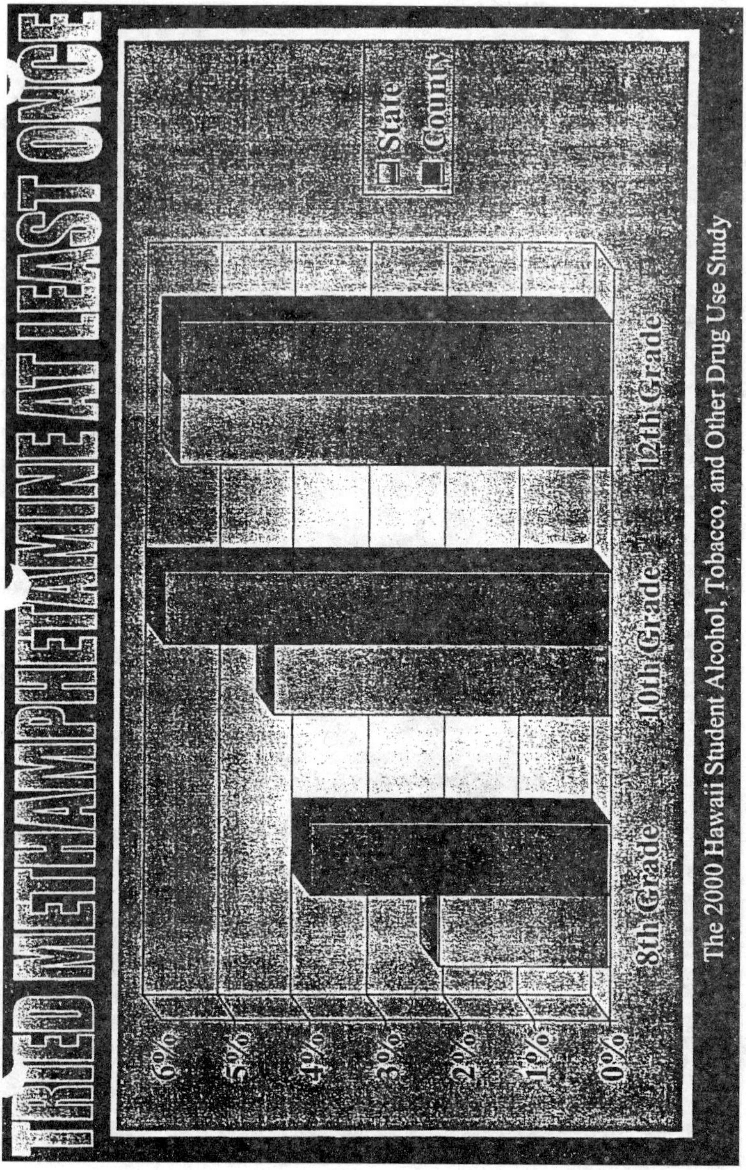
TRIED METHAMPHETAMINE AT LEAST ONCE
State
County
6%
5%
4%
3%
2%
1%
0%
8th Grade
10th Grade
12th Grade
The 2000 Hawaii Student Alcohol, Tobacco, and Other Drug Use Study

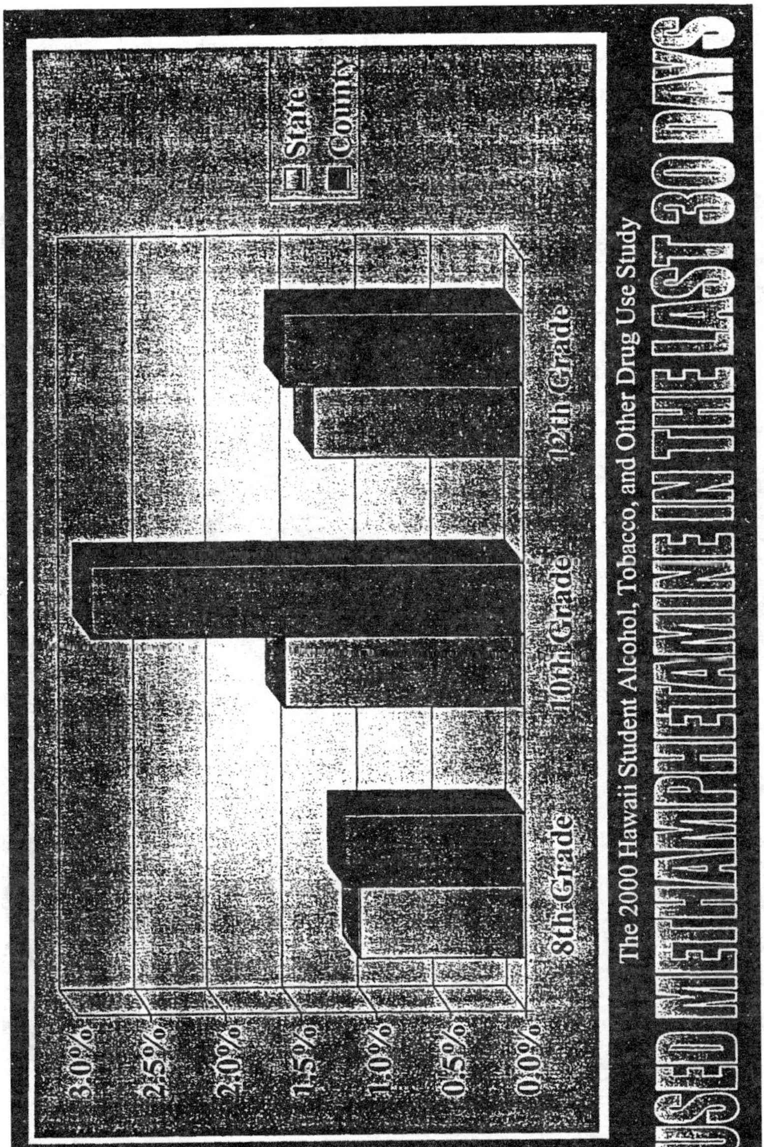
USED METHAMPHETAMINE IN THE LAST 30 DAYS
The 2000 Hawaii Student Alcohol, Tobacco, and Other Drug Use Study
3.0%
2.5%
2.0%
1.5%
1.0%
0.5%
0.0%
8th Grade
10th Grade
12th Grade
State
County

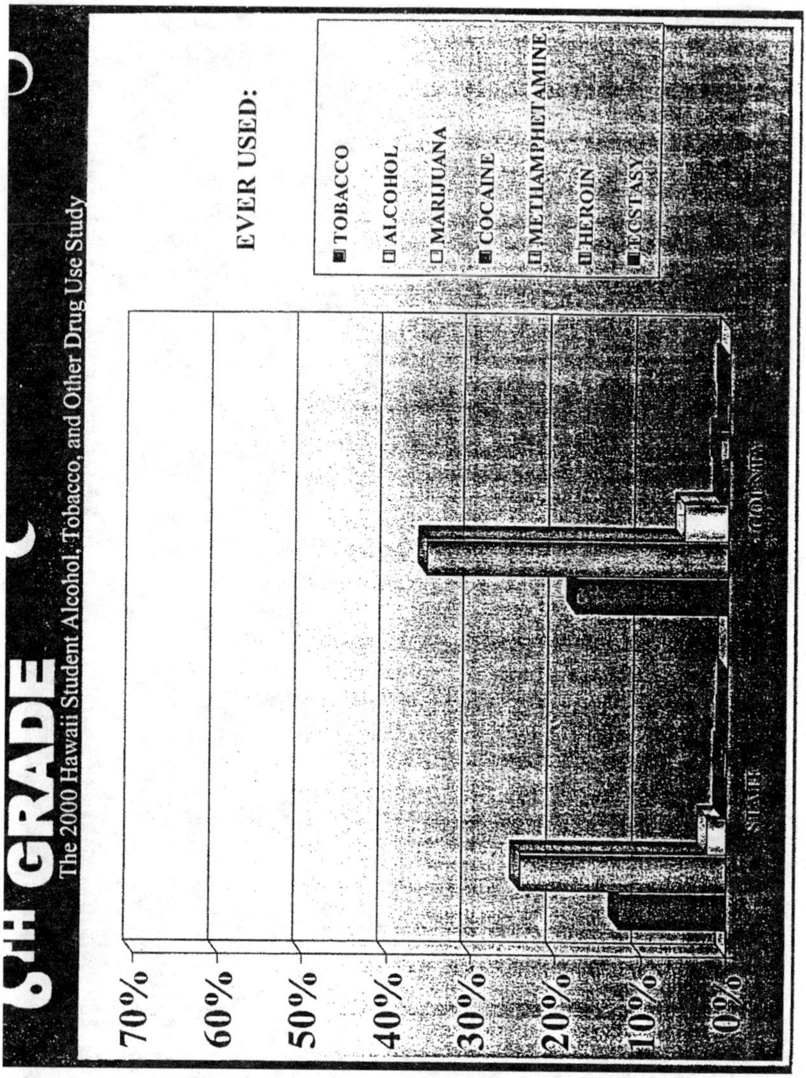
GRADE
The 2000 Hawaii Student Alcohol, Tobacco, and Other Drug Use Study
EVER USED:
TOBACCO
ALCOHOL
MARIJUANA
COCAINE
METHAMPHETAMINE
HEROIN
ECSTASY
70%
60%
50%
40%
30%
20%
10%
0%
STATE
COUNTY

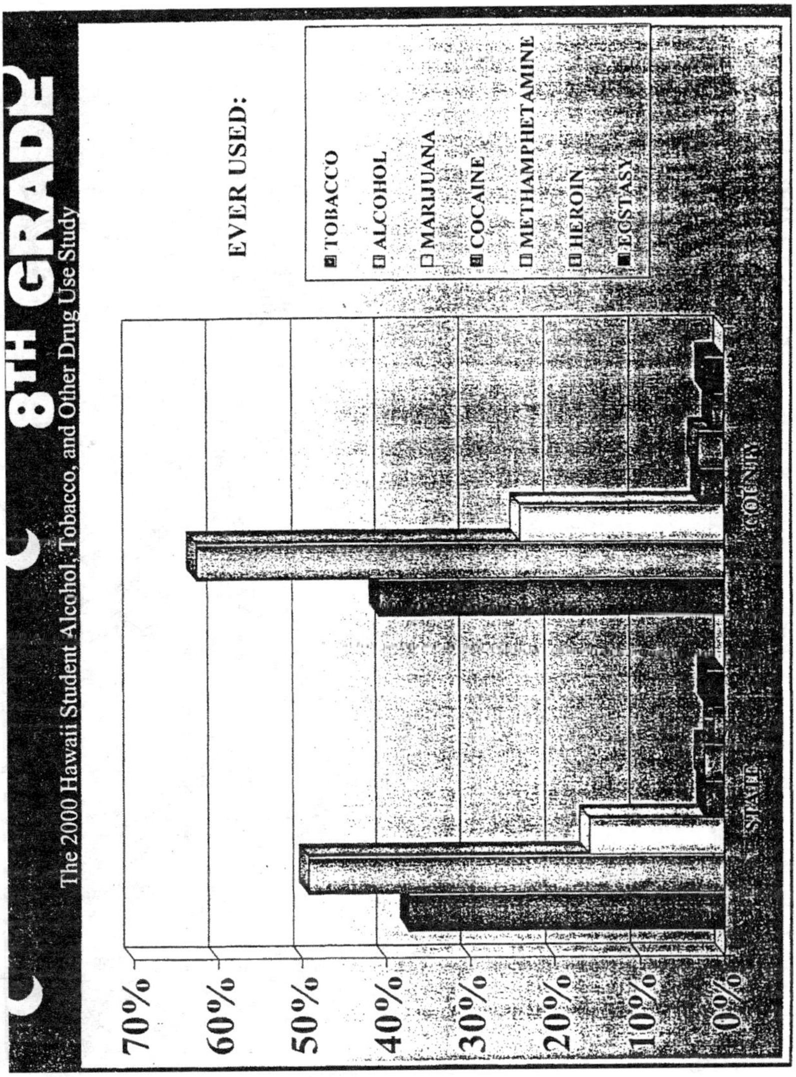
8TH GRADE
The 2000 Hawaii Student Alcohol, Tobacco, and Other Drug Use Study
EVER USED:
TOBACCO
ALCOHOL
MARIJUANA
COCAINE
METHAMPHETAMINE
HEROIN
ECSTASY
70%
60%
50%
40%
30%
20%
10%
0%
STATE
COUNTY

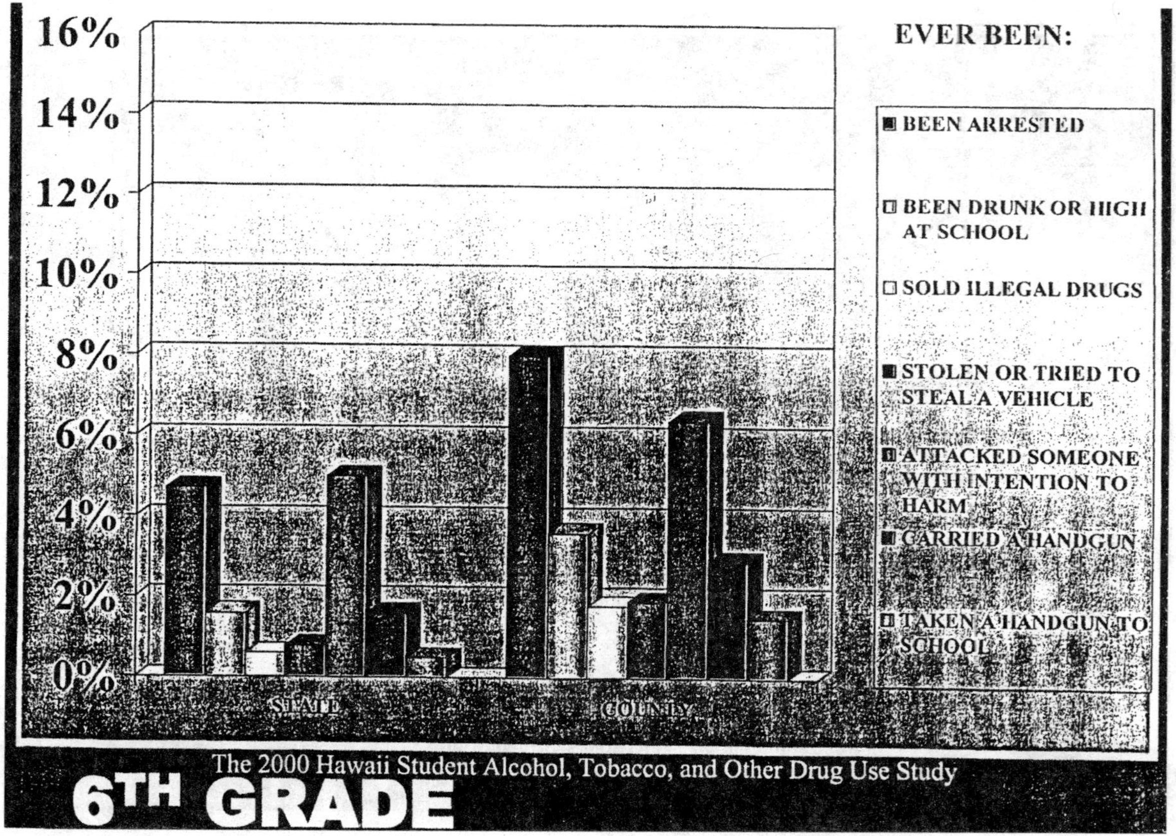
16%
14%
12%
10%
8%
6%
4%
2%
0%
STATE
COUNTY
EVER BEEN:
BEEN ARRESTED
BEEN DRUNK OR HIGH AT SCHOOL
SOLD ILLEGAL DRUGS
STOLEN OR TRIED TO STEAL A VEHICLE
ATTACKED SOMEONE WITH INTENTION TO HARM
CARRIED A HANDGUN
TAKEN A HANDGUN TO SCHOOL
The 2000 Hawaii Student Alcohol, Tobacco, and Other Drug Use Study
6TH GRADE

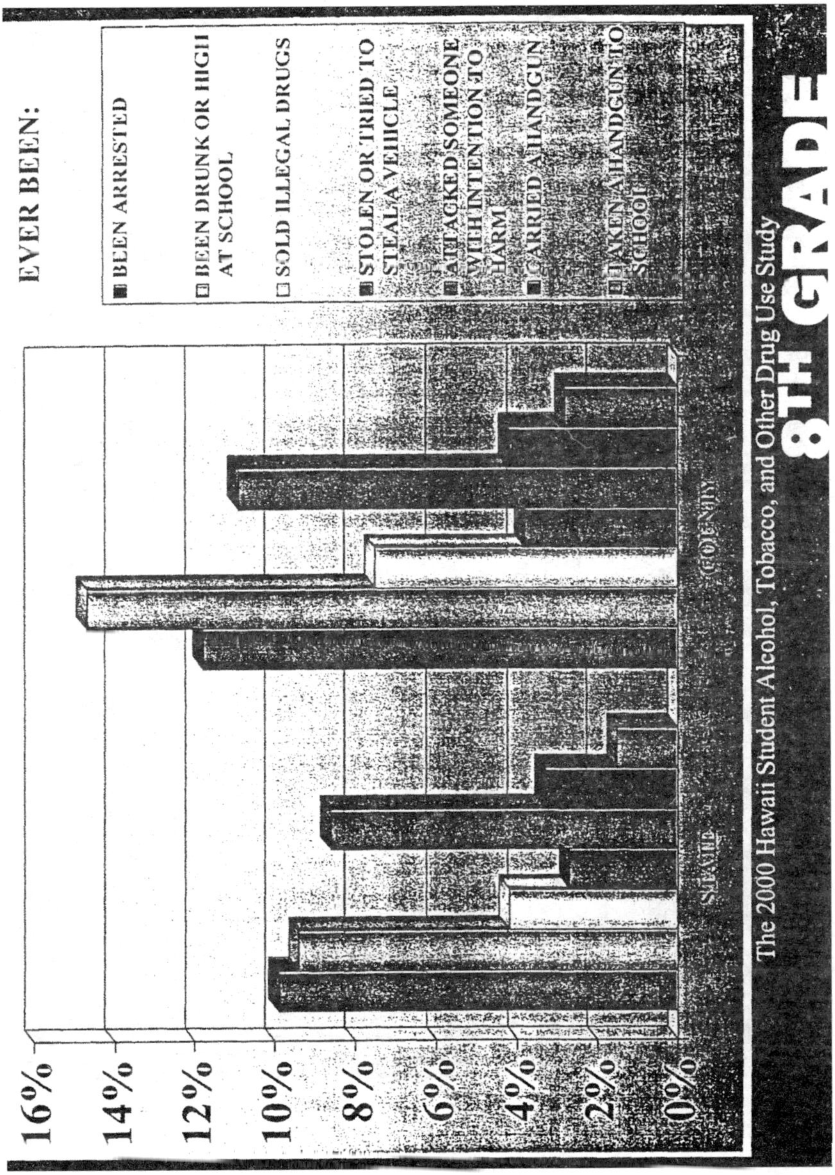
EVER BEEN:
BEEN ARRESTED
BEEN DRUNK OR HIGH AT SCHOOL
SOLD ILLEGAL DRUGS
STOLEN OR TRIED TO STEAL A VEHICLE
ATTACKED SOMEONE WITH INTENTION TO HARM
CARRIED A HANDGUN
TAKEN A HANDGUN TO SCHOOL
16%
14%
12%
10%
8%
6%
4%
2%
0%
The 2000 Hawaii Student Alcohol, Tobacco, and Other Drug Use Study
8TH GRADE

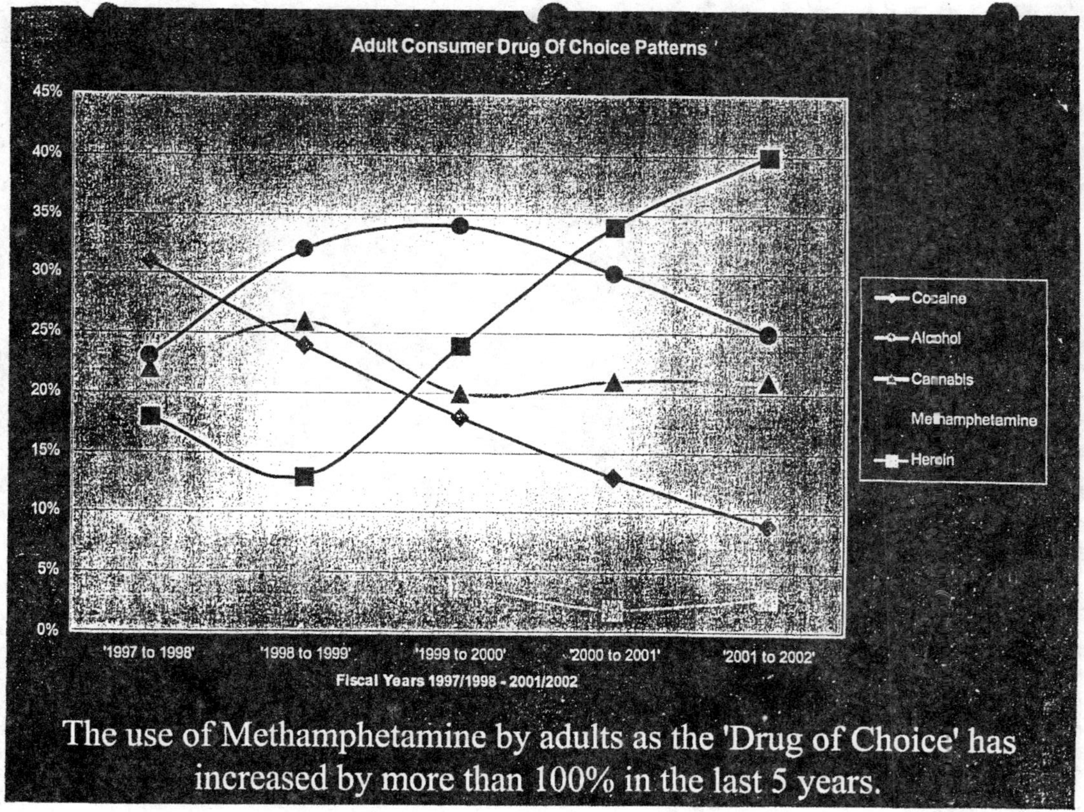
Adult Consumer Drug Of Choice Patterns
45%
40%
35%
30%
25%
20%
15%
10%
5%
0%
'1997 to 1998'
'1998 to 1999'
'1999 to 2000'
'2000 to 2001'
'2001 to 2002'
Fiscal Years 1997/1998 - 2001/2002
Cocaine
Alcohol
Cannabis
Methamphetamine
Heroin
The use of Methamphetamine by adults as the 'Drug of Choice' has increased by more than 100% in the last 5 years.

Methamphetamine related admissions to publicly funded facilities in Hawaii have increased by over 60% in the last 5 years.

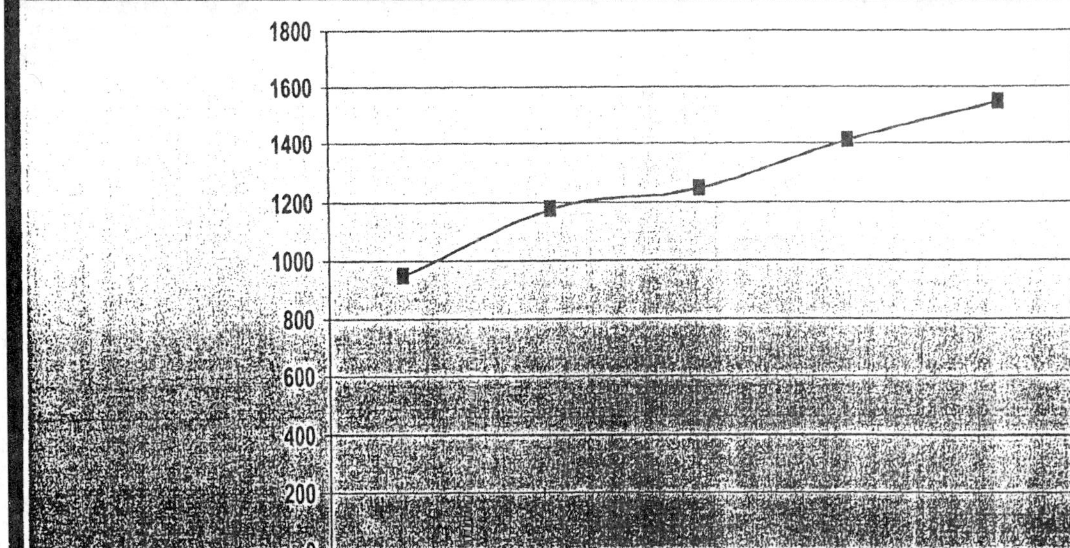

	1996	1997	1998	1999	2000
Methamphetamine Related Admissions to Publicly Funded Facilities in Hawaii	944	1175	1243	1417	1548

Source: U. S. Department of Health and Human Services, Substance Abuse and Mental Health Services Administration, Treatment Episode Data Set.

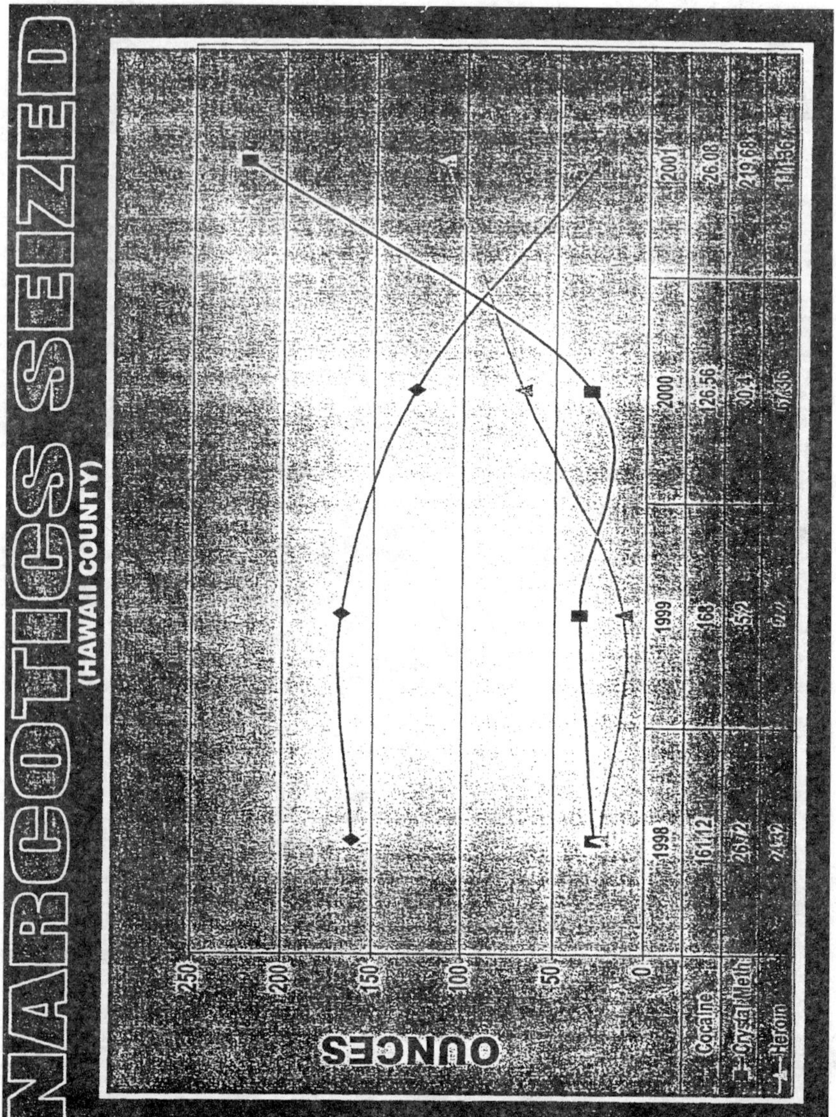
NARCOTICS SEIZED
(HAWAII COUNTY)
OUNCES
250
200
150
100
50
0
1998
1999
2000
2001
Cocaine 161.12 168 126.56 26.08
Crystal Meth 26.72 35.2 30.4 219.68
Heroin 24.32 67.36 111.56

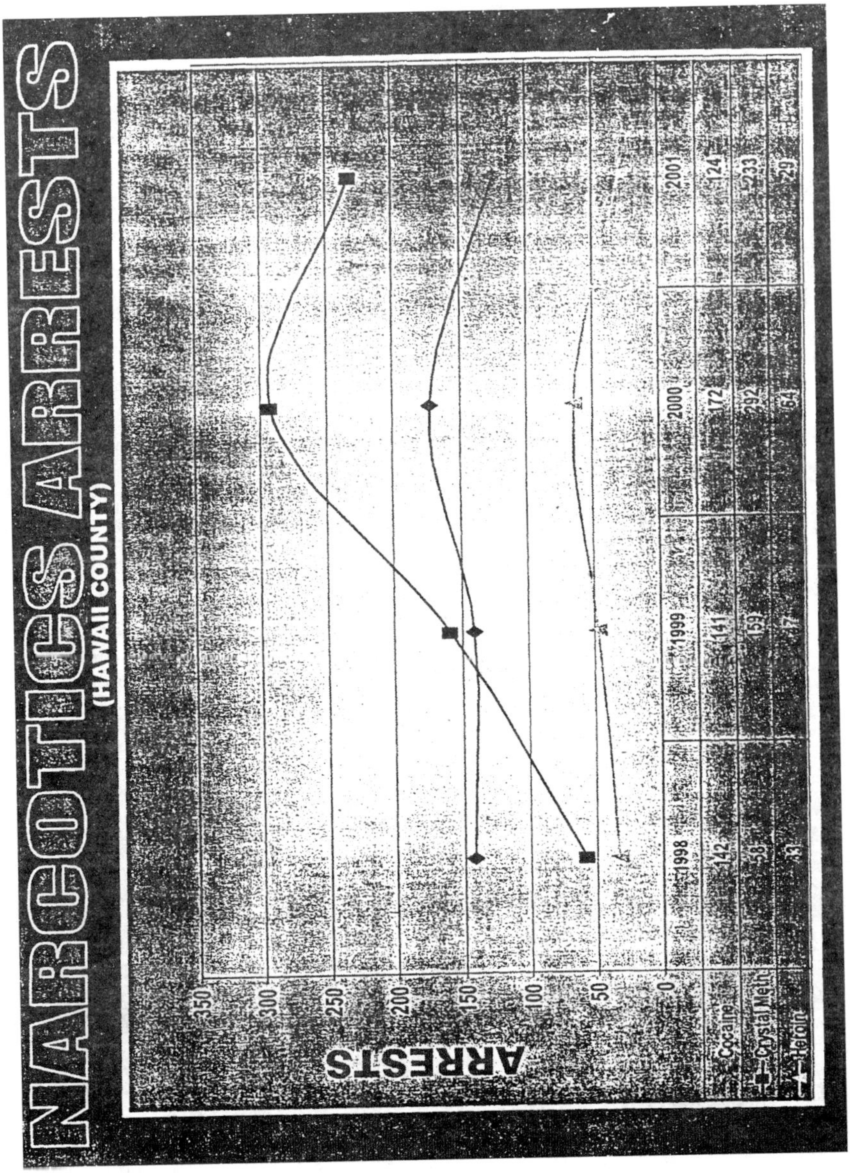
NARCOTICS ARRESTS
(HAWAII COUNTY)
ARRESTS
350
300
250
200
150
100
50
0
1998
1999
2000
2001
Cocaine 142 141 172 124
Crystal Meth 58 159 292 233
Heroin 33 47 64 29

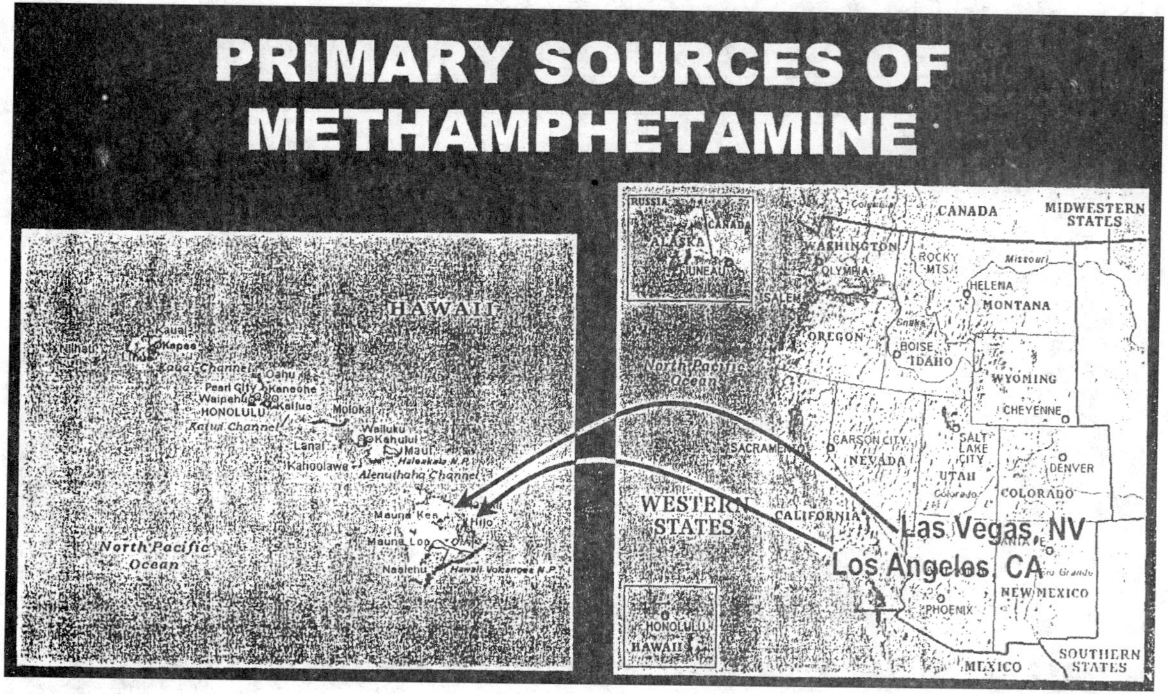
PRIMARY SOURCES OF
METHAMPHETAMINE
HAWAII
Kauai
Kauai Channel
Oahu
Pearl City
Kaneohe
HONOLULU
Kailua
Kaiwi Channel
Molokai
Wailuku
Kahului
Lanai
Maui
Kahoolawe
Alenuihaha Channel
Mauna Kea
Hilo
Mauna Loa
Naalehu
Hawaii Volcanoes N.P.
North Pacific
Ocean
RUSSIA
CANADA
ALASKA
JUNEAU
CANADA
MIDWESTERN
STATES
WASHINGTON
OLYMPIA
ROCKY
MTS.
Missouri
HELENA
MONTANA
SALEM
OREGON
BOISE
IDAHO
North Pacific
Ocean
WYOMING
CHEYENNE
CARSON CITY
NEVADA
SACRAMENTO
SALT
LAKE
CITY
UTAH
DENVER
COLORADO
WESTERN
STATES
CALIFORNIA
Las Vegas, NV
Los Angeles, CA
NEW MEXICO
PHOENIX
HONOLULU
HAWAII
MEXICO
SOUTHERN
STATES

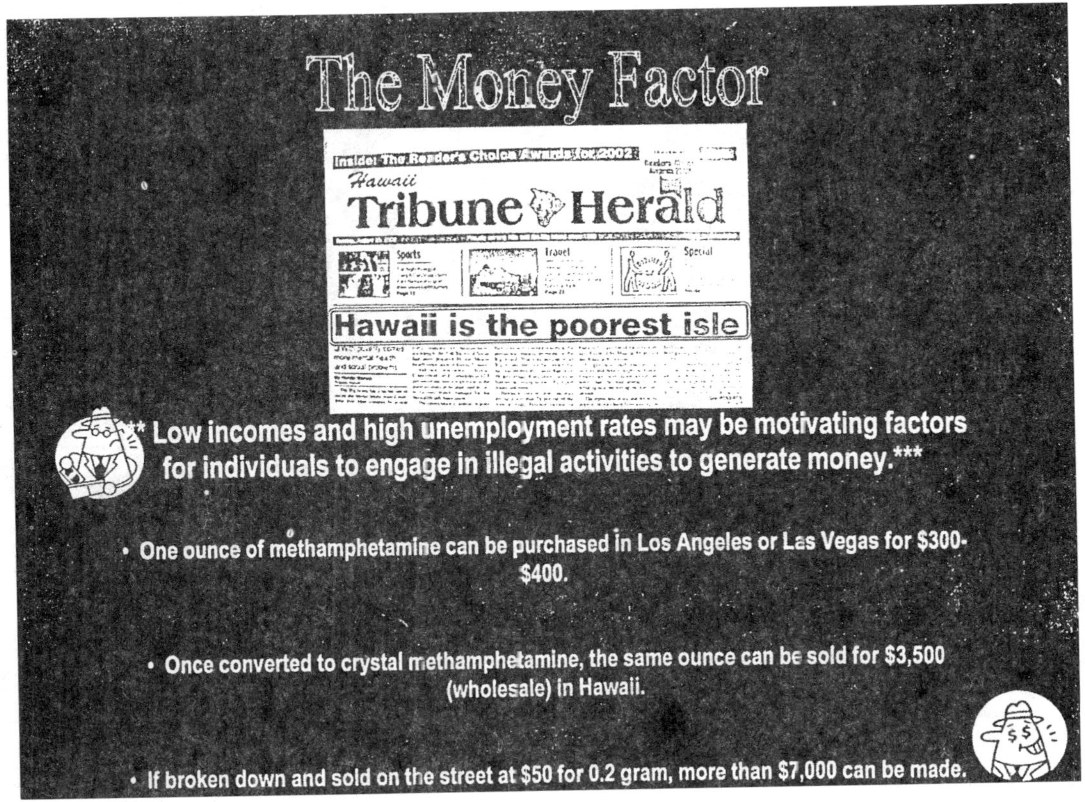
The Money Factor
Inside: The Reader's Choice Awards for 2002
Hawaii Tribune Herald
Sports
Travel
Special
Hawaii is the poorest isle
*** Low incomes and high unemployment rates may be motivating factors for individuals to engage in illegal activities to generate money.***
• One ounce of methamphetamine can be purchased in Los Angeles or Las Vegas for $300-$400.
• Once converted to crystal methamphetamine, the same ounce can be sold for $3,500 (wholesale) in Hawaii.
• If broken down and sold on the street at $50 for 0.2 gram, more than $7,000 can be made.

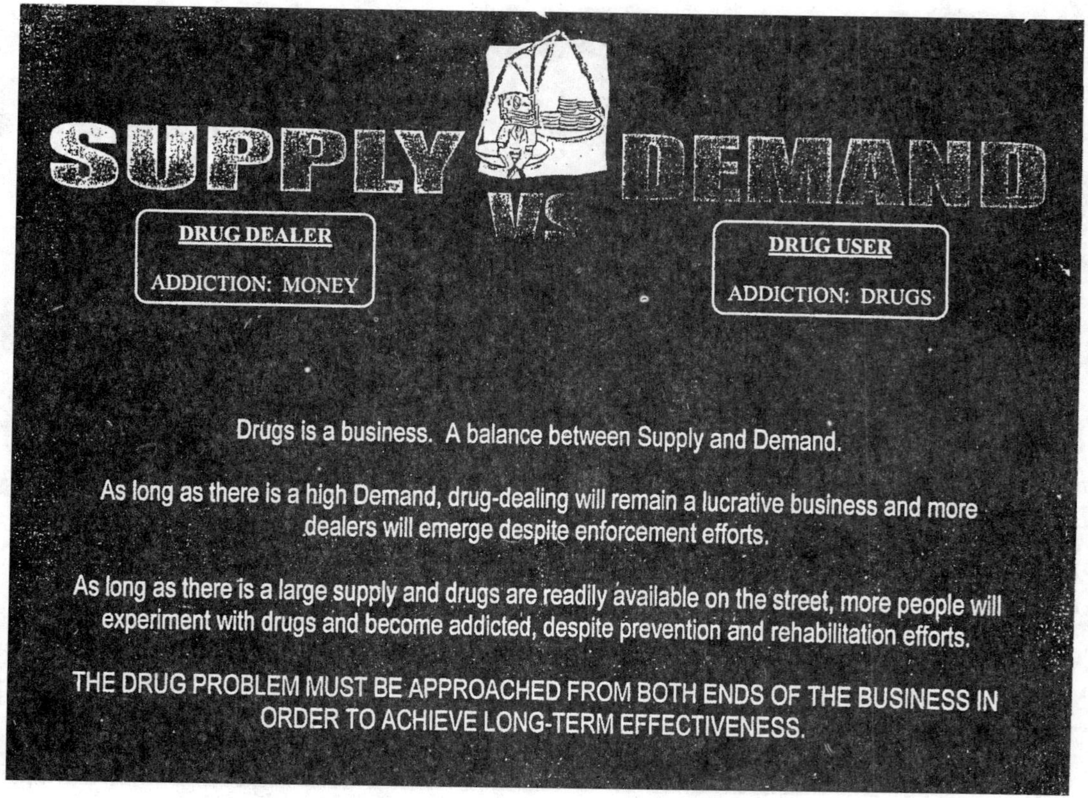
SUPPLY VS DEMAND
DRUG DEALER
ADDICTION: MONEY
DRUG USER
ADDICTION: DRUGS
Drugs is a business. A balance between Supply and Demand.
As long as there is a high Demand, drug-dealing will remain a lucrative business and more dealers will emerge despite enforcement efforts.
As long as there is a large supply and drugs are readily available on the street, more people will experiment with drugs and become addicted, despite prevention and rehabilitation efforts.
THE DRUG PROBLEM MUST BE APPROACHED FROM BOTH ENDS OF THE BUSINESS IN ORDER TO ACHIEVE LONG-TERM EFFECTIVENESS.

In a continued effort to improve the quality of life for the citizens of Hawaii County, we must draw upon every available resource and enlist the assistance of all Federal, State and County agencies in a collaborated attempt to mitigate the current drug epidemic that now threatens the future of our community.

HAWAII ISLAND METH SUMMIT I
AUGUST 27, 2002
ATTENDEES

Lynnese	Acia	Neighborhood Watch Program	Kailua-Kona
Richard	AhYo	Public Safety-Kulani	Hilo
Cookie	Akau-Gaspar	Hui Malama Ola Na 'Oiwi	Kamuela
Chris	Alameda	PARENTS, INC.	Hilo
Riki May	Amano	Judiciary	Hilo
Susan	Ancheta	Judiciary	Hilo
Bruce	Anderson	Dept. of Health	Honolulu
Mark	Ansel		Kapaau
Sidney	Aoki		Kealakekua
James	Arakaki	County of Hawaii	Hilo
Darlene	Araki	Hilton Waikoloa Village	Waikoloa
Lincoln	Ashida	County of Hawaii	Hilo
Naomi	Ashman		Kailua-Kona
Virginia	Aste	Na Poe Hoa Aina	Pahoa
Dorothee	Auldridge	Hawaii Island YMCA	Kamuela
Aley	Auna, Jr.	Judiciary	Kailua-Kona
Ryan	Aurellio	The Orchid at Mauna Lani	Kohala Coast
Debra	Barra	KCH	Kealakekua
Patti	Barry	Hale Ola Ka'u	Ocean View
Bob	Barry	Neighbohood Watch	Ocean View
Kay	Bauman	Public Safety	Honolulu
Lilian	Beaufrere	Kona Heavens Neighborhood Watch	Kailua-Kona
Don	Bebee	Family Support Services-West HI	Kailua-Kona
Jeannette	Bento	Queen Liliuokalani Children's Ctr.-Kona	Kamuela
Leomi	Bergknut	Hawaii Community College	Hilo
Lisa	Best	Kahakai Community Watch Program	Pahoa
Allysyn	Bezilla	Alu Like, Inc.	Hilo
Chad	Blair	Honolulu Weekly	Honolulu
Diane	Blanchard	Dept. of Human Svcs.	Hilo
Lani	Bowman	TEAM Kohala	Hawi
Janice	Brencick		Kamuela
Ken	Brooks	Waikoloa Baptist Church	Waikoloa
Gregory	Brosseau	Ka'u Adult Mental Health Clinic	Naalehu
Tom	Brown	County of Hawaii	Hilo
Doc	Buyers		Papaikou
Randy	Cabral		Pahala
Apolinario	Cabudol	Ka'u Rural Health Community Assoc.	Pahala
Margaret Ann	Cabudol	Ka'u Rural Health Community Assoc.	Pahala
Brandee	Cachola	Office for Social Ministry	Hilo
Healani	Cahill	Queen Liliuokalani Children's Ctr.	Kailua-Kona
Reggie	Camacho	Insights to Success, Inc.	Kailua-Kona
John	Carroll	Hawaii Community College	Hilo
Kelaukila	Carter	Hui Ho'ola O Na Nahulu O Hawaii	Pahoa
Bernard	Carvalho	St. Joseph Catholic Community	Hilo
Rick	Castberg	University of Hawaii at Hilo	Hilo
Cory	Causey	Family Support Services-West HI	Hawi
Diane	Chadwick	HI Community Foundation	Kamuela
Roger	Christie	The Hawaii Cannabis Ministry	Hilo
Aaron	Chung	County of Hawaii	Hilo
Brenda	Constine	Big Island Public Center	Hilo
Patti	Cook	Waimea Community Association	Kamuela
Darlene	Crawford	Waikoloa Community Response	Waikoloa
Kathleen	Damon	University of Hawaii, West Hawaii	Kealakekua

Lois-ellin	Datta	Datta Analysis	Waikoloa
Tom	Davies		Kailua-Kona
Nadia	Davies	Dept. of Education	Kailua-Kona
John	Dawrs	Hawaii County Police Dept.	Hilo
James	Day	Hawaii County Police Dept.	Hilo
Olani	Decker	Kanu O Ka 'Aina	Kamuela
John	DeFries	Hokulia	Kailua-Kona
Stewart	DelaCruz	Turning Point for Families	Kailua-Kona
Dan	DeLuz, Jr.	Thy Word Ministries	Hilo
Doreen	DeSilva	The Orchid at Mauna Lani	Kohala Coast
Maulili	Dickson	Waimea Family YMCA	Kamuela
Susan	Doyle	Aloha United Way	Honolulu
Florence	Dunn-O'Neal	Mental Health Center	Hilo
Michael	Ebesugawa	Public Defender's Office	Hilo
Gloria	Egle-Garbutt	BISAC	Hilo
Leningrad	Elarionoff	County of Hawaii	Hilo
Marge	Elwell	County of Hawaii	Naalehu
Susan	Emerson-McCree	Dept. of Human Svcs.	Kealakekua
Patricia	Engelhard	County of Hawaii	Hilo
Les	Estrella	St. Joseph Catholic Community	Hilo
Cindy	Evans		Waikoloa
Ivan	Faxon	Hilo Care	Hilo
Robert	Fernandez	DLNR-Conservation & Resources Enforcement	Honolulu
Gerald	Ferro		Hilo
Leialoha	Filoteo	Ke Ala Lokahi	Hilo
Christina	Fisher	County of Maui	Kula
William	Fisher		Kailua-Kona
Joseph	Florendo	Judiciary	Kealakekua
Tara	Flynn	Health Works Under the Banyan	Pahoa
Andrew	Ford	DLNR	Hilo
Edwin	Freitas	County of Hawaii	Hilo
David	Frior	University of Hawaii	Honolulu
Loretta	Fuddy	Dept. of Health	Honolulu
Mel	Fujino	County of Hawaii	Kealakekua
Letty Jane	Galloway	Queen Liliuokalani Children's Ctr.	Hilo
Bromson	Gambell	SRM	Kamuela
David	Garcia	Queen Liliuokalani Children's Ctr.-Kona	Kailua-Kona
Ulunui	Garmon	Edith Kanaka'ole Foundation	Hilo
David	Gaud	DLNR-Conservation & Resources Enforcement	Honolulu
Michael	Gibson	Hamakua Health Center	Kamuela
Arlene	Gillett		Pahoa
Carol	Gilliland	Kona Community Hospital	Kealakekua
Barbara	Gleeson		Kailua-Kona
Kawena	Gomes		Kamuela
Tamara	Gouveia	CRI	Kailua-Kona
Thomas	Gouveia, III	CRI	Holualoa
Jonathan	Gradie	STI	Honolulu
Carlene	Greenlee	Dept. of Human Svcs.	Hilo
Beverley	Grogan	Mental Health Association	Keaau
Carole	Gruskin	Child & Family Service	Kealakekua
Corinne	Gushiken	Judiciary	Hilo
Jerry	Hackett	Ka'u Rural Health Community Assoc.	Keaau
Kaiana	Haili	Ke Kahua Pa'a	Hilo

Helene	Hale	Hawaii State Legislature	Pahoa
Harold	Hall	Pacific Institute	Kamuela
Eric	Hamakawa	Hawaii State Legislature	Honolulu
Elizabeth	Hannah	Dept. of Human Svcs.	Kailua-Kona
Grayson	Hashida	Hawaii Island Humane Society	Kailua-Kona
Wendell	Hatada	County of Hawaii	Hilo
Paula	Helfrich	HI Island Economic Development Bd.	Hilo
Peter	Hendricks	Hawaii County Police Commission	Kamuela
Marni	Herkes	Kona-Kohala Chamber of Commerce	Kailua-Kona
Robert	Herkes		Volcano
Thomas	Hickcox	Hawaii County Police Dept.	Hilo
Zachary	Higa	Judiciary	Hilo
Peggy	Hilton	Dept. of Human Svcs.	Hilo
Dean	Hiraki	Judiciary	Hilo
Ron	Hochuli		Kamuela
Patricia	Hoffman	YMCA Family Visitation Center	Kailua-Kona
Peter	Hoffmann	Waikoloa Village Assn.	Waikoloa
Brad	Hollinger	Baha'is of South Kohala	Waikoloa
Claire	Hollinger	Baha'is of South Kohala	Waikoloa
Fred	Holschuh	Hilo Medical Center, ER	Honokaa
Joseph	Huttenlocker	The Salvation Army, Kona Corps	Kailua-Kona
Bryan	Hyatt	East Hawaii Clinic	Hilo
Edmund	Hyun	Public Safety-Hawaii Intake	Hilo
Ronald	Ibarra	Judiciary	Kealakekua
Charlene	Iboshi	County of Hawaii	Hilo
Lorraine	Inouye	Hawaii State Legislature	Hilo
Beryl	Iramina	Public Safety-HCCC	Hilo
Wallace	Ishibashi, Jr.	ILWU Local 142	Hilo
Julie	Jacobson	County of Hawaii	Hilo
Debra	Javar	Ka'u Rural Health Community Assoc.	Naalehu
Haunani	Joaquin	Edith Kanakaole Foundation	Hilo
Donnalyn	Johns	Big Island Substance Abuse Council	Hilo
Pilialoha	Johnson	Na Maka Haloa	Hilo
Thomas	Kaaiai	Safe and Drug Free	Honolulu
Robert	Kaaua	Hawaii County Police Dept.	Hilo
Dixie	Kaetsu	County of Hawaii	Hilo
Kalani	Kahalioumi	Coalition For A Drug Free Hawaii	Honolulu
Rita	Kahalioumi	Judiciary	Kealakekua
Maxine	Kahaulelio	Kealaula	Kamuela
Samuel	Kahele	The Bay Clinic, Inc.	Hilo
Jacqueline	Kalani	Dept. of Human Svcs.	Capt. Cook
Daniel	Kama	Hawaii County Police Commission	Mt. View
Mark	Kaminski	County of Hawaii	Hilo
Keith	Kamita	Public Safety-Narcotics Enforcement	Honolulu
Mona	Kanakamaikai	Turning Point for Families	Holualoa
Marshall	Kanehailua	Hawaii County Police Dept.	Hilo
Maile	Kanemaru	Weed and Seed	Honolulu
Kanoelani	Kanoho	County of Hawaii	Kealakekua
Lei	Kapono	Hawaii Community College	Hilo
Becky	Kawaihae	Aha Punana Leo-UHH	Hilo
Eric	Kawamoto	DLNR	Hilo
David	Kawauchi	Hawaii County Police Dept.	Hilo
Jonah	Kelekolio	Alu Like, Inc.	Hilo

Moana	Kelii	Dept. of Human Svcs.	Hilo
Harry	Kepa'a	Pahoa Family Health Center	Pahoa
Jay	Kimura	County of Hawaii	Hilo
Guy	Kitaoka	Judiciary	Kailua-Kona
Warren	Kitaoka	Judiciary	Kailua-Kona
Stefan	Koehler	Divine Faith Ministries	Ocean View
Russell	Kokubun	Hawaii State Legislature	Honolulu
Harold	Kolo	CRI	Kailua-Kona
Edward	Kubo	U.S. Attorney's Office	Honolulu
Kevin	Kunz	Kona Addiction Services	Kailua-Kona
Janet	Lang	HI Community College Crisis Response	Hilo
Wally	Lau	Neighborhood Place of Kona	Kailua-Kona
Stephanie	Launiu	The Bay Clinic, Inc.	Hilo
Ted	Leaf	Kona Crime Prevention Committee	Kailua-Kona
Bobby Jean	Leithead-Todd	County of Hawaii	Hilo
Andrew	Levin	County of Hawaii	Hilo
Pamela	Lichty	ACLU of Hawaii	Honolulu
Randal	Like	Hui Ho'ola O Na Nahulu O Hawaii	Pahoa
Patrick	Linton	Five Mountains Hawaii	Kamuela
Arthur	Logan	HI National Guard	Honolulu
Tarey	Low	DLNR-Conservation & Resources Enforcement	Lihue
Donald	Lupien	Access Capabilities, Inc.	Kailua-Kona
Rodney	Maeda	Judiciary	Kailua-Kona
Bruce	Makarewicz	Advanced Drug Testing Svc.	Kailua-Kona
Christina	Malinguis	Big Island Public Center	Hilo
Wesley	Margheim	BISAC	Hilo
Valerie	Mariano	Dept. of the Attorney General	Honolulu
Vivian	Mark	Dept. of Education	Hilo
David	Marquez	Insights to Success, Inc.	Kailua-Kona
Janet	Marrack	Family Support Services-West HI	Kailua-Kona
Jeannette	Martin	Five Mountains Hawaii	Kamuela
Craig	Masuda	County of Hawaii	Hilo
Bert	Masuoka	Office of Youth Services	Honolulu
Manuel	Mattos	Pahoa Sacred Heart Church	Keaau
Richard	McDowell	Kona Community Hospital	Kealakekua
Kalani	Mills	County of Hawaii	Hilo
Aolani	Mills	Judiciary-Adult Probation	Kailua-Kona
Pat	Mitchell	BISAC	Kealakekua
Billy	Mitchell	Mana Christian Ohana	Kamuela
Gervin	Miyamoto	U.S. Attorney's Office	Honolulu
Barry	Mizuno	HIEDB	Pahoa
David	Monahan		Kohala
Valdete	Moncreaff	PARENTS, INC.	Hilo
Melissa	Moniz	Keaukaha Community Association	Hilo
Lonnie	Morgan	BISAC	Kealakekua
Daniel	Morimoto		Kamuela
Liane	Moriyama	Dept. of the Attorney General	Honolulu
Steve	Morrison	Hilo Medical Center	Hilo
Clifford	Motta	Dept. of Human Svcs.	Hilo
Jackie	Murai	Judiciary	Hilo
Wil	Murakami	Dept. of Education	Kailua-Kona
Charles	Nahale	DLNR	Hilo
Ronald	Nakamichi	Hawaii County Police Dept.	Hilo

Greg K.	Nakamura	Judiciary	Hilo
Abigail	Napeahi	Alu Like, Inc.	Hilo
Richard	Nelson, III	Governor's Office-West Hawaii	Kailua-Kona
Paradise	Newland	Planet Puna	Pahoa
Lynn	Nicks	Dept of Human Svcs.	Hilo
Tamah-Lani	Noh	HI National Guard	Honolulu
Kelden	Ogawa	Public Safety-Kulani	Hilo
Darryl	Oliveira	County of Hawaii	Hilo
Jon	Olson	Puna Traffic Safety	Pahoa
Stanton C.	Oshiro	Law Offices of Stanton Oshiro	Hilo
Andrew	Ovenden	University of Hawaii at Manoa	Honolulu
Derek	Pacheco	Hawaii County Police Dept.	Hilo
Michael	Palazzo	Public Safety-OCCC	Honolulu
Lorrin	Pang	Maui District Health Office	Wailuku
Alan	Parker	County of Hawaii	Hilo
Leroy	Pasalo	Judiciary	Hilo
Steven	Pavao	Boys and Girls Club	Hilo
Pauline	Pavao	The Salvation Army	Hilo
Andi	Pawasarat-Losalio	Bridge House	Kailua-Kona
Kristi	Payne	A New Harvest Fellowship	Waikoloa
Howard	Pe'a	Alu Like, Inc.	Hilo
Karen	Perreira	Turning Point for Families	Hilo
Karen	Perreira	TPFF	HIlo
Thomas	Pinhey	University of Hawaii at Hilo	Hilo
William	Pink	DOJ/INS/Investigations	Honoluly
Nancy	Pisicchio	County of Hawaii	Kailua-Kona
Jewel	Post	Dept. of Education	Kamuela
Linda	Price	Child & Family Service	Kealakekua
Regina	Purinton	PARENTS, INC.	Hilo
Edwin	Rapozo	Hawaii County Police Dept.	Hilo
John	Ray	Waimea Community Association	Kamuela
Gina	Ready	BISAC	Kailua-Kona
Monty	Richards, Jr.	Kahua Ranch, Ltd.	Kamuela
Rhonda	Robinson		Kailua-Kona
Laurie Jo	Rogers	Destinations in Paradise LLC	Waikoloa
George	Roldan	Waimea Community Association	Kamuela
Gordon	Roque	Waikoloa Land Company	Waikoloa
Norma	Ross	USDA-ARS-PBARC	Hilo
Mitchell	Roth	County of Hawaii	Hilo
Donna	Ruden	The Salvation Army Task Force	Kailua-Kona
Gary	Safarik	County of Hawaii	Hilo
Jann	Saiki-Morimoto	Kona Adult Probation	Kailua-Kona
Ted	Sakai	Public Safety	Honolulu
Allen	Salavea	County of Hawaii	Hilo
Ernest	Saldua	Hawaii County Police Dept.	Hilo
Dorene	Santangelo	Ka'u Rural Health Community Assoc.	Keaau
Tiffany	Santos	Public Safety-Kulani	Hilo
Sandra	Schutte	Judiciary	Hilo
Gary	Shimabukuro	Laulima Hawaii	Honolulu
Alan	Shinn	Coalition For A Drug Free Hawaii	Honolulu
Julian	Shiroma	Hawaii County Police Dept.	Hilo
Richard	Smith	Simple Office Solutions	Kailua-Kona
Janet	Snyder	County of Hawaii	Hilo

Nancy	Soderberg	Dept. of Education	Kealakekua
Rueben	Soriano	Adult Probation	Hilo
Danielle	Spain	BISAC	Hilo
Andrea	St. Clair	Waikoloa Sub. Abuse Rehab. & Recovery Prog.	Kamuela
Glenda	Sugi	Judiciary	Kealakekua
Jean	Sunderland	Five Mountains Hawaii	Kapaau
Nani	Svendsen	TEAM Kohala	Hawi
Ruth	Tachibana	Judiciary	Hilo
Paul	Takehiro	Hui Ho'ola O Na Nahulu O Hawaii	Pahoa
Roy	Takemoto	County of Hawaii	Hilo
Shari	Tasaka	Public Safety	Honolulu
Sherrie	Taylor	Community of Christ	Kamuela
Likeke	Teanio	DASH	Hilo
Jane	Tocta	County of Hawaii	Hilo
Michelle	Teuber	PARENTS, INC.	Hilo
James	Texeira	Solid Rock Ministries	Kailua-Kona
Angela	Thomas	Good Beginnings Alliance	Kamuela
Derek	Tolentino	Hilton Waikoloa Village	Waikoloa
Kate	Tolentino	Dept. of Education	Kamuela
Karl J.	Toubman	Waimea Natural Health Center	Kamuela
Karen	Uemura	Hawaii Electric Light Company, Inc.	Hilo
Thomas	Varese	ACT Team	Hilo
Paula	Vickery	Community Care Services	Hilo
Sharon	Vitousek	Five Mountains Hawaii	Kamuela
Matilda	Vradenburg	Waikoloa Community Church Youth Ministries	Waikoloa
Alan	Walker	Kupulau Meadows Community Assn.	Hilo
Pat	Walker	Turning Point for Families	Hilo
Lynn	Walton	Kona Community Hospital	Kealakekua
Henry	Wana	Big Island Public Center	Hilo
Deborah	Ward	University of Hawaii at Hilo	Hilo
Carol	Warner	Judiciary	Kailua-Kona
Jamal	Wasan	Waikoloa Sub. Abuse Rehab. & Recovery Prog.	Waikoloa
Candace	Watson		Waikoloa
Larry	Weber	Hawaii County Police Dept.	Hilo
Kealoha	Wells		Kailua-Kona
William	Wenner	Private Practicioner	Volcano
Ramona	West	North Hawaii Community Hospital	Waikoloa
MaryJo	Westmoreland	Kapiolani Child Protection Ctr.	Kailua-Kona
Richard	White	DLNR	Hilo
Elaine	Wilson	Dept. of Health	Kapolei
Dominic	Yagong	County of Hawaii	Hilo
Leah	Yanagi	County of Hawaii	Hilo
Burnalyn	Yee	HCEOC	Hilo
Lynn	Yokoyama	Big Island Public Center	Hilo
Layne	Yoshida	Public Defender's Office	Hilo
Peter	Young	County of Hawaii	Kailua-Kona

2002 Hawaii Island Meth Summit Recommendations & Survey Results

SURVEY RESULTS (Top Recommendations)

Back to 2002 Hawaii Island Meth Summit

DOMAINS

(CJ) Criminal Justice, (ED) Education, (SG) State Government, (LE) Law Enforcement, (PA) Public Awareness, (TX) Treatment, (Y) Youth

RANKED IN TOP 10 FOR BOTH

Rec #	Dom		Imp Avg	Imp Rank	Feas Avg	Feas Rank
16	CJ	Conduct outreach to judges to include them in future summits and other planning factors.	4.47	5	4.19	2
76	LE	Expand community policing efforts.	4.56	1	4.18	3
102	TX	Establish training programs for residential rehab/treatment personnel.	4.40	10	4.06	8
145	Y	Publicize youth activities in the newspaper, radio announcements, and postings at school.	4.40	10	4.21	1

Back to Top

RANKED IN TOP 20 FOR BOTH

Rec #	Dom		Imp Avg	Imp Rank	Feas Avg	Feas Rank
15	CJ	Secure funding from the State to create drug courts.	4.54	2	3.93	17
43	SG	Pass legislation to make laws/sentences stricter for drug dealers that sell to or use youths for distribution.	4.39	15	4.04	10

85	PA	Educate families through a public awareness campaign about where the public can go to go for services.	4.39	15	4.10	7
94	PA	Involve grassroots organizations (Boys and Girls Club, seniors, faith organizations) in the drug education effort.	4.37	20	4.16	4
128	Y	Write a comprehensive plan for providing alternative activities and safe places for youth.	4.40	10	3.92	20
129	Y	Identify usable facilities for youth recreation and do a cost analysis for remodeling or building new facilities.	4.38	18	3.86	30
133	Y	Create a mentor program using adults and other youth as positive role models for youth.	4.38	18	3.91	22
134	Y	Implement culturally based, positive after-school activities such as skill-building programs and hands-on education (sailing, gardening, etc.).	4.49	3	4.01	12
135	Y	Create a program for youth that involves job training and shadowing, entrepreneurial activities, and the creation of internship opportunities.	4.48	4	4.00	13

Back to Top

TOP 30 FOR BOTH

22	ED	Develop, through the Department of Education, a mandatory drug curriculum for all grades on a consistent basis.	4.47	5	3.90	23
23	ED	Create a cross-sector task force to implement a comprehensive public educaiton plan that reaches out to children, funding sources, families, professionals, teachers, social workers, judges, etc., through the media, the Internet, and recovering addicts.	4.40	10	3.86	30
101	TX	Create a prison drug treatment facility (for users only) to teach anger management, vocational, parenting and life skills, in a safe environment.	4.40	10	3.88	26
127	TX	Create programs that incorporate one-on-one counseling with parent and child when drug problems are prevalent in the family.	4.42	9	3.90	23
137	Y	Hold a youth summit to identify kids' needs.	4.32	27	4.11	6

Back to Top

Back to Top

2002 Hawaii Island Meth Summit Recommendations & Survey Results

SURVEY RESULTS (in Original Order - by Domain)

Business Communities Criminal Justice Education Faith Community Law Enforcement Public Awareness State Gov't Treatment Youth

Back to 2002 Hawaii Island Meth Summit

Rec #	BUSINESS	Imp Avg	Imp Rank	Feas Avg	Feas Rank
1	Implement policies allowing flexible work hours for parents.	3.32	135	2.75	139
2	Work with employers to develop a mandatory work-place training curriculum on drug abuse.	4.06	71	3.73	50
3	Create a multi-agency body to design a master plan for economic development within rural/depressed communities.	3.98	82	3.41	103
4	Forge a partnership with the private sector to solve transportation, facility and resource development problems (give tax credits, etc.)	4.05	74	3.35	111

Back to Top

Rec #	COMMUNITIES	Imp Avg	Imp Rank	Feas Avg	Feas Rank
5	Engage the Hawaii Community Foundation to provide a .5 FTE position to identify all available public and private funding.	3.88	90	3.75	47
6	Organize Ice Summits and/or awareness fairs in every community.	4.25	38	4.14	5
7	Have the Community Empowerment Organization (CEO) organize communities by coordinating Neighborhood Watch groups, Business Watch groups and community associations, and building community capacity to problem-solve.	4.06	71	3.81	40

8	Identify an agency, or individual to facilitate a community-government forum.	3.66	116	3.62	65
9	Plan and conduct grant-writing education training for organizations.	3.82	98	3.87	28
10	Establish a list of motivational speakers and create a bureau to book them for events in schools, business, and other organizations.	3.88	90	3.82	38
11	Establish parenting and literacy classes for young families.	4.23	42	3.87	28
12	Develop a grassroots community-based initiative to address community involvement/networking and create a database.	3.87	94	3.48	92
13	Organize a committee to plan regular community-based events promoting a drug/alcohol-free environment and building pride in the community.	4.19	47	3.88	26
14	Bring together existing inter-agency committees (e.g. DVIAT, CJC, treatment community, CWS) and incorporate into larger coalition.	4.04	76	3.64	63

Back to Top

Rec #		Imp Avg	Imp Rank	Feas Avg	Feas Rank
	CRIMINAL JUSTICE				
15	Secure funding from the State to create drug courts.	4.54	2	3.93	17
16	Conduct outreach to judges to include them in future summits and other planning forums.	4.47	5	4.19	2
17	Repeal mandatory sentencing in order to allow for treatment (judicial discretion, individual sentencing).	3.79	101	3.4	105
18	Pass legislation to shorten the timeline for prosecution (currently six months to two years to get a case together).	4.33	25	3.54	79

Back to Top

Rec #		Imp Avg	Imp Rank	Feas Avg	Feas Rank
	EDUCATION				
19	Create a coalition to address funding for ice education and prevention programs.	4.27	35	4.05	9
20	Delegate a percentage of forfeiture proceeds to ice programs.	4.27	35	3.86	30
21	Perform random drug searches at schools (i.e.., drug dogs).	3.68	114	3.11	127
22	Develop, through the Department of Education, a mandatory drug curriculum for all grades on a consistent basis.	4.47	5	3.90	23
23	Create a cross-sector task force to implement a comprehensive public education plan that reaches out to children, funding sources, families, professionals, teachers, social workers, judges, etc. through the media, the Internet, and recovering addicts.	4.40	10	3.86	30

24	Create more career shadow programs, Rotary Vocational Service Committees, and stronger school-to-work programs.	4.01	78	3.60	70
25	Seek grant funding (Legislature, private foundation) for a substance counselor position or program in DOE.	4.12	57	3.59	72
26	Seek grant funding for education of professionals in best practices by DOH (Hawaii District Health Office) in conjunction with Big Island community hospitals.	3.79	101	3.51	85
27	Integrate drug education for teachers into curriculum while they are getting their degrees.	4.16	51	3.80	41
28	Develop flyers and brochures to make parents aware of drug problems among younger age groups.	3.95	86	3.95	15

Back to Top

FAITH COMMUNITY

Rec #		Imp Avg	Imp Rank	Feas Avg	Feas Rank
29	Use faith groups to educate congregations through substance abuse videos.	4.00	80	4.02	11
30	Create an internship program with universities and faith-based organizations to do in-home visits and reach out to families most affected by ice.	3.87	94	3.44	100
31	Coordinate Parks and Recreation Department with faith-based organizations.	3.30	137	3.07	131
32	Allow non-proselytizing, faith-based organizations the same access to funding as non-profit, secular groups.	3.15	140	2.90	136
33	Involve faith-based organizations by identifying needs that they could meet and approaching them for assistance.	3.96	85	3.77	44

Back to Top

STATE GOVERNMENT

Rec #		Imp Avg	Imp Rank	Feas Avg	Feas Rank
34	Create permission waivers allowing agencies to share information to better collaborate.	4.30	30	3.64	63
35	Dedicate taxes to meth program (e.g., alcohol, cigarettes).	4.09	62	3.46	96
36	Expand the bus system and do island-wide planning for transportation.	4.34	23	3.49	89
37	Coordinate cultural sensitivity and competence training for agencies dealing with the public.	3.75	107	3.55	76
38	Appoint community coordinators/liaisons in government agencies.	3.78	105	3.45	99
39	Increase general funding through the state lottery.	3.13	141	2.61	141

40	Create a position for a tech person to research and access funding/grant opportunities.	3.62	118	3.33	112
41	Lobby Congress to increase the number of DEA/federal agents (currently only one on the Big Island).	4.11	59	3.58	74
42	Implement a restorative justice system to expand or create recreational facilities, incorporating community service assignments, and prison day-releases.	4.09	62	3.52	82
43	Pass legislation to make laws/sentences stricter for drug dealers that sell to or use youths for distribution.	4.39	15	4.04	10
44	Create one web site for all agencies to promote interagency cooperation.	3.82	98	3.74	48
45	Pass legislation to balance funding of private/public schools.	3.09	143	2.58	143
46	Pass legislation to cut red tape for small business owners and lower the cost of doing business.	3.55	127	2.92	135
47	Pass legislation to mandate parenting skills classes in order to receive a marriage license	3.23	138	2.34	145
48	Pass legislation to implement a tax break for families to enter into community services together.	3.32	135	2.74	140
49	Open up the Federal grant process to allow direct application by non-profits.	3.73	110	3.23	118
50	Create local political subdivisions to decentralize government on Big Island.	3.11	142	2.51	144
51	Form a government subcommittee to seek funding/assets to develop communication to and from the community.	3.37	132	3.05	133
52	Pass legislation to give a tax break to large companies who provide employment to recovering addicts.	3.70	112	3.00	134
53	Have each district develop a public-private partnership under the island-wide strategic plan..	3.59	122	3.18	120
54	Ensure that the prosecutor's office continues developing a comprehensive communication network using technology to bring jurisdictions together.	4.04	76	3.61	69
55	Pass legislation to provide tax breaks to employers who provide childcare.	3.97	84	3.32	113
56	Require agency partnerships in order to acquire funding.	3.52	129	3.16	122
57	Work with the state to donate unoccupied land for building of Safe Houses.	4.07	68	3.37	110
58	Select an agency that oversees all programming and designates who shall provide which service.	3.07	144	2.59	142
59	Work with the County of Hawaii to seek accreditation standards for employees (State and County) work in areas affected by the drug problem.	3.59	122	3.09	128
60	Work with the Department of Public Safety to draft legislation to regulate chemical purchases in 2003 Legislative Session.	4.07	68	3.62	65
61	Apply for grants (through community groups, foundations, pharmaceuticals, manufacturers) and identify other sources of	4.05	74	3.38	108

	funding (e.g. wealthy homeowners along Kohala Coast) to fund rehab centers and training within the corrections system.				
62	Increase social services that go into homes and assess situation and family environment.	4.07	68	3.23	118
63	Pass legislation to create state tax credits for people/employers who volunteer their time.	3.69	113	3.17	121
64	Provide a local county jitney service to address transportation issues.	3.74	108	3.09	128
65	Increase treatment in jails (funding through grants).	4.37	20	3.79	42
66	Implement a tax on precursor chemicals.	3.48	131	3.08	130
67	Create a voucher system for private commercial transportation.	3.53	128	3.07	131
68	Adopt School and Community Based Management (SCBM) model in state agencies.	3.21	139	2.87	138
69	Set up a central government clearinghouse of the private/nonprofit sector with newsletter and website.	3.57	126	3.38	108
70	Pass State legislation to return the Adult Mental Health Division, the Child and Adolescent Mental Health Division, an the Alcohol and Drug Addiction Division to a single organization with a unified infrastructure.	3.88	90	3.29	115

Back to Top

Rec #	LAW ENFORCEMENT	Imp Avg	Imp Rank	Feas Avg	Feas Rank
71	Seek community support and involvement with law enforcement as volunteers.	4.11	59	3.54	79
72	Create a Cadet program that offers college credit.	3.59	122	3.16	122
73	Implement a media campaign to increase public awareness of the role of law enforcement and the need for increased manpower.	3.87	94	3.58	74
74	Implement a specialized enforcement/prosecution effort to eliminate drug use by bringing in temporary additional police personnel to assist in cleaning up trouble spots.	4.19	47	3.70	56
75	Redirect police funds from marijuana eradication towards ice education and eradication.	3.74	108	3.49	89
76	Expand community policing efforts.	4.56	1	4.18	3
77	Work with the County Council to approve addition funds for officers dedicated to drug interdiction.	4.36	22	3.84	33
78	Work with the Police Chief and district heads to reassign officers based on community need, to make the best use of personnel for the problem.	4.31	29	3.76	45
79	Expand the number of police beats.	4.09	62	3.40	105
80	Re-hire retired officers for certain tasks.	3.63	117	3.32	113
81	Have law enforcement create a separate Hard Drug Task Force.	3.79	101	3.40	105

82	Develop a clear process on reporting and have law enforcement educate communities on procedures, standards of evidence, etc. so citizens' efforts can be more effective (e.g., run an "Ask Mr. Policeman" column in newspapers).	3.93	87	3.73	50

Back to Top

Rec #		Imp Avg	Imp Rank	Feas Avg	Feas Rank
	PUBLIC AWARENESS				
83	Identify public/private funding for media campaign; use private media as partners.	4.06	71	3.73	50
84	Implement a media campaign to strengthen families/family values; involve the media, public leaders (e.g., the Mayor), and local organizations.	4.08	67	3.67	60
85	Educate families through the public awareness campaign about where the public can go to go for services.	4.39	15	4.10	7
86	Develop a "media team" to publicize/recognize the good things that youth do, using the media as lead resources; including newspaper, radio and television.	4.20	45	3.92	20
87	Incorporate a weekly newspaper column including a "Hall of Shame" and a "Hall of Success".	3.01	145	2.89	137
88	Disseminate information through church papers, neighborhood newsletters, schools, and radio programs when various audiences are listening.	4.09	62	3.83	37
89	Develop multi-cultural educational materials and distribute to specific sectors of the community, i.e., churches, schools, preschools, businesses.	3.90	88	3.69	57
90	Implement a media campaign that increases knowledge of the system process, including child protective services, police, courts, etc.	3.98	82	3.76	45
91	Expand resources and outreach by creating videotapes and other materials for home education.	3.68	114	3.46	96
92	Develop a resource guide and make it more accessible to churches, PTAs, schools, families, businesses, etc.	4.17	50	3.93	17
93	Designate DOE, DOH, DHS, and DOJ as lead agencies in public education.	3.60	120	3.29	115
94	Involve grassroots organizations (Boys and Girls Club, seniors, faith organizations) in the drug education effort.	4.37	20	4.16	4
95	Implement a media campaign aimed at pharmacies including brochures, mailings, etc.	3.34	134	3.15	124
96	Establish business partnerships to include educational information on consumer products, such as milk cartons or juice and soda cans.	3.62	118	3.29	115
97	Create an Internet clearinghouse of information about the ice problem; include statistics used at the Summit.	4.01	78	3.89	25

98	Create a community drama team to raise awareness of the ice problem.	3.52	129	3.52	82

Back to Top

Rec #	TREATMENT	Imp Avg	Imp Rank	Feas Avg	Feas Rank
99	Expand ADAD funding to include treatment for un-incarcerated users.	4.29	32	3.74	48
100	Use forfeiture money to fund drug treatment in prison.	4.09	62	3.62	65
101	Create a prison drug treatment facility (for users only) to teach anger management, vocational, parenting and life skills, in a safe environment.	4.40	10	3.88	26
102	Establish training programs for residential rehab/treatment personnel.	4.40	10	4.06	8
103	Create a program for job shadowing between agencies and treatment counselors.	3.72	111	3.46	96
104	Establish a collaborative partnership between all relevant service providers (those who deal with drug abuse, violence, physical/mental/sexual abuse); create a forum to share ideas.	4.24	39	3.84	33
105	Build in-patient and out-patient drug facilities for meth users.	4.34	23	3.53	81
106	Establish a residential treatment facility for dual diagnoses on the island.	4.43	7	3.59	72
107	Educate stockholders (Federal and State government, private organizations, etc.) on the importance of cultural competency in providing treatment.	3.99	81	3.65	62
108	Develop Federal/State/private funding partnership to fully fund Big Island demonstration programs to address the lack of treatment facilities.	4.16	51	3.68	59
109	Establish a cultural healing center as part of follow-up care and relapse prevention.	381	100	3.48	92
110	Develop licensing standards for treatment programs through the Department of Health.	3.83	97	3.55	76
111	Work with the State Insurance Commissioner to call to study group to examine best practices for insurance reimbursement for substance abuse treatment and make policy recommendations to the Legislature.	3.90	88	3.50	87
112	Hold community meetings hosted by police department and substance abuse facilities to educate the community about services, availability, the meth problem, public safety concerns, and how to make referrals to services.	4.22	43	3.94	16
113	Encourage the State Alcohol and Drug Abuse Branch to have all mental health service providers integrate substance abuse treatment.	4.14	54	3.62	65
114	Extend the timeframe for treatment coverage.	4.43	7	3.69	57

115	Implement a distance learning VTC system to train treatment personnel.	3.88	90	3.48	92
116	Work with Hawaiian Airlines and Aloha Airlines to donate free airline coupons for travel to treatment facilities off the island.	3.76	106	3.12	126
117	Create a central database of statistics, organizations, providers, resources, funding opportunities, etc. which his available to all (agencies, public, etc.).	4.16	56	3.73	50
118	Increase health insurance provision for drug treatment to provide adequate care.	4.39	15	3.44	100
119	Educate neighborhoods about recovery homes "in their back yard" and find houses in neighborhoods that will accept recovering persons (prevent NIMBY).	4.20	45	3.41	103
120	Have the government and insurance companies fund assessment centers and drug treatment at all give Hawaii County hospitals/facilities.	4.26	37	3.42	102
121	Expand integrated case management program to provide access to treatment at all levels of abuse.	4.19	47	3.5	76
122	Implement outreach treatment programs where caseworkers go into the community instead of people coming to them.	4.21	44	3.52	82
123	Provide transportation to treatment by grant-funded shuttles that pick up patients at home and take them to the facility.	4.24	39	3.51	85
124	Develop a strategy for including Ho`oponopono in the treatment process.	3.79	101	3.66	61
125	Identify effective national prevention models and determine concrete ways to adapt them to Hawaii.	4.32	27	3.82	38
126	Streamline referral programs to improve monitoring and treatment.	4.30	30	3.78	43
127	Create programs that incorporate one-on-one counseling with parent and child when drug problems are prevalent in the family.	4.42	9	3.90	23

Back to Top

Rec #		Imp Avg	Imp Rank	Feas Avg	Feas Rank
	YOUTH				
128	Write a comprehensive plan for providing alternative activities and safe places for youth.	4.40	10	3.92	20
129	Identify usable facilities for youth recreation and do a cost analysis for remodeling or building new facilities.	4.38	18	3.86	30
130	Implement a media campaign to foster volunteer support for youth programs.	4.14	54	3.71	54
131	Solicit mor efunding (State, Federal, County, private) for transportation for youth to positive activities.	4.28	33	3.60	70
132	Create a committee to oversee youth-designed "first Nights" for New Year's Eve.	3.58	125	3.49	89

133	Create a mentor program using adults and other youth as positive role models for youth.	4.38	18	3.91	22
134	Implement culturally based, positive after-shool activities such as skill-building programs and hands-on education (sailing, gardening, etc.).	4.49	3.	4.01	12
135	Create a program for youth that involves job training and shadowing, entrepreneurial activities, and the creation of internship opportunities.	4.48	4	4.00	13
136	Implement a media campaign that trains youth in creating public service announcements about meth.	4.12	57	3.84	33
137	Hold a youth summit to identify kid's needs.	4.32	27	4.11	6
138	Involve youth as participants in County and Parks and Recreation decision-making.	4.10	61	3.71	54
139	Implement a 'Kids in Recovery' program (Sobriety High).	4.24	39	3.93	17
140	Have high school cheerleaders promote a drug-free message during half-timne through a special performancfe.	3.36	133	3.50	87
141	Use capital improvement funds to build youth centers.	4.16	51	3.47	95
142	Assign a government (County) employee "Kid Czar" to ntetwork with private service organizations to develop partnerships.	3.60	120	3.14	125
143	Identify and engage peer counselors for children of recovering addicts.	4.33	25	3.84	33
144	Sponsor youth activities such as boat jams, drag races, clubs, ice blocking, and swimming.	4.28	33	3.96	14
145	Publicize youth actiivites in the newspaper, radio announcements, and postings at school.	4.40	10	4.21	1

Back to Top

Back to 2002 Hawaii Island Meth Summit

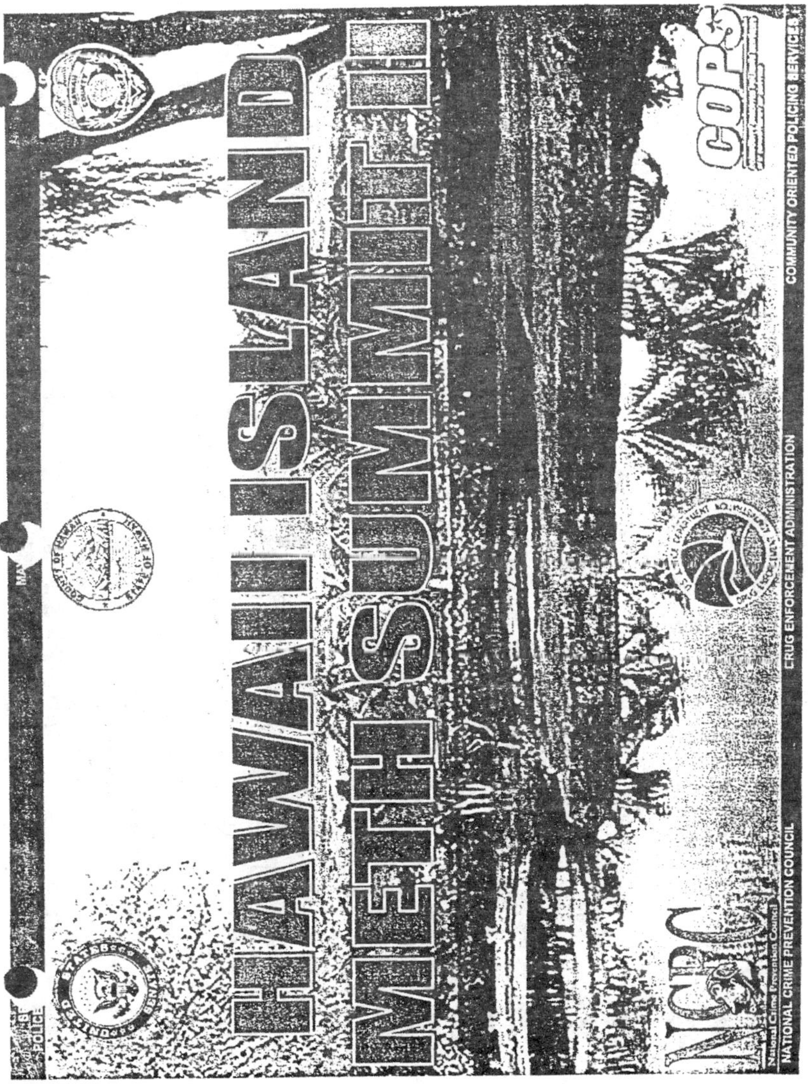
HAWAII ISLAND
METH SUMMIT!
NCPC
NATIONAL CRIME PREVENTION COUNCIL
DRUG ENFORCEMENT ADMINISTRATION
COPS
COMMUNITY ORIENTED POLICING SERVICES

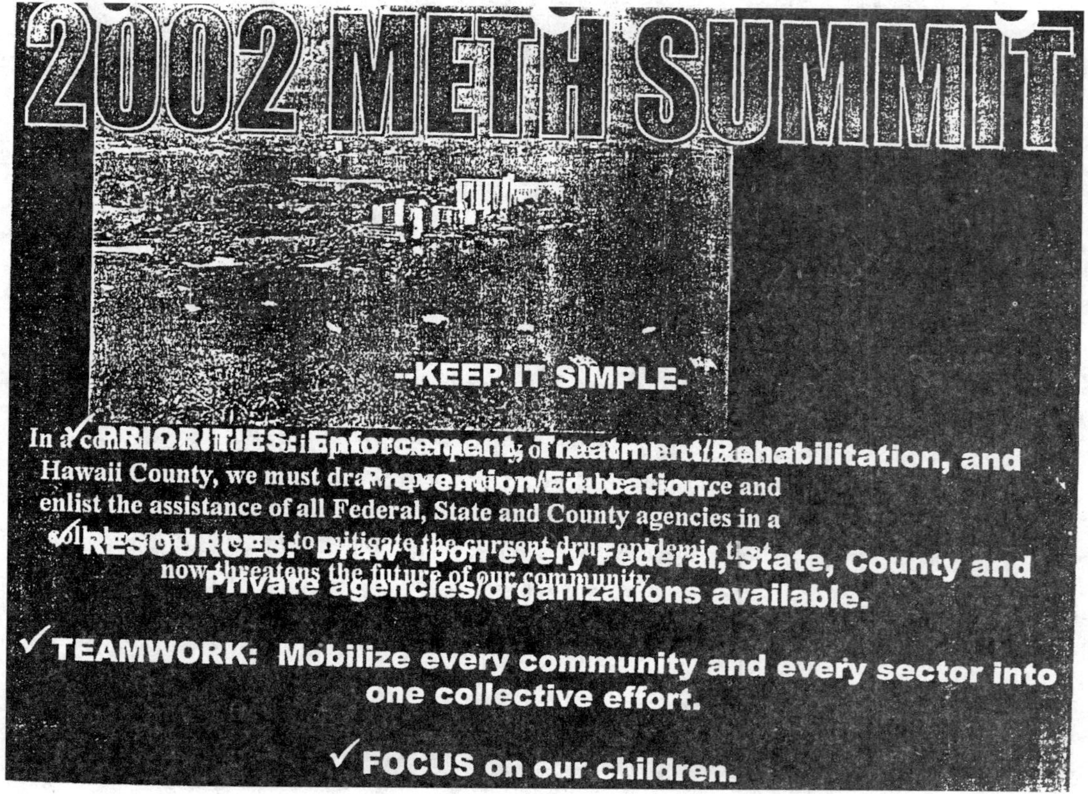
2002 METH SUMMIT
--KEEP IT SIMPLE-
PRIORITIES: Enforcement, Treatment/Rehabilitation, and Prevention/Education.
enlist the assistance of all Federal, State and County agencies in a
RESOURCES: Draw upon every Federal, State, County and Private agencies/organizations available.
TEAMWORK: Mobilize every community and every sector into one collective effort.
FOCUS on our children.

From January to June 2003, the Hawaii County Police Department has conducted search warrants on 37 Ice Houses and 49 vehicles island-wide, making 123 arrests and seizing 11.2 lbs of crystal methamphetamine.

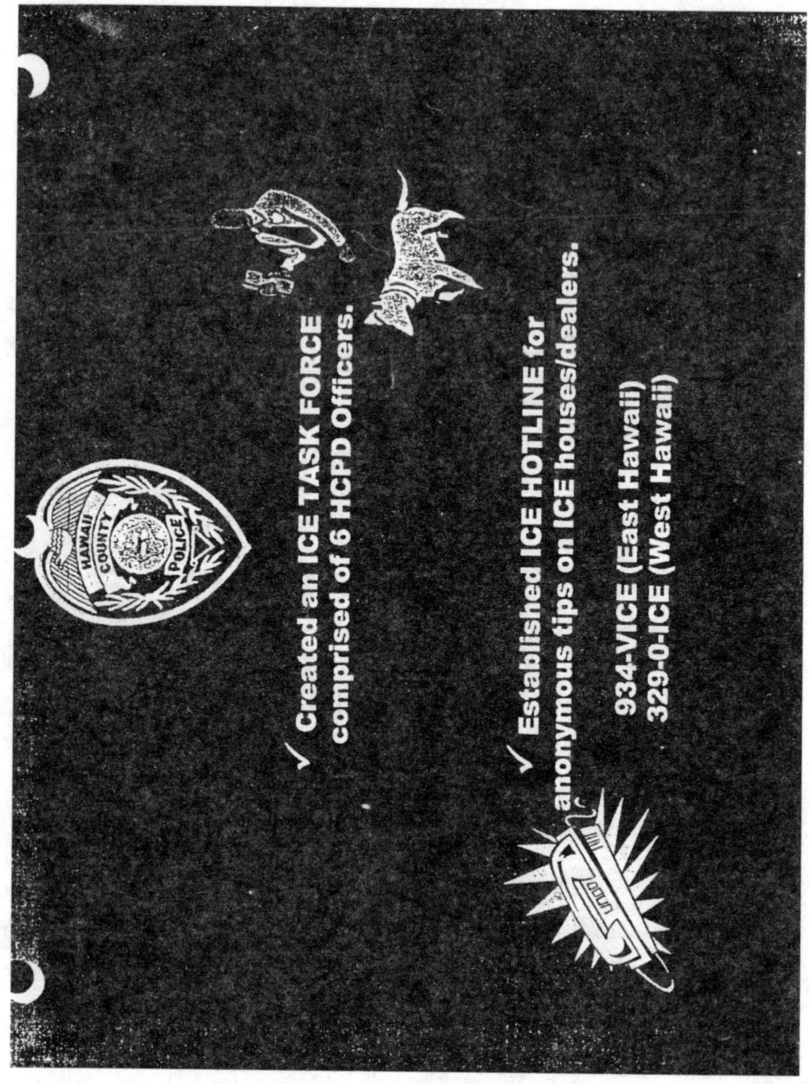
HAWAII
COUNTY
POLICE
✓ Created an ICE TASK FORCE comprised of 6 HCPD Officers.
✓ Established ICE HOTLINE for anonymous tips on ICE houses/dealers.
934-VICE (East Hawaii)
329-0-ICE (West Hawaii)

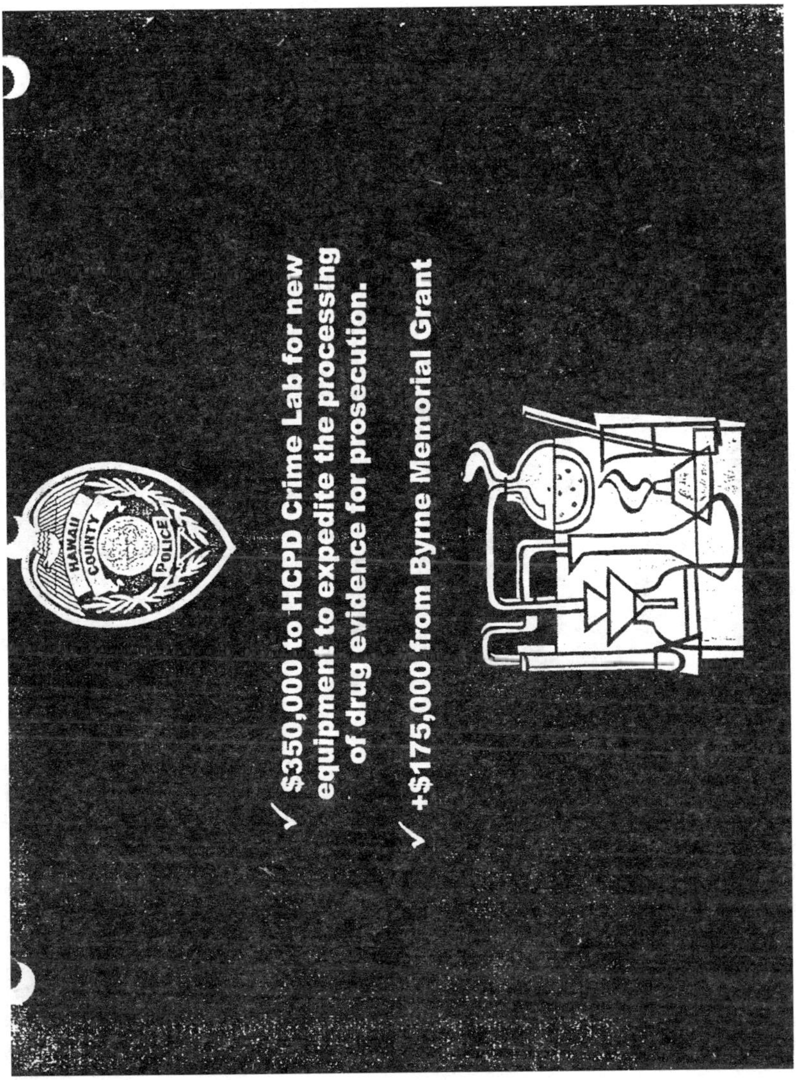
HAWAII COUNTY POLICE
$350,000 to HCPD Crime Lab for new equipment to expedite the processing of drug evidence for prosecution.
+$175,000 from Byrne Memorial Grant

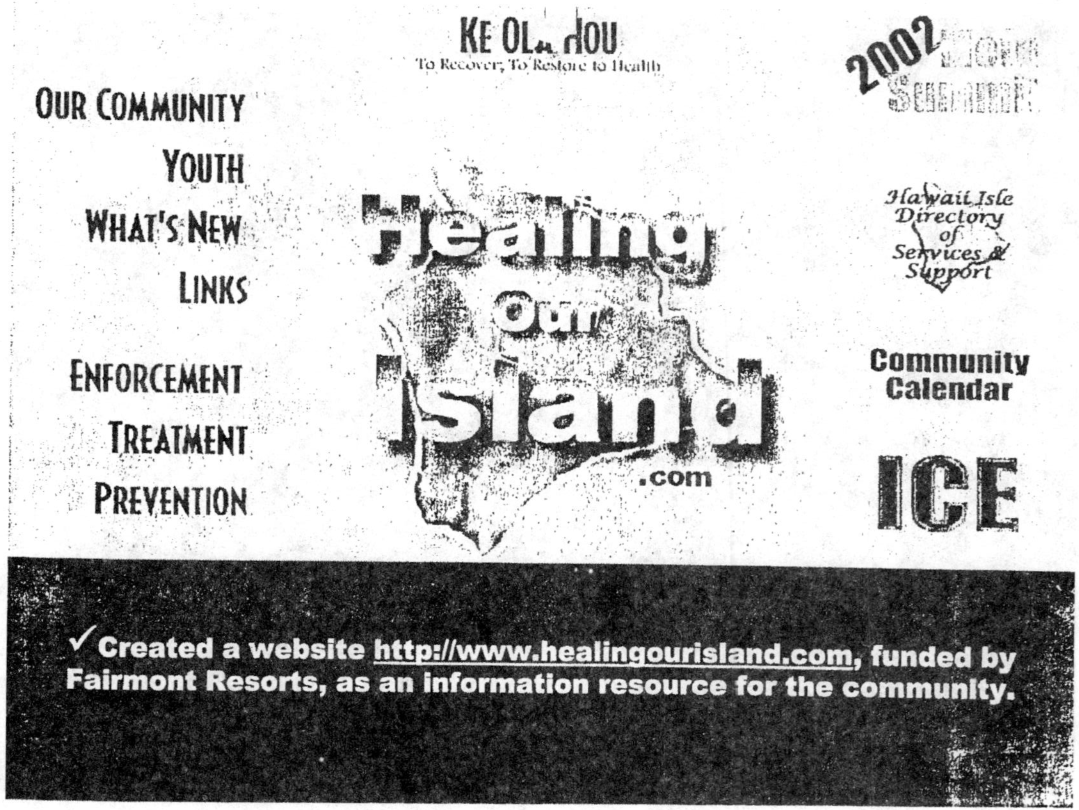
KE OLA HOU
To Recover, To Restore to Health
OUR COMMUNITY
YOUTH
WHAT'S NEW
LINKS
ENFORCEMENT
TREATMENT
PREVENTION
Healing Our Island .com
2002
Hawaii Isle Directory of Services & Support
Community Calendar
ICE
✓Created a website http://www.healingourisland.com, funded by Fairmont Resorts, as an information resource for the community.

Hawaii National Guard - Counterdrug Program: Increased personnel from 2 to 4 assigned to Hawaii County.

Counterdrug personnel provide assistance to law enforcement agencies in conducting drug interdiction operations and provide drug demand reduction services to the community.

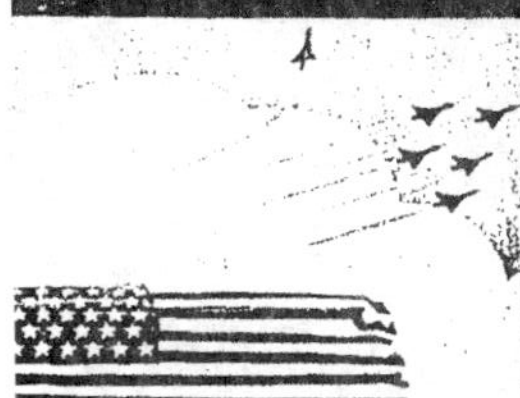

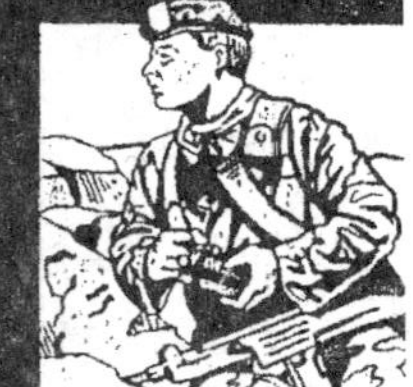

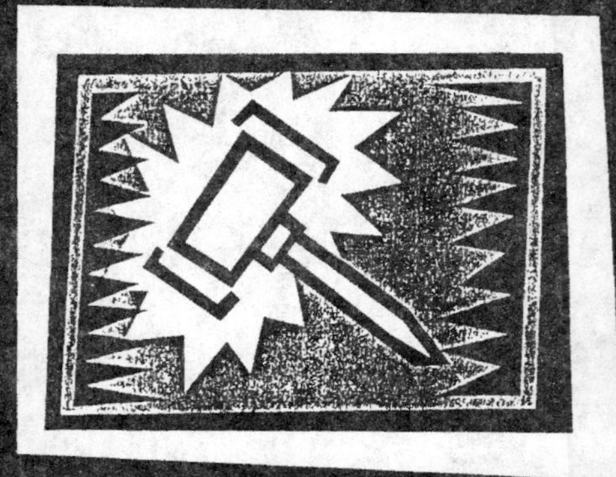

Drug Court established for both adult and juvenile drug courts in East and West Hawaii.

Established Drug Nuisance Abatement Unit in the Office of the Attorney General.

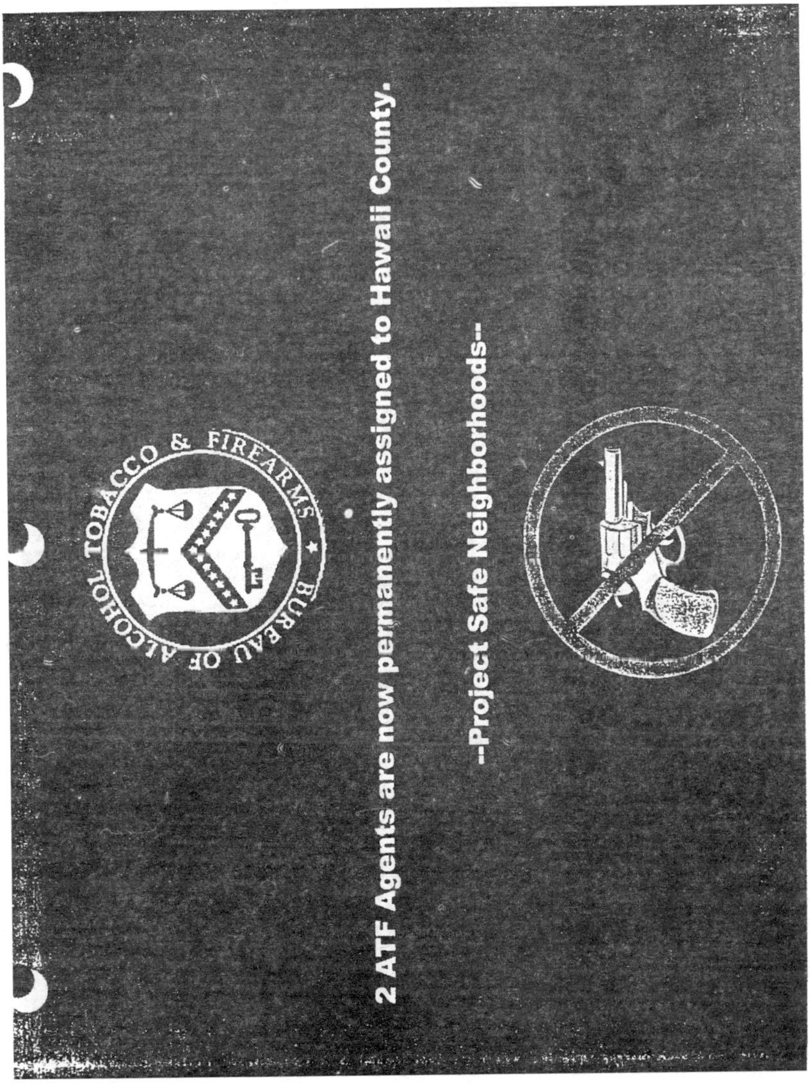
BUREAU OF ALCOHOL TOBACCO & FIREARMS
2 ATF Agents are now permanently assigned to Hawaii County.
--Project Safe Neighborhoods--

U.S. JUSTICE DEPARTMENT
DRUG ENFORCEMENT ADMINISTRATION

1 additional DEA Agent will be assigned to Hawaii County for a total of 2 Agents, effective October 2003.

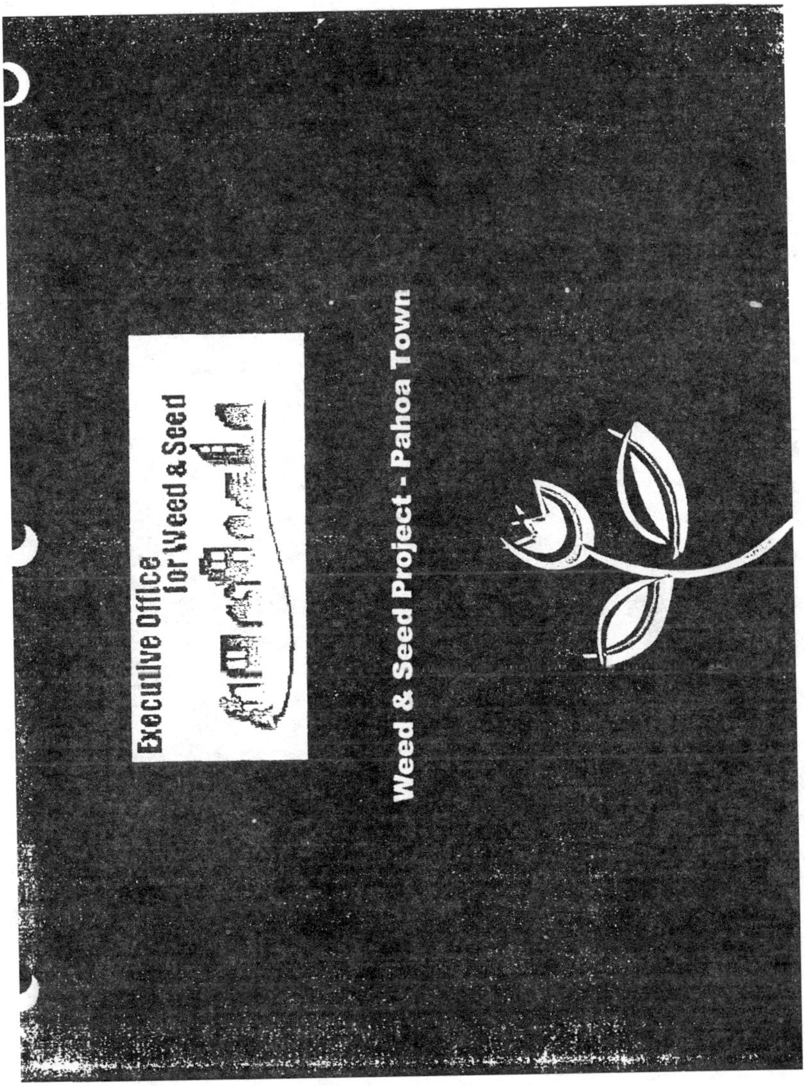
Executive Office
for Weed & Seed
Weed & Seed Project - Pahoa Town

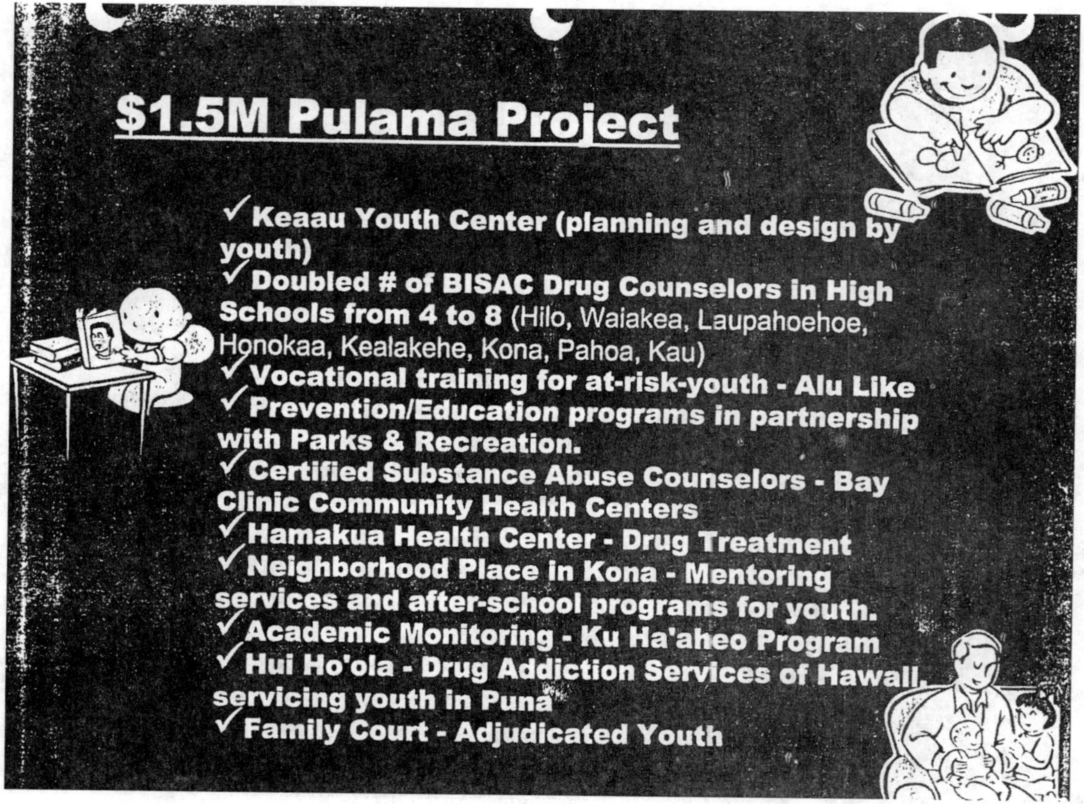
$1.5M Pulama Project
✓Keaau Youth Center (planning and design by youth)
✓Doubled # of BISAC Drug Counselors in High Schools from 4 to 8 (Hilo, Waiakea, Laupahoehoe, Honokaa, Kealakehe, Kona, Pahoa, Kau)
✓Vocational training for at-risk-youth - Alu Like
✓Prevention/Education programs in partnership with Parks & Recreation.
✓Certified Substance Abuse Counselors - Bay Clinic Community Health Centers
✓Hamakua Health Center - Drug Treatment
✓Neighborhood Place in Kona - Mentoring services and after-school programs for youth.
✓Academic Monitoring - Ku Ha'aheo Program
✓Hui Ho'ola - Drug Addiction Services of Hawaii, servicing youth in Puna
✓Family Court - Adjudicated Youth

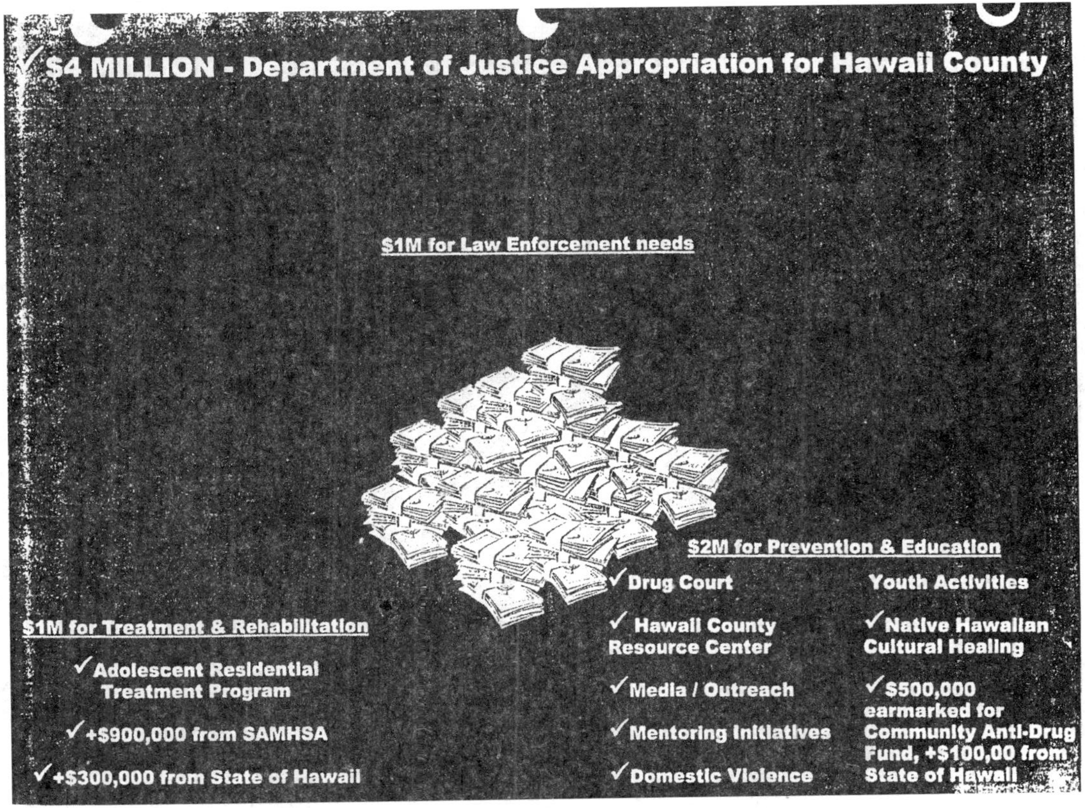
✓$4 MILLION - Department of Justice Appropriation for Hawaii County
$1M for Law Enforcement needs
$1M for Treatment & Rehabilitation
✓Adolescent Residential Treatment Program
✓+$900,000 from SAMHSA
✓+$300,000 from State of Hawaii
$2M for Prevention & Education
✓Drug Court
✓Hawaii County Resource Center
✓Media / Outreach
✓Mentoring Initiatives
✓Domestic Violence
Youth Activities
✓Native Hawaiian Cultural Healing
✓$500,000 earmarked for Community Anti-Drug Fund, +$100,00 from State of Hawaii

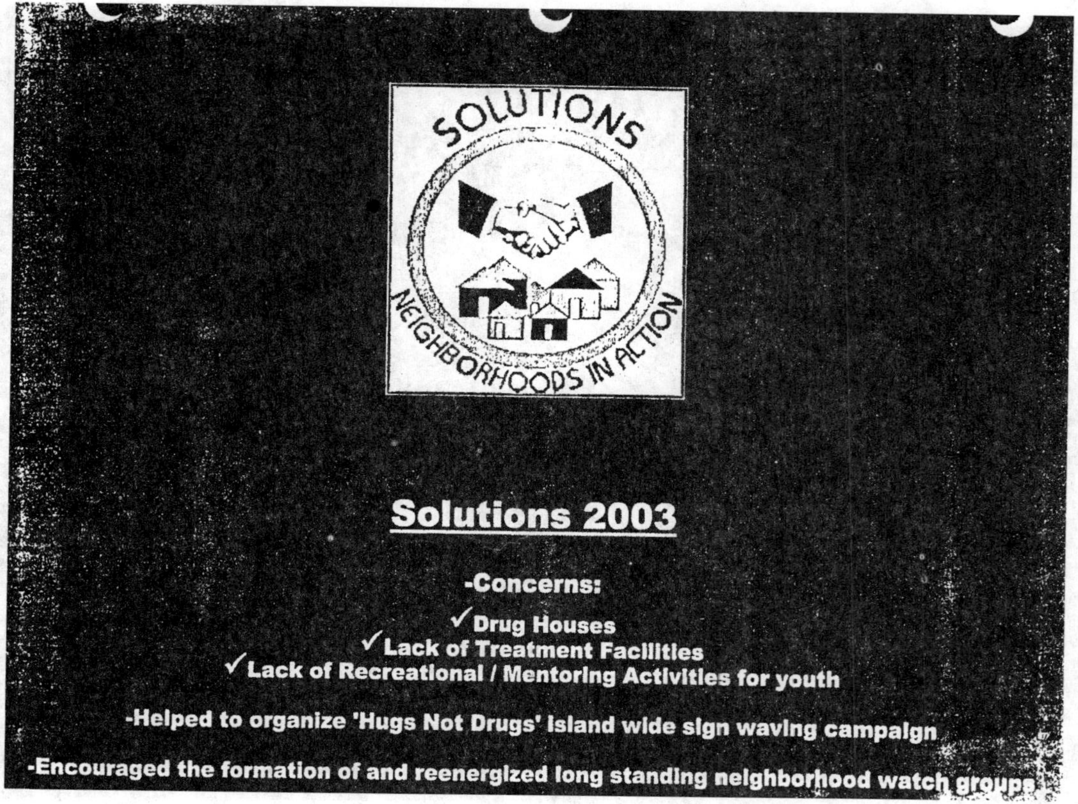
SOLUTIONS
NEIGHBORHOODS IN ACTION
Solutions 2003
-Concerns:
✓Drug Houses
✓Lack of Treatment Facilities
✓Lack of Recreational / Mentoring Activities for youth
-Helped to organize 'Hugs Not Drugs' Island wide sign waving campaign
-Encouraged the formation of and reenergized long standing neighborhood watch groups

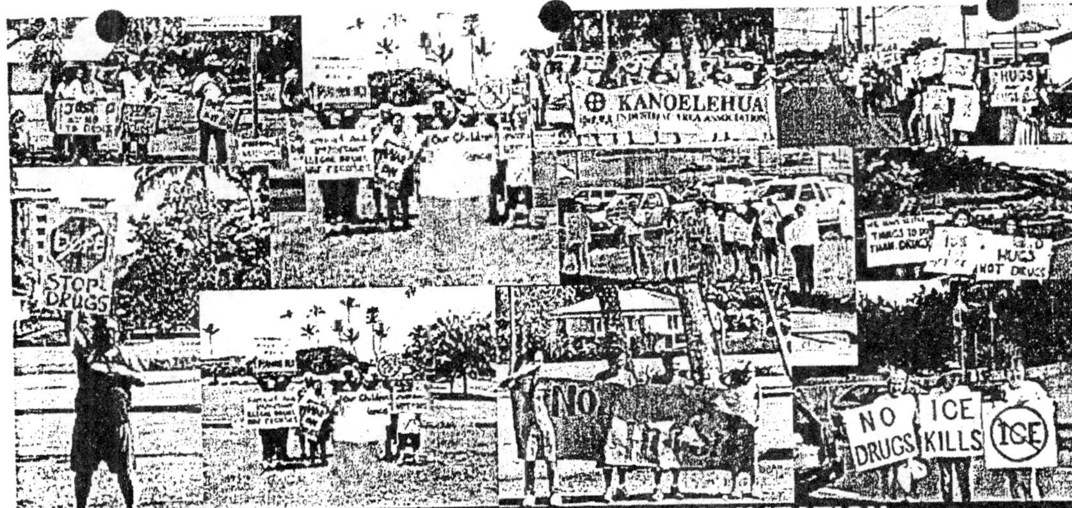

COMMUNITY INVOLVEMENT & MOBILIZATION

✓Faith Against Drugs - Clean and Sober Houses

✓Power of Choice and CRI

✓North Hawaii Drug-Free Coalition

✓65+ BREAKING ICE Performances in schools and in the community

✓Ice Breakers Anti-Drug Event @ Kailua-Kona

✓Increased Drug Awareness presentations given around the Big Island to schools, businesses, civic organizations, and communities by members of the Hawaii County Police Department, Hawaii National Guard - Counterdrug Program, Mayor's Office, and Laulima Hawaii (Gary Shimabukuro)

✓"The War on ICE" public education program, Ch. 55

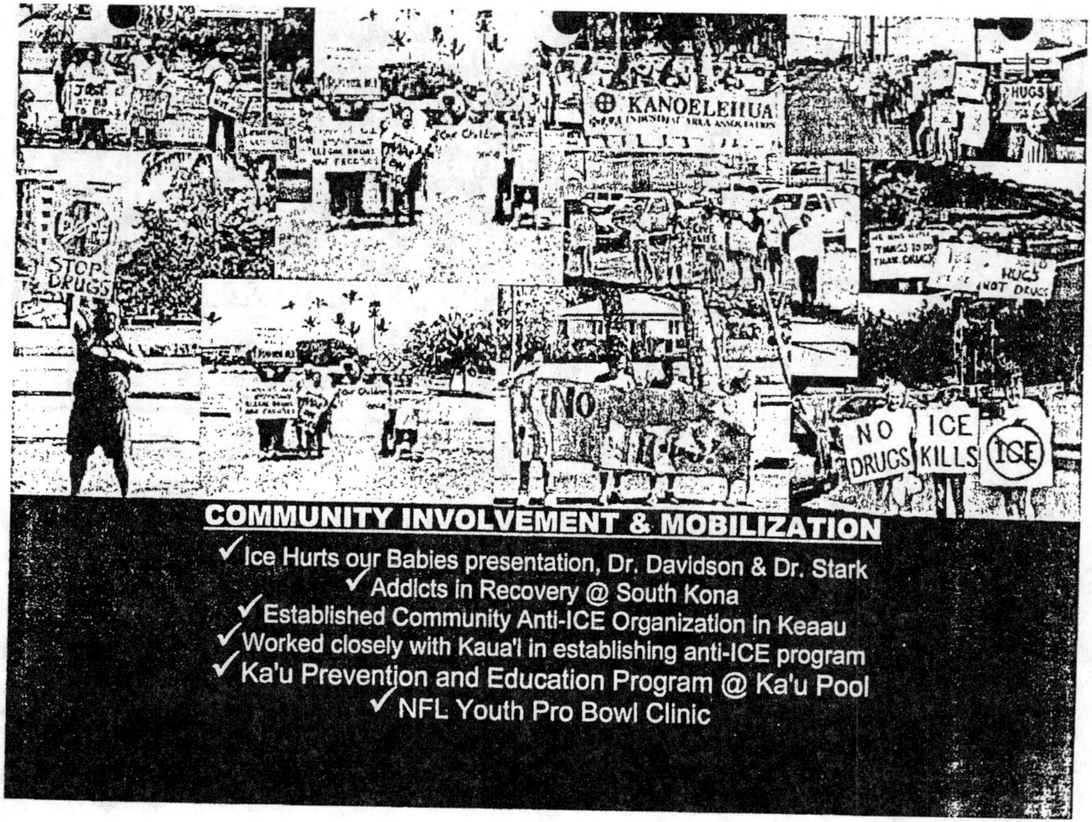
STOP DRUGS
KANOELEHUA
NO DRUGS
ICE KILLS
COMMUNITY INVOLVEMENT & MOBILIZATION
✓Ice Hurts our Babies presentation, Dr. Davidson & Dr. Stark
✓Addicts in Recovery @ South Kona
✓Established Community Anti-ICE Organization in Keaau
✓Worked closely with Kaua'i in establishing anti-ICE program
✓Ka'u Prevention and Education Program @ Ka'u Pool
✓NFL Youth Pro Bowl Clinic

THE YEAR AHEAD

2003 - 2004

- Legislative session in January
- State Drug Summit in September
- Increase Treatment Options
- Establish an Adolescent Residential Treatment Facility and Program
- Follow Through on Summit Recommendations and Priorities
- Maintain Community Effort and Momentum
- Support Community Based Initiatives - Key to Sustainability
- Transportation
- Increase Youth Activities and Mentoring
- IMPLEMENTATION

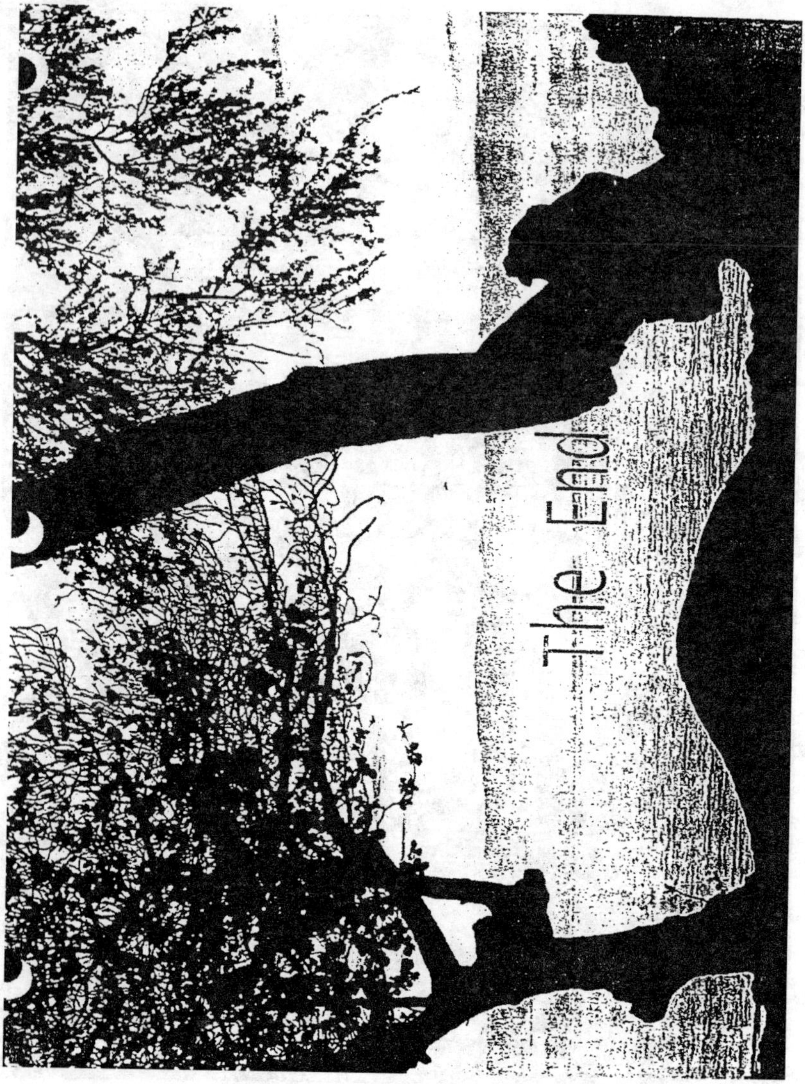
The End

HAWAII ISLAND METH SUMMIT II
AUGUST 25, 2003
ATTENDEES

Lovi	Acob	Office for Social Ministry	Hilo
Melodie	Aduja	State of Hawaii	Honolulu
Cookie	Akau-Gaspar	Hui Malama Ola Na Oiwi	Kamuela
Maria	Andaya	Pulama Project	Hilo
Havinne	Anderson	Aloha United Way 211	Honolulu
Douglas	Andrews	Judiciary	Honokaa
Mark	Ansel		Kapaau
Sidney	Aoki	Kona CRI	Kailua-Kona
Sandra	Apo-Silva	Pulama Project	Hilo
James	Arakaki	County of Hawaii	Hilo
Lincoln S. T.	Ashida	County of Hawaii	Hilo
Ginny	Aste	Na Poe Hoa Aina	Pahoa
Dorothee	Auldridge	YMCA	Kamuela
Mary	Auvil	DOE	Honokaa
Debra A.	Barra	Kona Community Hospital	Kealakekua
Patti	Barry	Hale Ola Kau	Ocean View
Bob	Barry	Neighborhood Watch	Ocean View
Marge	Bartelt	DHS/CWS	Kurtistown
Don	Bebee	Family Support Svcs. West HI	Kailua-Kona
Jeannette	Bento	Queen Liliuokalani Children's Ctr.	Kailua-Kona
Leomi	Bergknut	Hawaii Community College	Hilo
Lisa	Best	Kahakai Neighborhood Watch	Pahoa
Allysyn	Bezilla	Alu Like Inc.	Hilo
Diane	Blanchard	DHS/CWS	Hilo
James	Boetcher	Dept. of Public Safety	Hilo
Lani	Bowman	TEAM Kohala	Hawi
Steve	Bradford	Neighborhood Watch	Kamuela
Janice	Brencick	Aloha Clinic	Kamuela
Tom	Brown	County of Hawaii	Hilo
Larry	Burnett	HIETA	Honolulu
Elizabeth	Bush	Hamakua Health Center	Honokaa
Antonio	Carrisal	JC Posse Outreach Ministery	Hilo
Juanita	Carrisal	JC Posse Outreach Ministery	Hilo
Kelaukila	Carter	DASH	Pahoa
Bernard	Carvalho	St. Joseph Catholic Community	Hilo
Craig	Carvalho		Keaau
Ed	Case	Representative	
Susan	Caseria	County of Hawaii	Hilo
Cory	Causey	TEAM Kohala	Hawi
Diane	Chadwick	Hawaii Community Foundation	Kamuela
Verna	Chartrand	Care Hawaii Inc.	Kailua-Kona
Roger	Christie	Hawaii Cannabis Ministry	Hilo
Lucille	Chung	North Hilo Community Council	Hilo
Matthew	Claybaugh	Marimed Foundation	Kaneohe
Joel	Cohen		Kukuihaele
Brenda	Constine	PARENTS, Inc.	Hilo
Lisa	Cook	DASH	Honolulu
Patti	Cook	Power of Choice, Waimea	Kamuela
Sandy	Daniels	DOE	Kailua-Kona
Lois-ellin	Datta	Datta Analysis	Captain Cook
Wendell	Davis		Kailua-Kona
Doreen	DeSilva	The Fairmont Orchid	Kohala Coast
Char	Donat	TEAM Kohala	Kapaau
Fran	Duntz	Kapiolani Child Protection Center	Kailua-Kona

Michael	Ebesugawa	Office of the Public Defender	Hilo
Gloria	Egle	BISAC	Hilo
Leningrad	Elarionoff	County of Hawaii	Hilo
Samuel	Elbertson	Bridgehouse	Kailua-Kona
Marge	Elwell	Naalehu Main Street	Naalehu
Susan	Emerson McCree	DHS/CPS	Kealakekua
Leinaala	Enos	Queen Liliuokalani Children's Ctr.	Naalehu
Les	Estrella	Faith Against Drugs	Hilo
Cindy	Evans	Hawaii State Legislature	Honolulu
Ivan	Faxon	Care Hawaii Inc.	Hilo
Violette	Fedora		Kamuela
Leialoha	Filoteo	Turning Point for Families	Hilo
Joseph	Florendo	Judiciary	Kealakekua
Edwin	Flores	Volunteer Legal Services HI	Honolulu
Michael	Flynn	Health Works Under the Banyan	Hilo
Tara	Flynn	Health Works Under the Banyan	Hilo
Rory	Flynn	County of Hawaii	Hilo
Jim	Fraiser	Police Commission	Kamuela
Edwin	Freitas	County of Hawaii	Hilo
Chiyome	Fukino	Dept. of Health	Honolulu
Debra	Fuller	DOE	Pahoa
Maring	Gacusana	DOE	Pahoa
Joelouie	Genus	Five Mountains Hawaii	Kamuela
Barbara	Gleeson	Care Hawaii Inc.	Kailua-Kona
Gail	Gnazzo	Maui Youth & Family Services	Paia
Farrah-Marie	Gomes	The Catalyst Group, LLC	Honolulu
Robert	Gomes	Kau Rural Health Comm. Assoc.	Pahala
Phoebe	Gomes	Kau Rural Health Comm. Assoc.	Pahala
Tami	Gouveia		Kailua-Kona
Judy	Graham	YWCA	Kamuela
Beverley	Grogan	Mental Health Association	Keaau
Carole	Gruskin	Child and Family Service	Kealakekua
Colleen	Gundaker	Kau Ice Support Group	Naalehu
Pearl	Haili	Panaewa Neighborhood Watch	Hilo
Harold	Hall	Pacific Institute	Kamuela
Eric	Hamakawa	Hawaii State Legislature	Honolulu
Elizabeth	Hannah	DHS/CPS	Kailua-Kona
Sharon K.	Hassard	Faith Against Drugs	Hilo
Nancy	Hayes	DOE	Honokaa
Kevin	Hedlund	BISAC	Hilo
Pete	Hendricks	County of Hawaii	Kailua-Kona
Thomas	Hickcox	County of Hawaii	Hilo
Robert	Hickcox	County of Hawaii	Hilo
Zachary	Higa	Judiciary	Hilo
Peggy	Hilton	DHS	Hilo
Cyd	Hoffield	Bay Clinic	Hilo
Peter	Hoffman	Waikoloa Village Assn.	Waikoloa
Patricia	Hoffman	YMCA	Kailua-Kona
Tom	Hohler	VS Web Design	Kailua-Kona
Fred	Holschuh	County of Hawaii	Hilo
Brian	Hyatt	DASH	Hilo
Fred	Hyun	Dept. of Public Safety	Hilo
Josephine	Ibarra		Hilo
Earl	Ikeda	Puna/Kau Hongwanji	Keaau

Lorraine	Inouye	Hawaii State Legislature	Hilo
Beryl	Iramina	Dept. of Public Safety	Hilo
Wallace A.	Ishibashi	ILWU Local 142	Hilo
Mark	Ishiki	Hawaii National Guard	Honolulu
Bob	Jacobson	County of Hawaii	Hilo
Debra	Javar	Ka'u Hospital	Naalehu
Mark	Jernigan	Hawaii State Legislature	Honolulu
Alvin	Jitchaku	The Salvation Army	Hilo
Luana	Jones	Native Hawaiian Ed. Council	Pahoa
Thomas	Kaaiai	Pac. Resources for Ed. & Learning	Honolulu
Dixie	Kaetsu	County of Hawaii	Hilo
Rita	Kahalioumi	Judiciary	Kealakekua
Kalani	Kahalioumi	Pulama Project	Hilo
Maxine	Kahaulelio	Power of Choice, Waimea	Kamuela
Kelii	Kahele	Bay Clinic	Hilo
Jackie	Kalani	DHS/CWS	Captain Cook
Daniel	Kama	HICAC	Mt. View
Rhonda	Kamai-Kekela	Hui Malama Ola Na Oiwi	Keaau
Maile	Kanemaru	Weed & Seed	Honolulu
D. Lei	Kapono	Hawaii Community College	Hilo
Candace	Kauahi		
Dean	Kauka	Imiola Church	Kamuela
Mel	Kawahara	Judiciary	Hilo
Eric	Kawamoto	DLNR/DOCARE	Hilo
Darin	Kawazoe	Office of the Lieutenant Governor	Honolulu
Norman	Keamo	County of Hawaii	Hilo
Jonah	Kelekolio	Alu Like Inc.	Hilo
Nancy	Kelly	County of Hawaii	Hilo
Maggie	Kelly	Alcholics Anonymous	Kailua-Kona
Harry	Kepa'a	Bay Clinic	Hilo
Miulan	Kia	Panaewa Neighborhood Watch	Kurtistown
Ashley	Kierkiewicz	St. Joseph High School	Hilo
Richard	Kim	The Catalyst Group, LLC	Honolulu
Jay	Kimura	County of Hawaii	Hilo
Guy	Kitaoka	Judiciary	Kailua-Kona
Lari	Koga	Dept. of the Attorney General	Honolulu
Russell	Kokubun	Hawaii State Legislature	Honolulu
Midori	Kondo	Hilo Betsuin	Hilo
Robin	Krueger	DOE	Kapaau
Kevin	Kunz, M.D.	Kona Addictions Services	Kailua-Kona
Janet	Lang	Child & Family Service	Hilo
Wally	Lau	Neigborhood Place of Kona	Kailua-Kona
Andrew	Levin	County of Hawaii	Hilo
Randal	Like		Pahoa
Pat	Linton	Five Mountains Hawaii	Kamuela
Frank J.	Lopez	Dept. of Public Safety	Honolulu
Bill	Lucas	Kau Rural Health Comm. Assoc.	Ocean View
LaVerne	Lucero	Bay Clinic	Hilo
Donald	Lupien	Access Capabilities, Inc.	Kailua-Kona
Catherine	Luthe	Hamakua Health Center	Honokaa
Rodney	Maeda	Judiciary	Kailua-Kona
Valerie	Mariano	Dept. of the Attorney General	Honolulu
Aimee	Marquardt	Recovering Adict	Kealakekua
Jessanie	Marques	Kau Rural Health Comm. Assn.	Pahala

Trinidad	Marques	Kau Rural Health Comm. Assoc.	Pahala
David	Marquez	Kealakehe Ahupua'a 2020, Inc.	Kailua-Kona
Jan	Marrack	Family Support Svcs. West HI	Kamuela
Margaret	Masunaga	County of Hawaii	Kealakekua
Manuel S.	Mattos	Pahoa Sacred Heart Church	Keaau
Mark	McGuffie	King Kamehameha Kona Beach	Kailua-Kona
Charlene N.	Merritt	DASH	Hilo
William	Meyers	BISAC	Hilo
Aolani	Mills	Judiciary	Kealakekua
Eleanor	Mirakitani	Waikoloa Land Co.	Waikoloa
Corinne	Miyazu	Judiciary	Hilo
Melissa	Moniz	Keaukaha Community Assoc.	Hilo
Alice	Moon	DVIAT	Hilo
Ipo	Morgan	BISAC	Hilo
Lonnie	Morgan	BISAC	Hilo
Liane	Moriyama	Dept. of the Attorney General	Honolulu
Nancy	Moser	YWCA	Hilo
Kalani	Motta	DHS	Hilo
Jackie	Murai	Judiciary	Hilo
Wil	Murakami	DOE	Kailua-Kona
Irene	Nagao	Business Education Partnership	Hilo
Abbie	Napeahi	Alu Like Inc.	Hilo
Jeani	Navarro	Kalopa Enterprises, Inc.	Honokaa
Keith	Nealy	Earl Bakken Foundation	Hawi
Roy	Nishida	Kauai Mayor's Office	Lihue
Tamah-Lani	Noh	Hawaii National Guard	Honolulu
Clayrsse	Nunokawa	Hawaii Community Foundation	Honolulu
Darryl	Oliveira	County of Hawaii	Hilo
Jeannette	Oliver	Five Mountains Hawaii	Kamuela
Jon	Olson	Puna Traffic Safety Council	Pahoa
Stanton C.	Oshiro		Hilo
Ida	Otake	TEAM Kohala	Kapaau
Wendell	Paiva	County of Hawaii	Hilo
Alan	Parker	County of Hawaii	Hilo
Steven	Pavao	Boys & Girls Club Big Island	Hilo
Andi	Pawasarat	Bridgehouse	Kailua-Kona
Howard	Pe'a	Alu Like Inc.	Hilo
Cecilia	Poblete	Power of Choice	Kamuela
Valeria	Poindexter	Ookala Comm. Dev. Corp	Ookala
Regina	Purinton	PARENTS, Inc.	Hilo
Steven	Querobin	AFL-CIO	Hilo
Noelani	Quihano	DOE	Pahoa
John	Ray	Hawaii Leeward Planning Conf.	Kamuela
Larry	Reichner	DEA	Honolulu
Alvin	Rho	DOE	Kailua-Kona
Monty	Richards	Kahua Ranch	Kamuela
Laurie Jo	Rogers	Waikoloa Comm. Action Group	Waikoloa
Gordon	Roque	Waikoloa Land Co.	Waikoloa
Mitch	Roth	County of Hawaii	Hilo
Eric	Rouelle	The Fairmont Orchid	Kawaihae
Donna J.	Ruden	The Salvation Army	Kailua-Kona
Gary	Safarik	County of Hawaii	Hilo
Jann	Saiki-Morimoto	Judiciary	Kailua-Kona
Karen	Sakoda	Big Island Visitors Bureau	Hilo

Jose	Salinas	The Fairmont Orchid	Kohala Coast
Dorene	Santangelo		Keaau
John	Santangelo		Keaau
Jan	Sears	Waikoloa Comm. Action Group	Waikoloa
Donni	Sheather	State Incentive Grant	Kamuela
Gary	Shimabukuro	Laulima Hawaii	Honolulu
Julian	Shiroma	County of Hawaii	Hilo
Shawn	Slater	DOE	Pahoa
Kehau	Sloan	Keaau Community Coalition	Keaau
Andy	Smith	Governor's Liaison-East Hawaii	Hilo
Richard	Smith	Simple Office Solutions	Kailua-Kona
Janet	Snyder	County of Hawaii	Hilo
Rueben	Soriano	Judiciary	Hilo
Mary	Souza	The Fairmont Orchid	Waikoloa
Danielle	Spain	BISAC	Hilo
Michael	Spain	BISAC	Hilo
Angela	Spiegelman	TEAM Kohala	Hawi
Glenda	Sugi	Judiciary	Kealakekua
Nani	Svendsen	TEAM Kohala	Hawi
Deborah J.	Swanson	Waikoloa Village Assoc.	Waikoloa
Sandra	Takamine	DOE	Hilo
Kelvin	Taketa	Hawaii Community Foundation	Honolulu
Sandra	Taosaka	DOE	Kealakekua
Phyllis	Tarail		Kukuihaele
Cheryl	Taupu	Bridgehouse	Kailua-Kona
Lawrence	Terlep, Jr.	DLNR/DOCARE	Hilo
Angela	Thomas	Good Beginnings Alliance	Kamuela
Chris	Tolley	DEA	Honolulu
Alvin	Tuifagu	Bridgehouse	Kailua-Kona
Reginald	Une	Dept. of Public Safety	Hilo
Christine	Van Bergeijk	Hawaii Community Foundation	Honolulu
Thomas	Varese		Hilo
Jill	Vasconcellos	Hui Malama Ola Na Oiwi	Capt. Cook
Matilda	Vradenburg	Waikoloa Church Youth Ministries	Waikoloa
Eileen	Wagatsuma	DOE	Hilo
Lynn	Walton	Kona Community Hospital	Kealakekua
Deborah J.	Ward	4-H Youth Development Program	Hilo
Jamal	Wasan	Waikoloa Comm. Rehab Program	Waikoloa
Richard	West	HIEDB	Hilo
Mary Jo	Westmoreland	Kapiolani Child Protection Center	Kailua-Kona
Elaine	Wilson	Dept. of Health	Kapolei
Lee	Wilson	Verizon	Hilo
Dean	Yamamoto	Dept. of Public Safety	Honolulu
Leah	Yanagi	County of Hawaii	Hilo
Lynn	Yokoyama	Big Island Public Center	Hilo
Gary	Yoshiyama	HGEA	Hilo
Joydee	Young	DASH	Hilo

THE HAWAI'I ISLAND METH SUMMIT 2
August 25, 2003
Waikoloa Marriott

GROUP RESULTS

There were 9 sectors with a total of 16 groups:

a. Legislators
b. Prevention and Education
c. Faith-based
d. Community
e. Business
f. Treatment
g. Social Services
h. Law Enforcement
i. Judiciary

The question posed to the groups was "Based on what you have heard today and what you know about the drug problem on the Big Island, what challenges face YOUR SECTOR and what are you willing to do about it?" To obtain a list of challenges, affinity charting was used where each group brainstormed challenges, clustered like ideas, named each cluster of challenges and voted for the top 2 priority challenges. The challenges are listed in order of priority.

Starting with the top priority, each group was then asked "What are you willing to do about this challenge facing your sector?" Action steps were then solicited using the "who is going to do what by when" process.

GROUP 1 – LEGISLATORS

CHALLENGES

1. Financial Resources – 9 votes
   - Funding for treatment
   - Funds to help the drug program
   - More money to develop and maintain facility
   - Tracing the money
   - Funding
   - Public health nursing funding
2. Programs – 8 votes
   - For the kids
   - More recreational possibilities
   - Inadequate treatment facilities
   - Mid-elementary school awareness program

3. Law enforcement – 3 votes
   - Enforcement maintaining rights
   - Create new laws from summit recommendations
   - Importation of ice from California and elsewhere via air cargo, mail, harbors (no searches)
   - Amending criminal laws
   - Change existing statutes that will conform to Federal law
4. Economic development – 2 votes
   - Need for jobs
   - Economy
   - Bring in clean industry
5. Strategy – 2 votes
   - Agreeing on priorities
   - Develop consensus priorities
   - Community accessible information system
   - Assessing program effectiveness
   - Unwilling to try new things
   - Coordinate the Hawaii Drug Control Strategy Summit
   - Write the Hawaii Drug Control Strategy: A New Beginning

ACTION STEPS

1. Financial resources
   - A. By 12/31/03, Lorraine Inouye will follow up regarding SB 1305 and all other bills relating to drugs to assure release of funding from the Governor for those programs such as substance abuse, domestic violence, etc.
   - B. By 03/31/04, Eric Hamakawa will consider an amendment to the statute regarding adults selling drugs to minors. The amendment will include a financial penalty.
   - C. By 12/31/03, Melodie Aduja (State Legislature) and Fred Holschuh (County Council) will follow up with congressional delegation regarding increase or continuation of federal funds.
   - D. On an ongoing basis, Andy Levin will lobby State Legislature for more treatment funding.
   - E. By 01/31/04, Lorraine Inouye will introduce a bill to use Tobacco Funds and/or cigarette tax to fund ice programs to guarantee sustainability.
   - F. By the end of today, Fred Holschuh will speak with Dr. Fukino, DOH Director, on increase Public Health Nursing funding to do preconception counseling.
   - G. On an ongoing basis, Leningrad Elarionoff will seek private funding.
   - H. On an ongoing basis, State and County Legislative Auditors will monitor spending of funds appropriated for specific districts for program effectiveness.
   - I. By 01/31/04, Lorraine Inouye will introduce a bill to codify Public Health Nursing into the Hawaii Revised Statutes.
   - J. On an ongoing basis, Rory Flynn will follow up with the County Dept. of Transportation regarding Federal DOT funds.

2. Programs
   A. By 9/30/03, Fred Holschuh will follow up with Billy Kenoi regarding Federal monies so all areas get their allocation to extend County programs and he will also follow up with County Parks & Recreation.
   B. On an ongoing basis, Leningrad Elarionoff will encourage his community to participate in programs.
   C. By 11/30/03, Cindy Evans will approach the Dept. of Education superintendent and Legislature Education chair to integrate drug education awareness programs to each grade level.
   D. By 9/30/03, Fred Holschuh will ask Billy Kenoi for a Council briefing on summit follow up.
   E. On an ongoing basis, Fred Holschuh will lobby County Council regarding County grantees having a drug crisis intervention as part of their program.
   F. On an ongoing basis, Rory Flynn and Fred Holschuh will develop a way to monitor the effectiveness of initiatives.
3. Law enforcement
   A. By 12/31/03, Lorraine Inouye will follow up with Ed Kubo on a constitutional amendment regarding walk and talk and wiretapping.
   B. By 12/31/03, Lorraine Inouye will work with Ed Kubo on how our laws relate to all incidences regarding reporting ice use, dealing ice, etc.
   C. By 12/31/03, Lorraine Inouye will follow up with Ed Kubo regarding his statement on "threshold" (amount of substance).

GROUP 2 – PREVENTION/EDUCATION

CHALLENGES

1. Lack of awareness of the problem and a need to increase the information presented in the schools, willing to risk bringing in information – 8 votes
2. Expand services to retain students
3. Increase caretaker/parent involvement at home and school
4. Retain cultural relevance to all stakeholders – 3 votes
5. Replace "No Drugs" with positive community activities and messages from media
6. Building trust between educators and students
7. Schools need to be ready to collaborate with community efforts (top down willlingness) – 2 votes
8. Community building, getting commitment – 2 votes
9. K-12 drug prevention curriculum – 1 vote
10. Foster homes/therapeutic homes for "learning ready" students with a liaison to addicted parent – 1 vote
11. Faith-based working partnership with schools
12. Special education is "dumping ground" for education to the detriment of LD kids
13. Teachers need better specific strategies to work with these kids and families
14. Interaction of teachers with sober addicts to gain understanding
15. How the community can formulate positive message by increasing activities, drug free environments, etc. – 1 vote
16. Increase parent component of reading, home visits, newsletters – 3 votes
17. Schools cannot do it all
18. Drug testing would also require increase in treatment programs – 2 votes
19. Drug testing is controversial
20. Events need to include whole community – 2 votes
21. Need to hear more from recovering people
22. Identify student and offer increased options within the school system to retain them in school – 3 votes
23. Confidentiality issues can be a challenge
24. Re-empowering parents – 1 vote
25. What if parents are the users?

ACTION STEPS

1. Lack of awareness of the problem and a need to increase the information presented in the schools.
   A. Breaking ice video in production for use by teachers on their own schedule – Family Support Service/CRI by November 2003
   B. Find presenters to come to educate teachers how to recognize and handle drug problems – BISAC, MD, CRI, Gary Shimabukuro, NA presentations, school principals by October 2003
   C. Target counselors for education first so they can help student and family – District office, complex superintendents
   D. Find or develop grade appropriate drug education – SRS, PE dept. heads, Kam Schools, health resource teachers, Alu Like, current, on-going

2. Expand services to retain students
   A. Same actions steps as #1
3. To increase parent/caretaker involvement at home and school
   A. Make educational sessions convenient for families
4. To replace "No Drugs" with positive community activities and positive messages in the media
   A. Emphasize after-school, free activities from 3-7 p.m. – RFPs for 501(c)(3)'s
   B. Actively support community efforts

GROUP 3 – PREVENTION/EDUCATION

CHALLENGES

1. Lack of community resources to deal with substance abuse treatment and intervention – 12
   - Big problem, limited resources
   - Voluntary evaluation, participation
   - Need more time
2. Lack of education regarding substance abuse – 12 votes
   - Develop curriculum
   - Drug education
   - To provide quality and effective drug education (prevention) to our schools
   - Pregnancy education
   - Consistent, relevant education
   - Poor parenting skills
   - Positive education
   - Lack of time to share information with teachers and try to motivate them to implement
   - Finding trained instructors
   - Substance abuse counselors need higher education to deal with ice
   - Not enough personnel trained in substance abuse
   - Encourage more CSACs in non-profits
3. No youth treatment – 6 votes
   - Residential treatment for youth
   - Help kids directly
   - Support youth residential
   - Organize youth groups
   - Join with like-minded people
4. Personal intervention needs for further support – 5 votes
   - Family project sessions
   - Continuous support groups for recovering addicts
   - Sponsor newcomers (CMA addicts)
5. Privacy as barrier – 1 vote
   - Parental consent

ACTION STEPS

1. Lack of community resources to deal with substance abuse and intervention
   A. Continue to provide information to community in newspaper
   B. Share accurate, current information
      - justice system, Feds
      - support groups
      - web sites to other media resources
      - CRI, Billy Kenoi
      - look at community needs
      - CRI directory in East and West Hawaii media

-

C. Develop ways for awareness to happen
   - use resource booklet e.g. Waimea Power of Choice, Kona Neighborhood Place, blue flier
   - work proactively with teens
   - DOE identify resource distribution of services
   - Sept. '03 Counselor training
   - Care Hawaii Inc. Office # 326-2283
   - Kealakehe High School – Sandy Daniels help teachers implement health standards in classroom
   - Debra Fuller will develop a resource booklet for East Hawaii

D. Develop community-based outreach programs

E. Establish a sustainable protocol for recovering users
   - develop guidelines
   - find help at AA, NA and other programs that have recovery steps for addicts

F. Get involved in community response to ice

2. Lack of education relating to substance abuse

A. Train more personnel in substance abuse

B. Encourage more CSACs in non profit organizations. – 4000 hours of direct services needs to apply to take test

C. Involve more local residents

GROUP 4 – FAITH-BASED ORGANIZATIONS

CHALLENGES

1. Congregation awareness – 11 votes
   - Consistent, relevant education
   - Getting members of congregation involved outside our church
   - Educate and provide service opportunities
   - Personal and group awareness through education
   - Real awareness
   - Education, rehabilitation, prevention
   - Outreach through written and spoken messages
   - Educating faith communities
   - More treatment centers
   - Share my experience, strengths and hope in meetings
   - Motivating those active in the disease
2. Utilization of faith-based organizations – 10 votes
   - Church = multitudinal resource
   - Availability for help
   - How to mobilize community volunteers
   - Get churches involved
   - Continue to serve
   - No specific program in the church for addict
3. Youth activities, center – 5 votes
   - Youth activities
   - Inform youth and parents
   - Youth activity center
   - Youth facility
4. County collaboration – 4 votes
   - County relationships, networking
   - Unorganized in resources
   - County red tape
5. Honor the individual, especially the addict – 2 votes
   - Prohibitionist mentality
   - The community needs to reach out to ice addicts
   - Accepting addicting persons – fear, ignorance by parishioners, fear of condemnation by addicts
   - Respect each other
   - Demonstrate openness

ACTION STEPS

1. Congregation awareness
   A. Educational materials
   B. Testimonies, speakers
   C. Workshops
   D. Advise of dangers, i.e. theft of tools of mentors
   E. Start with capacity building of board members of church by getting on agenda of next board meeting and continue at other meetings. Go to church business meetings to present ideas.

F. Pastors, elders, and church member representative of a community (interfaith) meet regularly to discuss problem to reach community. Work together as one. Faith Against Drugs.
G. Report of results of Meth Summit through faith web-site is being worked on
H. Educate churches on how they can help to decrease their fears
I. Educate church members, policy makers, clergy about the problem – what is the problem, who are the abusers, how you can help, whole recovery process is using spiritual strengths
J. Find out what other churches are doing – get a list of services "Faith Against Drugs"
K. Get testimony from abusers after church is accepting. It takes an addict to accept an addict. Identify abusers and involve them in leadership.
L. Bahai has holy book – addiction is a substitute for spirituality. Welcome beacon-safe haven

2. Utilization of faith-based services
A. Introduce to country living – learn about God & nature
B. Exercise class – body tempo maintenance
C. Live foods health workshop and eventually motivate person to recovery to lead classes
D. Participation from church to help person find a job, advocate for them, i.e. take to appointments. Give hope & support to increase self confidence
E. Go to <u>all</u> churches to learn what are programs in place now
F. Survey congregation to find what skills they have that they can share and teach
G. List resources of all churches & accessible to everyone
H. Trained Baha'i youth workshop that can go into community and reaches youth with presentation, i.e. social issues like abuse, addiction
I. Create recovery ministries within the church
J. 12 step Christ-centered regeneration meetings: evaluates people and their needs, including Ohana
K. Be speaker on radio, luncheons-share what you are doing
L. Faith-based model is first place to give forgiveness & amnesty to ice user without condoning the use
M. Meet their daily needs: clothing, shelter, provide transportation
N. Immediate response to children, i.e. CPS involved
O. Contact people:
   - Healthworks, Under the Banyan, Michael/Tara Flynn – 934-7837
   - Les Estrella, Faith Against Drugs – 934-7852
   - Roger Christie – 961-0488
   - JC Posse, Outreach Ministry of New Hope Keaukaha – 936-8015 (h), 981-0747(b)
   - Antonio/Juanita Carrisal, Baha'i Faith South Kohala – 883-8584

GROUP 5 – COMMUNITY

CHALLENGES

1. Community apathy/non-involvement – 14 votes
   - Community communication
   - Community participation
   - Lack of values
   - Public awareness and involvement
   - Denial/apathy
   - Show your aloha
   - Non participation
   - Lack of awareness
   - Must get involved
   - Shame factor in getting help
   - Increased criminal activity
   - Help eliminate source
   - Parent/family involvement
   - Saving our youth
2. Education – 10 votes
   - Saving our youth
   - Promote cultural connectivity
   - Comprehensive education in schools
   - What to do
   - People are uneducated
   - Trainable work force retention sustaining effort

ACTION STEPS

1. Community apathy/non-involvement
   A. Involving County Parks for youth-based activities
   B. Contacting community and getting them involved
   C. Getting youth involved to get their parents involved
   D. Educate NIMBY
   E. Work on community needs/interests that keys on prevention
   F. Partnering with government to restructure P&R system to meet community needs – community facilities not available to community for free
   G. Keeping parks/recreational areas alcohol-free
   H. Hosting alcohol-free events for families
   I. More immediate government involvement
   J. Stay committed to challenges
   K. Assessment of existing facilities
2. Education
   A. Communication through newsletters and various readily available media
   B. K-12 drug curriculum
   C. Youth involvement in drug education
   D. Government should have a drug policy master plan
   E. Drug "ice" education for teachers
   F. Parent education through coalitions, unions, work site/business
   G. School-wide drug education working with student/faculty using lots of visuals
   H. Rebuilding values

GROUP 6 – COMMUNITY

CHALLENGES

1. Youth activities – 10 votes
   - Community center
   - Teen activities
   - Work with children in church
   - Youth opportunity
   - Create positive leisure atmosphere for youth
   - Increase amount of school activities for youth
   - Youth activities/transportation
   - Activities for kids after-school/summer
2. Community mobilization – 9 votes
   - Drug traffic intelligence gathering
   - Community organization
   - Community drug (ice) awareness
   - Community mobilization
   - Ice scare media campaign targeting youth
   - Find a trained coordinator to direct community resources against drugs
3. Education – 6 votes
   - Leadership training
   - Parenting classes
   - Substance abuse education at 4th-5th grades
   - Substance abuse advocacy training
   - Educate families about ways to help a loved one who is using
4. Transportation – 3 votes
   - Hele-on transportation for youth of rural areas
   - Transportation to existing programs for kids
   - Transportation to treatment

ACTION STEPS

1. Youth activities
   A. Youth center – infrastructure and staff
   B. Using existing P&R facilities
   C. Partner and network
   D. Identify individuals/resources in each community
   E. Involve youth in community meetings, faith-based and school programs
   F. Mentoring
2. Community mobilization
   A. Community organizing
   B. Drug awareness
   C. Medical/physical complications
   D. Positive action
   E. Leadership training – process oriented
   F. Block watch
   G. Partnering with County, State, non-profit, non-govt., faith
   H. HIRHA will educate on legislative process by December

I. Waikoloa will network with other partners to develop a skateboard park in conjunction with community center by December
J. 4-H is willing to share education curriculum on an ongoing basis
K. Hilo Wooden Boat does sailing, building, education
L. Hilo Youth Center will partner with faith-based organization for youth activities, involving drug prevention
M. YWCA Hilo will start prevention education for middle school girls in January
N. Waikoloa Neighborhood Pot Luck to be held with an education program
O. North Hawaii Community Learning Center will do youth mentoring
P. County mentoring – network together to get additional money
Q. Establish a newsletter/email/communication network – request County to provide the list of attendees
R. Ka'u Resource Center and Distance Learning has wellness program (HEROS), education and prevention programs

GROUP 7 – COMMUNITY

CHALLENGES

1. Lack of community accountability/involvement – 9 votes
   - General social acceptance of drug use/abuse
   - Awareness of the problem
   - Close relatives don't want to turn him/her in
   - Community involvement
   - Unwilling to be involved/fear of involvement
   - Lack of volunteer support
   - Changing prevailing attitudes
   - Participation of community
   - Personal ownership
   - Motivation of community members to be involved
2. Treatment and rehabilitation – 8 votes
   - Lack of on-island treatment
   - Adolescent treatment
   - Treatment within our community
   - Detox
   - Lack of safe homes
   - More programs to help parents deal with child who comes out of treatment
3. Transportation – 6 votes
   - Transportation for young people
   - Transportation for recovering addicts
4. Lack of supportive community programs – 6 votes
   - Lack of intervention resources
   - Lack of foster homes
   - Knowing what works
   - Youth centers
   - Capacity building
   - Melding the haves with the have-nots to empower themselves
   - Instituting "culturally sensitive" education programs
   - Getting fun activities and curricula to out of school care providers, volunteers, mentors and how do we get kids to come
   - Need park development/skateboard park
5. Lack of media coverage/resources – 6 votes
   - Not enough media
   - Media/communication
   - Getting message out!
6. Economic development – 5 votes
   - Economy/employment
   - Need economic development/large certified kitchen
7. Funding – 1 vote
   - Funding – seek more Federal funding
8. Lack of law enforcement – 1 vote
   - Lack of law enforcement

ACTION STEPS

1. Lack of community accountability/involvement
   A. Educate the community about ice through regular community meetings:
   - Melissa (Keaukaha) will schedule periodic meetings by 9/1
   - Ka'u partners (38 organizations) scheduling community education. Next one is on 10/15. Ongoing weekly meetings
   - Kea'au have recovering addicts testimony outreach (Ka'u, Keaukaha)
   - www.hawaiicounty resource – Angela to contact Karin at West Hawaii,Hawaii Tribune Herald and Laura Dierenfield at North Hawaii News by 8/26 to make sure website is publicized

   B. By 8/31/03, Team Kohala to contact all newspapers on-island to see how a weekly space can be donated/dedicated to community "ice" updates

   C. By the end of today, Angela will speak with faith-based community in attendance at summit to ask if they would speak to their congregations to increase awareness
   - Clergy to discuss/network at their meetings to strategize message to get out
   - Ask clergy to approach their congregation (bulletins and verbally) with a message to include resources, Hawai'i County web-sites, phone numbers for vice, hotline)
   - Prosecutor's office pulling together list of all faiths in East Hawaii to form a coalition and educate them. Pat, Sidney and Aloha to polist list by 9/30/03. Product will be out by the end of the year. Melissa and Aloha part of planning process which is happening now

   D. Make a list of "5" simple things that everyone can do to get involved:
   - Attend community education programs and bring your kids, friends, colleagues
   - Make signs with your kids for "sign waving" (i.e. this is a "drug-free house"). Option to put it in your yard.
   - Be a Hero – work with your police dept. Call the anonymous vice hotline if you know of an ice house/dealer
   - Support your State and County representatives
   - Talk to your kids about ice
   - Talk to your friends and have them pass on the ice awareness message
   - Walk the talk
   - Befriend a child outside of your family/volunteer to be a mentor
   - Support someone coming out of recovery, make an extra effort to support their recovery
   - Form/start/join a neighborhood watch group

GROUP 8 – BUSINESS

CHALLENGES

1. Education/awareness – 14 votes
   - Close knit family (in same business) hesitate to report on each other
   - Lack of focus/awareness for collective campaign for educational programs for businesses, i.e. stronger approach collectively
   - Lack of knowledge on how bad the problem is and how it affects businesses
   - Treat as illness, not punitive
   - Lack of ability to provide information, confidentiality barrier (unions)
   - Workplace attitude
   - Affect those in poverty and those with jobs (no distinction on class)
   - "Drug business" established in businesses
   - Lack of education, connect with police
   - As a high profile person, resources to tap into but probem kept secret and allows addicted persons access to tangible items
2. Coordination/collaboration – 10 votes
   - Lack of focus/awareness for collective campaign for educational programs for businesses, i.e. stronger approach collectively
   - Lack of cohesive campaign
   - Lack of coordination
   - Union and business (small and big) share in solution
3. Limited resources – 5 votes
   - Increasing difficulty in finding dependable employees
   - Rising cost of medical services
   - Limited resources, looking for ways after aware of problem to create answers
   - Insurance coverage doesn't adequately cover treatment program
   - Treatment program not in place
   - Don't have individual resources, union and businesses need to work together
   - Employers have problems, no tools. Unions have problems, also no tools
   - Economic problem/education problem, not individualized problem
   - Lack of police
4. Security/safety – 3 votes
   - Security, loss of product, theft
   - Tentativeness businesses have about bringing people with drug problems into their establishment (liability and risk), new and current employees
   - Street use/drug abuse has negative effect on business environment
   - Verbal abuse of staff from the public on drugs
   - "Drug business" established in businesses
   - Lack of police
5. Legal issues (perplexity) – 2 votes
   - Liability, work loss, absenteeism, quality of work
   - What can you ask a prospective employee? Drug test? Ask if they have substance abuse problem?
   - Lack of ability to provide information, confidentiality barrier (unions)

6. Programs – 0 votes
   - Treatment program not in place
7. Root causes = lack of jobs, education, economy – 0 votes

ACTION STEPS

1. Address education and awareness through collaboration and coordination
   A. Mary will create a list of those agencies that need volunteers and put up on healing our island web-site
   B. Fairmont Orchid will host a Health Education Awareness Campaign in 2004
   C. Fairmont Orchid will take advantage of educational resources such as: HCPD, Mayor's office, BISAC, Kahua 'Oihana and national unions
   D. Businesses/unions will encourage participation and/or support of community organizations
   E. Become personally educated
   F. John S. will hire more people with drug addiction problems in collaboration with others (agencies) and with increased education
   G. Gary Y. (HGEA) will increase awareness of what resources are available and coordinate with agencies in contact with ice, i.e. WIB, County level, etc.
   H. Lee of BISAC will initiate and coordinate a "Business Task Force" umbrella campaign
   I. Identify legislation to deal with issues affecting employers/employees and campaign for legislation
   J. Hawaii Leadership Series – community service component: 1/3 of group will be "hands-on" activity relative to ice use
   K. Work with labor for better drug policy for employees/employers
   L. Assist "marketer" with educational awareness (island-wide educational campaign)
   M. Big Island Women in Travel will take information back (1st step awareness program), i.e. B. Kenoi for them to then share with others

GROUP 9 – LAW ENFORCEMENT

CHALLENGES

1. Education/training – 18 votes
   - Double standards/other drugs
   - Community understanding of roles of law enforcement
   - How to identify use
   - Educating youth on drug prevention
   - Educating public on dangers of ice
   - Educating local law enforcement
   - Get associations/organizations involved
   - Participate in educating community
   - Requiring drug education in public schools
2. Legislation – 17 votes
   - New medical privacy law as barrier to effective treatment
   - Inability to use existing wiretap law
   - Hawaii Constitution is more liberal than U.S. Constitution which in turn gives criminals more rights
   - Major state constitutional amendments to bring parity between Feds and State to assist law enforcement
   - Increase effectiveness of law enforcement through legislative action to improve Walk and Talk, Knock and Talk, and Title III law
   - Making sense of all the community information on drug use, look for software tools to analyze information
3. Funding – 16 votes
   - Lack of manpower
   - Funding to support programs
   - Increase in manpower
   - Manpower to support enforcement efforts
   - Lack treatment services on neighbor islands
   - Additional funding by Federal govt. for educational programs
   - Letters to Congress lobbying for financial assistance for drug programs
   - Heavy caseload for probation and parole officers of substance abusers
   - Reduce property crimes committed by drug addicts
   - Lack of prosecutors focused only on high level drug defendents/organizations
   - Not enough people on my staff
4. Coordinated law enforcement – 10 votes
   - Supervision of enforcement activities from distance
   - Coordinating enforcement efforts between County/State/Federal agencies
   - Coordination of a planned law enforcement response
5. Criminal justice/public information – 7 votes
   - Accurate information for public
   - Id drug-related arrests in CJ system
   - Quick ID of offenders and past drug history
   - Provide support services (info, stats, arrest processing) to law enforcement
   - Reporting between govt. agencies, confidentiality problem
   - More emphasis in drug investigation involving ice

6. Treatment – 5 votes
   - Insurance coverage for △'s
   - Lack of treatment facilities, resources
   - Finding and providing effective treatment for offenders
   - Eliminate the combination of alcohol and drugs
7. Geography – 1 vote
   - Most of my staff on Oahu
8. Prison – 1 vote
   - Jail overcrowding
   - Increase in incarcerated population
   - Staff involvement in bringing in drugs
9. Community – 1 vote
   - Recruiting community-based individuals to mobilize to address the drug problem
   - Sustaining community involvement
   - Addressing community complaints with limited manpower
   - Lack of sufficient manpower in certain enforcement situations due to legal limitations by State courts
10. Assessment – 0 vote
    - Assessment of agency ability to address challenges

ACTION STEPS

1. Education/training
   A. By November 2003, Margaret will have Hawaii State Bar Assn. provide information in public schools
   B. By December 2003, Margaret and the Hawaii State Commission of the Status of Women will initiate a mentoring program
   C. By December 31, 2003, Mitch/DEA/PA will develop a Powerpoint presentation on the roles of law enforcement, State vs. Federal and provide presentation to Dept. of Education and Legislature
   D. By January 2004, Val from the AG office will provide community mobilization training on grant programs
   E. Ongoing, Larry and HIDTA will provide monthly local law enforcement training on the Big Island
   F. Ongoing, Norman and Bob from HPD will educate the community on the roles of law enforcement and public dangers of ice
   G. Jay and HIDTA will research software to analyze information and exchange information to law enforcement and community
   H. By August 2004, Charles will encourage all Pop Warner football coaches to attend drug seminar
2. Legislation
   A. By December 2003, Mitch/DEA/PA will develop a Powerpoint presentation on the roles of law enforcement, State vs. Federal and provide presentation to Legislature
   B. By August 2004, Jay K./LE coalition introduce major State Constitution amendments on differences between State and Federal laws
   C. In September 2003, HIDTA/AG/U.S. Attorney will attend a State Drug Summit and will address major State/Federal laws, medical privacy, increase effectiveness of law enforcement, change wiretap laws, too liberal Hawaii State Constitution

GROUP 10 – TREATMENT

CHALLENGES

1. Government – 5 votes
   - Lack of and need for government leadership in providing legislation for parity treatment/benefits for substance abuse/mental health
   - Government restraints keep investments away from ownership – no permanent facilities, mortgage on facilities not allowed by Feds
   - Insurance limits
2. Need for treatment facilities – 5 votes
   - Homes for the programs
   - Not enough treatment facilities
   - Need for adolescent centers in-patient and out-patient
   - Lack of resources
3. Family/community – 3 votes
   - Intervention with family, parent/family involvement
   - Loss of cultural values
   - Stigma and family denial about "private" problems
   - Needing more support for cultural aspect of the communities and ohana I work with
   - Youth lack of identity, spiritual emptiness
   - Community involvement
   - Fostering family involvement
   - Changing environment of home/community
4. Continuing after care – 2 votes
   - After care for adolescents, pre,during and post treatment
   - Transitioning after treatment
5. Funding – 1 vote
   - Long term stable funding
   - Limited function
   - Assistance in identifying and obtaining govt. funding
   - Lack of sufficient youth services
   - Accessibility to treatment
6. Vision/future – 0 votes
   - Need for children to become competent and expect a good future

ACTION STEPS

1. Government
   A. Kat Bradley will introduce bills, keep in touch with her, get phone number from 5 Mountains
   B. Brief legislators, take Kevin to educate them in joint session, in town rally
   C. Candice will represent groups' priority at 9/4 Waikoloa
   D. Lobbying, call/write letters, encourage public lobbying efforts
   E. Get legislator to introduce/reintroduce bill
   F. Ask Senator Russell Kokubun and Rep. Hamakawa to sponsor bill
   G. Open letter to the editor asking for parity

2. Need for treatment facility
   A. 2.2 million designated for 13-18 age group facility
   B. Turn drug houses into safe house, find support – faith based, 5 Mountain, 501(c)(3)
   C. Take small steps to realize facilities by:
      - spread the word, identify key people
      - encourage govt. support for facility
      - tap into the diverse cultures
      - make connections/integrate ancient wisdom
      - realize how were all in treatment
   D. Keep being the squeaky wheel –keep…keep..
   E. Tap into Weinberg/other funds
   F. Make sure money goes to treatment facility, not administration
   G. Create coalitions, like North Hawaii Drug-Free Coalition, to have a say in where money goes. Coalitions have more funding oppportunities
   H. Encourage shared use of existing facilities
   I. Keep attending meetings at grassroots level
   J. Take care of ourselves to keep strong and able to serve

GROUP 11 – TREATMENT

CHALLENGES

1. Seamless care
   - Transitional programs
   - Continuing care (seamless)
   - Support services
   - Activities and transportation to them
2. Partnerships
   - Importance of partnerships, separate principles-focus on problem
   - More community involvement
   - Need to fine tune goals between agencies
   - Shrink down goals to meet resources to eliminate burnout
   - Turnstile on DV and ice within criminal justice system
3. Funding
   - Need for on-going/long term funding
   - Grant writing organizations
   - Self sufficiency
4. Access to ice
   - Availability/easy access to ice

ACTION STEPS

1. Create seamless, continuing care-support services for clients in transition
   A. Survey needs/needs assessment - Sandra, Maria and Kalani
   B. Recovering community to share stories, support each other - Kelau and Kalani
   C. Court contact for community service - Sandra and Maria
   D. Identify all support services, i.e. AA, NA, etc. - Harry
   E. Empower families and individuals (i.e. Parent Project through Young Life) – Maria, Sandra
   F. Individualized treatment program/plans – Maria, Sandra thru BISAC
2. Kukakuka – Partnerships
   A. Create a data base, constantly updated – Kalani (email, name)
   B. Communication through talk story/networking – Sandra, Janice, Maria
   C. Share services/referrals - Kalani, LaVerne, Harry, Phyllis, Kaipulani, Kelau, Aunty Myra, Sandra, Maria and Janice
   D. Newsletters, hot line, community board – Harry, Cyd
   E. Participation of clients, their experiences – Kelau
   F. Utilizing existing web sites, i.e. healingourisland.com
   G. Letter writing campaigns to change legislation – Janice
   H. Utilizing existing services/resources

GROUP 12 – TREATMENT

CHALLENGES

1. Community/families – 7 votes
    - Lack of awareness
    - NIMBY – not here!
    - Unwillingness to see it's happening
    - Needs to be included in treatment
    - Needs to know how to help, what treatment is/isn't
    - Foster families need connections with affected families
    - Culturally appropriate
2. More residential facilities – 6 votes
    - Need $$$
    - Where put 'em
    - Lack trained staff
    - Bed space
    - Family services/babies
    - Family therapy too
    - Women's space
3. Education – 3 votes
    - Cultural
    - Age-appropriate
    - Family, public, community too
    - Doctors, CPS, judges, probation
    - Intermediate staff training
    - Trained mentors
    - Diversity of staff training
    - #4 can feel superior authority
4. More $$$
    - Can't expand (beds, staff, etc.)
    - More uniform pay scale for staff
    - More treatment days paid
    - Use what we have wisely
    - Avoid politics

ACTION STEPS

1. Community/family
    A. Community center, esp. adolescents in S. Kona, 6 months – Cheryl Taupu, Bridgehouse
    B. Family treatment idea, on drawing board, Feb. 2004 – Care Hawaii in East Hawaii
    C. Spreading the parent project, ongoing – Care Hawaii in East Hawaii
    D. Hold East and West community meetings with police, in 90 days – Regina, Danielle, Ipo, BISAC, Verna at Care Hawaii
    E. Extended, increased treatment in Puna, mid-October – Rhonda, Hui Malama
    F. Dr. Rick Delaney's treatment model, February – Regina @ Parents, Inc.
    G. Community response to ice in East Hawaii, February – Collaboration between Rhoda, Verna, Danielle, Ipo, and Regina

2. More treatment facilities
   A. Working on program, West Hawaii – Verna, West Hawaii Care Hawaii/BISAC Barb Rasale, case manager
   B. Support what's already happening – Regina
   C. Continue to serve present clients – Danielle
   D. Help with new adolescent treatment program – Danielle
   E. Support intensive treatment on BI – Care Hawaii
   F. Volunteer hours to Kona adolescent facility – Cheryl, Bridgehouse

GROUP 13 – TREATMENT

CHALLENGES

1. Lack of qualified personnel – 9 votes
   - Obtaining appropriate training for professionals
   - Find qualified counselors
2. Too short treatment – 5 votes
   - Not enough time
   - Need longer stay time
   - Need longer treatment time
   - Increasing length of stay in treatment
3. Education and awareness – 4 votes
   - Realize drug addiction
   - Better community understanding of addiction/disease
4. Lack of coordinated care – 4 votes
   - No resource/referral information
   - Connection with community groups
   - Collaborate for treatment
   - War coordination/leadership
   - Coordination of disciplines
5. Lack of money – 2 votes
   - Money
   - Shortage of funds
   - Need funding
6. Lack of adolescent and children treatment – 2 votes
   - No place to detox children in crisis
   - Unable to test kids who appear to have used
   - Lack of education for kids
   - Sustaining adolescent residential treatment funds
7. Lack of adult treatment – 2 votes
   - Not enough treatment services
   - No treatment programs
   - Need continuum of services - "residential treatment"
   - Expanding adult access to treatment
   - Managed care has too much control
8. Lack of transportation for treatment – 0 votes

ACTION STEPS

1. Lack of qualified personnel
   A. Training budget – DASH
   B. Now, approved practicuum site – BISAC, Assess capability
   C. Within 12 months, provide training site and trainer 2x a year for continuing required training on West side – Bridgehouse
   D. Within 3 months, invite Jamal/Dr. Kunz to train nurses on ice – Ka'u Hospital
2 Too short treatment
   A. Now, provide pre-treatment services – Access capability
   B. In Jan.-June 2004, ask ADAD for more than one therapeutic living stay per year – Bridgehouse

GROUP 14 – SOCIAL SERVICES

CHALLENGES

1. Inadequate staffing – 7 votes
   - Accountability to need
   - Lack of staff support – CRI
   - Not enough staff
   - Increasing caseload without increasing staff
   - Lack of trained/dedicated foster homes
2. Barriers to service – 6 votes
   - Family members' attitude
   - Lack of understanding/education
   - Open communication/collaboration with treatment
   - Community knowledge of available services
   - System "hopeless" attitude
3. Inadequate substance abuse prevention/treatment services
   - Available treatment services
   - Access to services
   - Accessibility to refer
   - Inadequate/not enough slots to refer clients to
   - Support for addicts' families
   - Lack of mother/infant residential
   - D/A assessment
   - Lack of business/youth mentoring

ACTION STEPS

1. Inadequate staffing
   A. Ongoing, approach State and local legislature through union/private sector – CWS Advisory Committee, Don Bebee, Marge Bartelt (pager 899-9777)
   B. By October, look into proposals and grant writing – Don Bebee, Donna Ruden, other group members contact Don if hear about grants/proposals
2. Barriers to services
   A. Ongoing, CRI group – Susan/Don
   B. Ongoing, education/awareness of services/problems – Havinne, 211, Sept. Ice Epidemic TV program
   C. Referrals to Crystal Meth Anonymous
   D. By October 31st, learning intake/discharge criteria, policies of different programs – Lovi
   E. By 11/30, Hui Laulima as resource to learn about other agencies/programs – Don

GROUP 15 – SOCIAL SERVICES

CHALLENGES

1. Treatment – 7 votes
   - Limited treatment resources
   - Lack of residential treatment
   - Drug treatment programs
   - Counseling program
   - Lack of medical insurance coverage to pay for length and level of treatment
   - Treatment/recovery takes longer than Federal Laws allows (one year) before termination of parental rights in CPS
   - No readily available treatment/medical level of care for all family members
2. Resources/funding – 5 votes
   - Funding in rural areas
   - Staff shortage
   - Funded coalition coordinator for DV
   - Transportation
3. Awareness – 4 votes
   - No public awareness campaign
   - Awareness of staff who are not substance abuse sensitive
   - Ice addiction is criminalized instead of being treated as a medical problem and treated accordingly
4. Elderly/seniors – 0 votes
   - Dependence on older adults for assistance
   - Crimes against elderly
5. Follow up/continuum of care – 0 votes
   - Continuum of care coordination
   - Supervised release – change in check in

ACTION STEPS

1. Treatment
   A. Develop treatment plan to include extended family and patient to include co-dependency awareness
   B. More extensive training for foster care providers
   C. Change language in contracts to provide education for extended family members
   D. Monitoring payments in accordance with contracts/agreements
2. Resources/funding
   A. RFP accessibility - DHS advertisements should be island-wide
   B. Clarify/streamline RFP process
   C. Collaboration between RFP applicants
   D. Coordinate effort with govt. agencies to match needs with resources

GROUP 16 – JUDICIARY

CHALLENGES

1. Treatment – 10 votes
   - Having enough treatment agencies for referrals (particular locations, esp. Ka'u, HOVE, etc.)
   - Lack of treatment programs
   - Treatment resources
   - Sober living houses
   - Residential treatment facility
   - Lack of specialized treatment alternatives
   - Minimal resources
   - Treatment in our probationers who are addicted
   - Treatment modalities for clients
   - Lack of treatment alternatives
   - Limited resources to accomplish mission
   - Lack of family and community support for offenders
   - Research and list non-traditional community support
2. Sentencing – 10 votes
   - Mandatory sentencing barrier to treatment
   - Parolee apathy
   - Getting clients to attend treatment
   - Prison overcrowding
   - Too lenient sentencing
   - Too many breaks for those not in compliance
3. Education – 8 votes
   - System changes with staff
   - Knowledge of addiction
   - Educating staff as well as clients
   - Ready access to information
   - Funding for additional staff
   - Updating the education programs regarding DUI-intoxicants referrals
4. Ice – 0 votes

ACTION STEPS

1. Treatment
   - A. Sober living houses
     - funding for, i.e. grants, etc.
     - contracts with existing sober living houses
     - contract more bed spaces
   - B. On 9/2, Aolani will speak with Warren about getting additional beds
   - C. Assess treatment options in our communities to identify gaps
   - D. Do adult matrix modeled after existing juvenile matrix for Hawaii Island – graduated interventions
   - E. Group 16 will meet to begin the process by video conferencing in Prosecuting Office in Hilo and Kona
   - F. Zach will collect names and phone numbers for Group 16
   - G. First meeting scheduled for 9/19 from 9-11 a.m.
2. Sentencing
   - A. Address sentencing options for ice, drug driven crime
   - B. Meet to discuss sentencing options on 9/19 from 9-11 a.m.

Solutions 2003: Neighborhoods in Action Drug Survey Report

survey was sent to 423 individuals on April26, 2003 and ended May 12, 2003 with 122 (29%) responses

Survey Results - Top Three Drug Issues

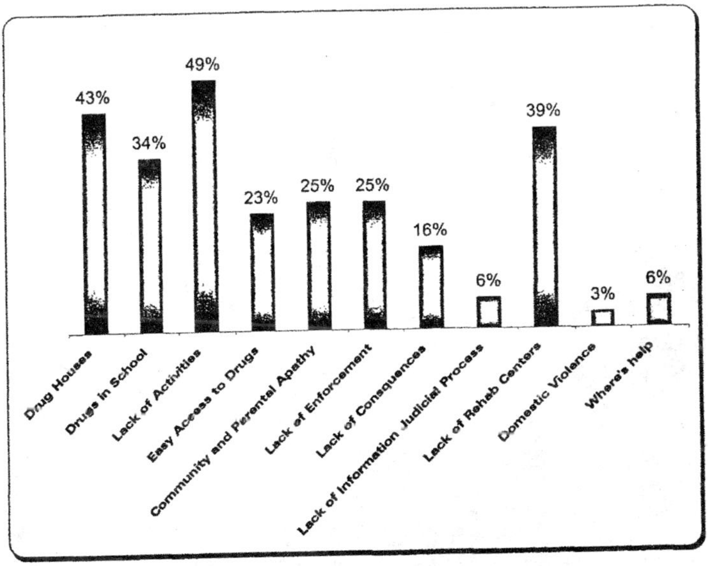

1 - Lack of Activities / Opportunities / Mentoring for Kids

2 - Drugs Houses

3 - Rehab Centers

ENCHANTED LAKES

KAILUA

MAUNAWILI

KAWAINUI

PŌHĀKUPU

WAIMĀNALO

KAILUA AREA
COMMUNITY PROFILE

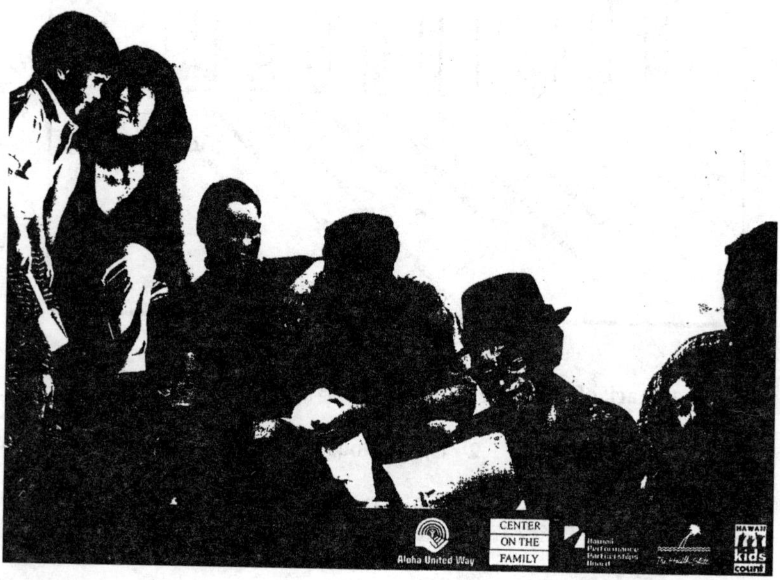

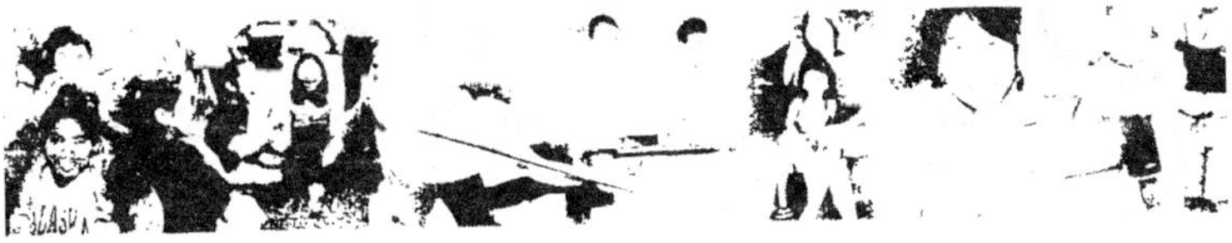

*I*NTRODUCTION

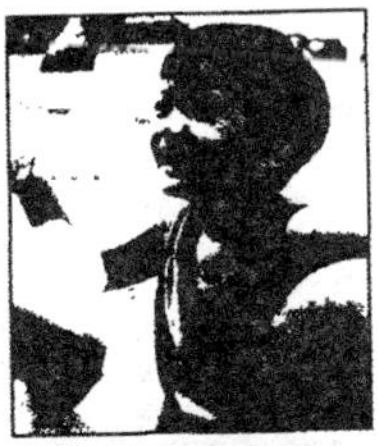

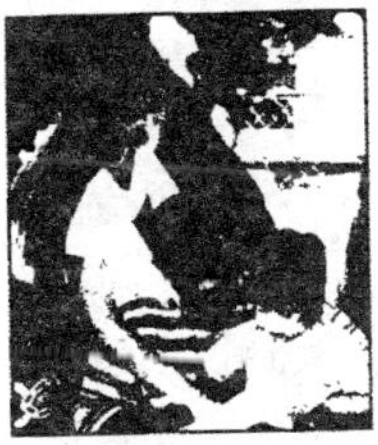

Hawai'i nō ka 'oi—Hawai'i the best—is a sentiment shared by many people in our island state. Those who have left and yearn to return home speak movingly about missing the best beaches in the world, delicious *local grinds* found no-where else, a mix of ethnicities at school, play, and work, and the *aloha* spirit that infuses even the smallest act. There are so many other things we can point to with pride:

- Hawai'i has the lowest rates of child deaths and teen deaths in the nation
- Life expectancy is higher in Hawai'i than anywhere else in the nation
- Three-fourths of Hawai'i's families eat dinner together 5 or more times a week
- More than 80% of Hawai'i's people feel they can rely on others in their community for help
- The average donation to charity is higher in Hawai'i at every income level when compared to mainland giving.

There are, of course, many serious problems that require our attention and action. Some of these may seem monumental and insurmountable, such as the problem of drug abuse, but Hawai'i's people, working together, have overcome major obstacles in the past and can do so in the future.

This is one of 43 community profiles developed by the Center on the Family that can be used as a resource to improve conditions for children and families in your neighborhood. The profiles provide data and information about the people who live in specific geographic areas encompassed by a public high school and all of its feeder intermediate and elementary schools. Factual information provides a good starting point for making informed decisions and plans for strategic action. We hope that this first-ever presentation of data at the school/community-complex level will provide you with a better understanding of your community and spur you to take action to keep Hawai'i *nō ka 'oi*.

*K*AILUA AREA

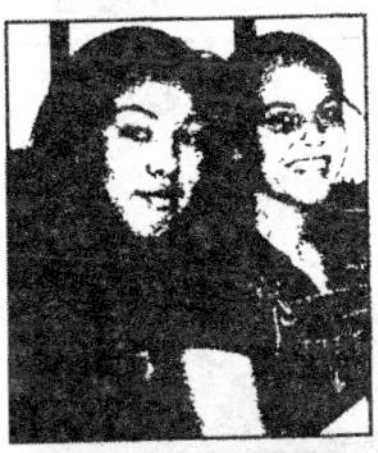

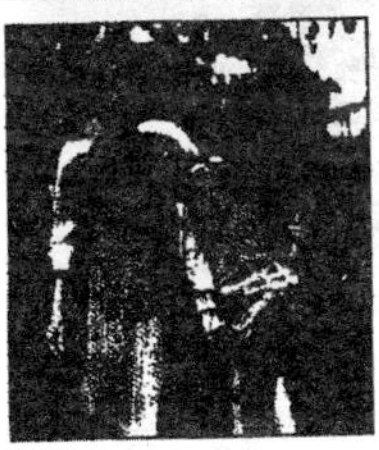

This area on the Windward Coast of O'ahu has over 28,000 residents and includes the neighborhoods of Enchanted Lakes, Kailua Heights, Maunawili, Kawainui, Pōhākupu, and Waimānalo. The median age of 37.8 is slightly higher than the State average, reflecting a larger proportion of residents between the ages of 35 and 64. The ethnic makeup is mixed, with just over 25% each of Caucasian, Asian, and bi- or multi-racial, as well as a relatively high proportion of Hawaiian and Part-Hawaiian (35.7%), and small percentages of other ethnicities.

A high percentage of adults in the Kailua Area has completed high school and college, and a high share of the teachers has advanced degrees. Compared to other communities Statewide, the per capita income is in the top 20% of all communities and home ownership is in the top 10%. However, the proportions of persons receiving Temporary Assistance to Needy Families (TANF) and families receiving food stamps are slightly higher than the State average.

A high percentage of parents believe the Kailua Area schools are safe, but fewer teachers agree. The percent of 3rd graders scoring below average on the SAT reading test exceeds that in two-thirds of other communities, but these children score closer to the State norm on the SAT math test. In a Statewide survey of 6th, 8th, 10th, and 12th graders, almost half of the adolescents from this area who responded reported a lack of interest in school. Public high school seniors rank in the bottom 15% for percent graduating. Nevertheless, the majority of high school seniors plan to attend college, and more than half of the adolescents surveyed here reported strong neighborhood and family satisfaction.

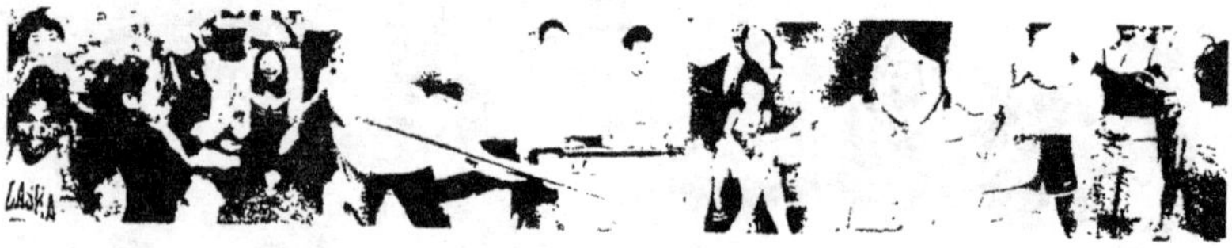

DEMOGRAPHICS

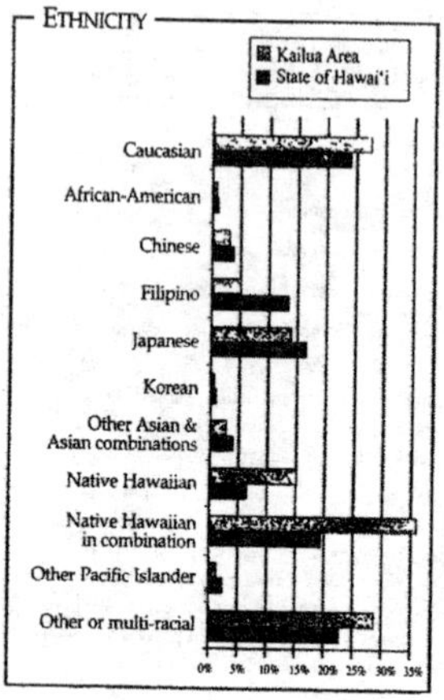

	KAILUA AREA	HONOLULU COUNTY	STATE OF HAWAI'I
Total Population	28,396	876,156	1,211,537
Median age	37.8	35.7	36.2
RACE AND ETHNICITY			
Percent choosing only 1 race	71.7%	80.1%	78.6%
Caucasian	27.3%	21.3%	24.3%
African-American	0.6%	2.4%	1.8%
Asian:	25.8%	46.0%	41.6%
Chinese	3.5%	6.1%	4.7%
Filipino	5.1%	14.2%	14.1%
Japanese	13.7%	18.4%	16.7%
Korean	0.7%	2.5%	1.9%
Other Asian and Asian combinations	2.9%	4.9%	4.2%
Other Pacific Islander	1.9%	3.2%	2.8%
Native Hawaiian	15.2%	5.6%	6.6%
Native Hawaiian in combination with 1 or more other races	35.7%	17.5%	19.8%
Some other race or choosing 2 or more races	28.9%	21.2%	22.7%

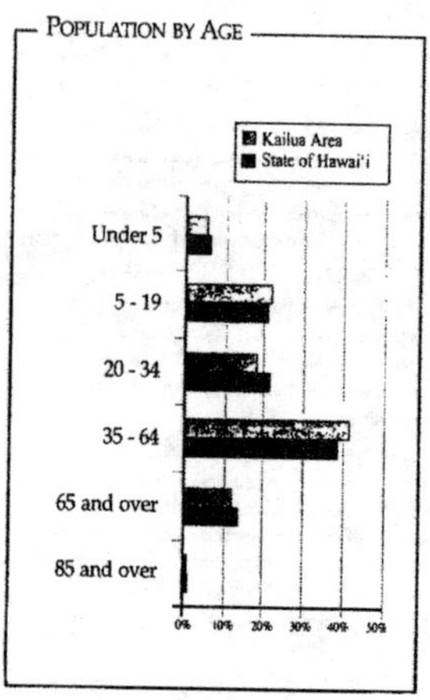

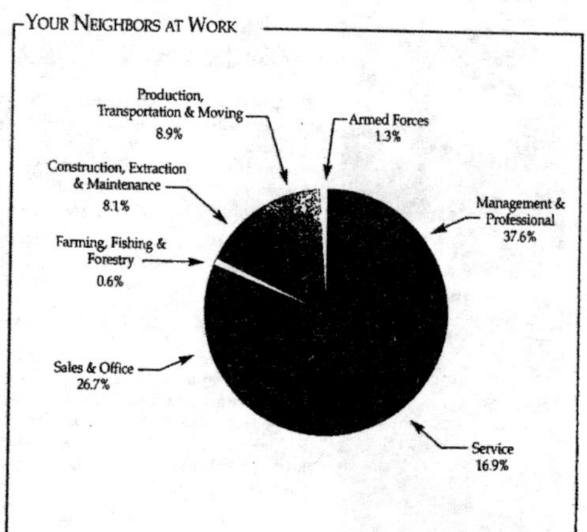

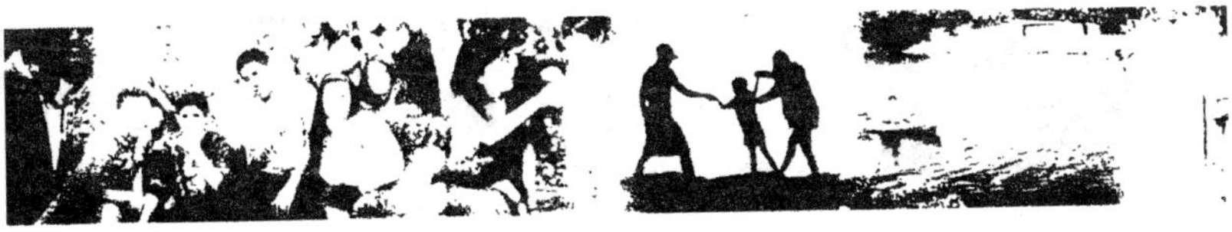

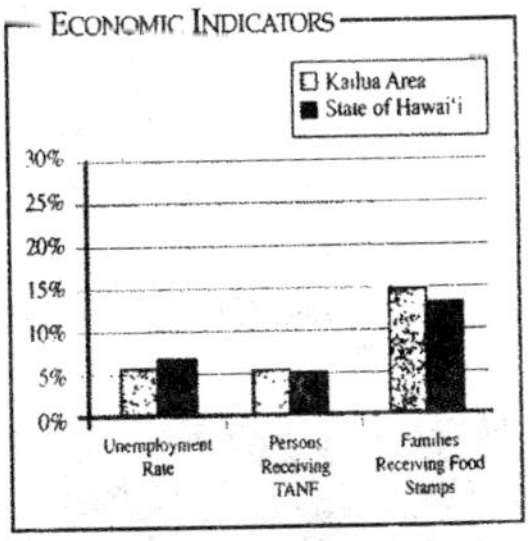

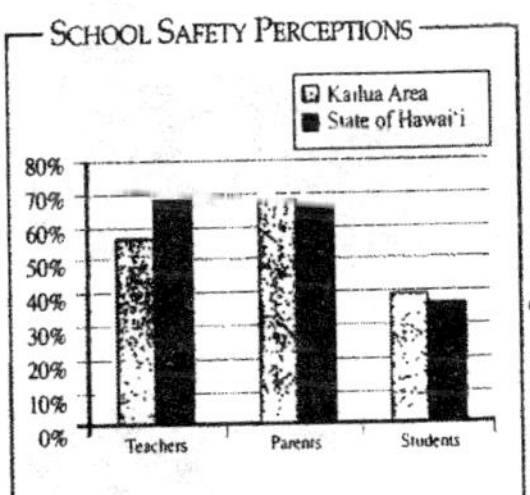

Percent of teachers, parents, and students who report their schools are safe

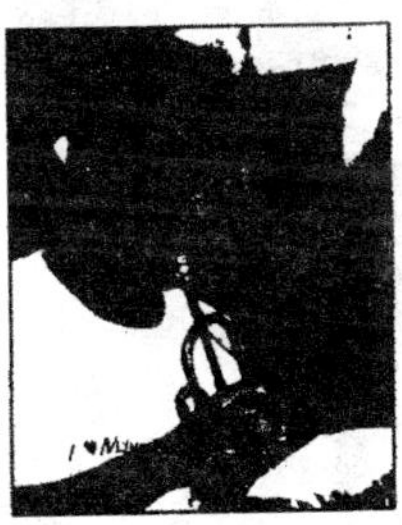

COMMUNITY

	KAILUA AREA	HONOLULU COUNTY	STATE OF HAWAI'I
Per capita income	$24,726	$21,998	$21,526
Home ownership - owner occupied housing units	78.5%	54.6%	56.5%
Residential stability - lived in same house from 1995-2000	69.4%	56.3%	56.8%
Residents who are U.S. citizens born in Hawaii	68.9%	55.8%	56.9%
New immigrants - foreign-born residents who entered Hawaii since 1990	2.1%	6.5%	6.0%
Residents over age 5 with language other than English at home	15.8%	28.9%	26.6%
Population over age 16 in the labor force	14,581	447,320	612,773
Civilian Unemployment	5.6%	6.2%	6.3%
Adults with high school diploma or higher	88.9%	84.8%	84.6%
Adults with Bachelor's Degree or higher	32.5%	27.9%	26.2%
*Adolescents reporting unsafe neighborhoods	47.1%	45.8%	43.9%
*Adolescents lacking close neighborhood ties	32.1%	38.7%	38.6%
Teachers with 5+ years at their school	66.0%	68.3%	66.4%
Teachers with advanced degrees	25.5%	17.9%	19.1%
Teachers reporting a safe school environment	57.0%	67.7%	68.2%

FAMILY

	KAILUA AREA	HONOLULU COUNTY	STATE OF HAWAI'I
Number of families	6,777	205,672	287,068
Families with children under age 18	38.8%	44.3%	45.0%
Families with children, headed by married couple	79.6%	77.4%	74.8%
Average household size	3.5	3.0	2.9
* Adolescents reporting close family ties	52.0%	45.0%	46.2%
Parents report checking child's homework and other public school involvement	63.3%	63.9%	63.2%
* Adolescents reporting poor parental supervision	44.6%	45.7%	46.3%
Parents feeling positive about students' safety	68.2%	68.7%	66.8%
Persons receiving Temporary Assistance to Needy Families (TANF)	5.9%	5.0%	5.4%
Families receiving food stamps	14.1%	12.2%	13.2%
Population ages 21-64 with disabilities	13.6%	16.8%	17.7%
Households lacking telephone service	0.7%	1.7%	2.0%

These data represent responses from 6th, 8th, 10th, and 12th graders from both public and private schools. Many communities had a higher proportion of young respondents and some communities had a low response rate overall. Age and sample size may affect the results.

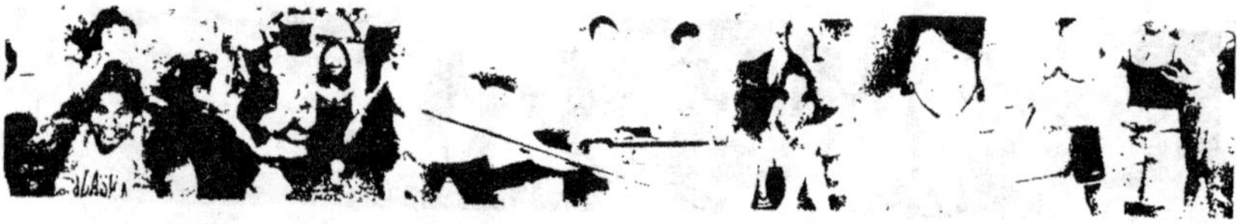

CHILDREN

	Kailua Area	Honolulu County	State of Hawai'i
K - 8 students with health insurance	93.4%	91.4%	90.3%
Child abuse rate per 1000 children	12	10	11
Children ages 0-5 living in poverty	5.6%	13.6%	15.4%
Children ages 0-5 with all parents in the labor force	67.3%	60.7%	61.8%
Children ages 3-5 enrolled in nursery school, pre-school, or kindergarten	75.6%	73.0%	72.7%
Children ages 6-8 with untreated tooth decay	36.2%	37.9%	36.0%
Students in public school program for limited English proficiency	3.3%	7.1%	6.3%
SAT Reading: 3rd graders scoring below average	21.2%	17.1%	17.8%
SAT Math: 3rd graders scoring below average	17.5%	18.1%	18.1%
Public school students in Special Education	13.4%	10.3%	11.0%
Public school 8th graders who feel safe at school	39.9%	36.5%	37.6%
* Adolescents reporting exposure to illicit drug use in their school and community	20.6%	12.4%	14.5%
* Adolescents reporting a lack of interest in school	47.3%	44.0%	45.3%
Teens age 16-19, not in school and not working	7.3%	7.9%	8.6%
Public school attendance	94.3%	93.7%	93.4%
Graduation rates of public school seniors	89.9%	94.8%	94.6%
Public school seniors with plans for 2 or 4 year college	83.1%	75.9%	74.8%
Percent accepted of the seniors with plans for college	56.6%	60.1%	58.5%

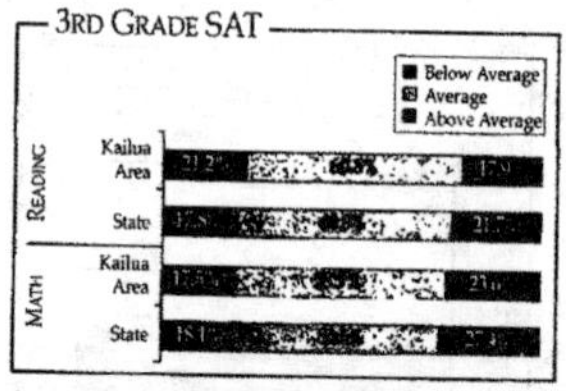

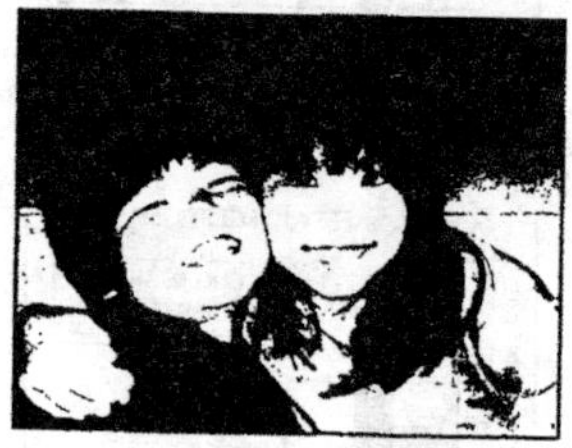

ELDERLY

	Kailua Area	Honolulu County	State of Hawai'i
Individuals age 65 & older living alone	16.6%	30.8%	31.8%
Individuals age 65 & older living in poverty	3.3%	7.4%	7.4%
Individuals age 65 & older with a disability	36.9%	40.4%	40.6%
Grandparents who live in the same household as their grandchildren under age 18	1,769	36,668	49,237
Grandparents responsible for the care of grandchildren with whom they live	23.2%	28.1%	28.5%

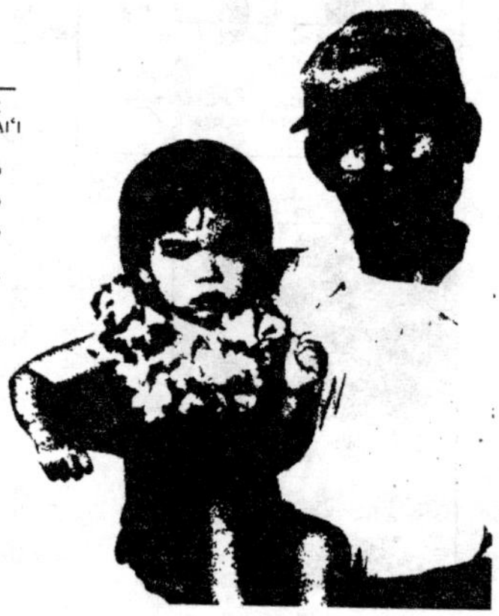

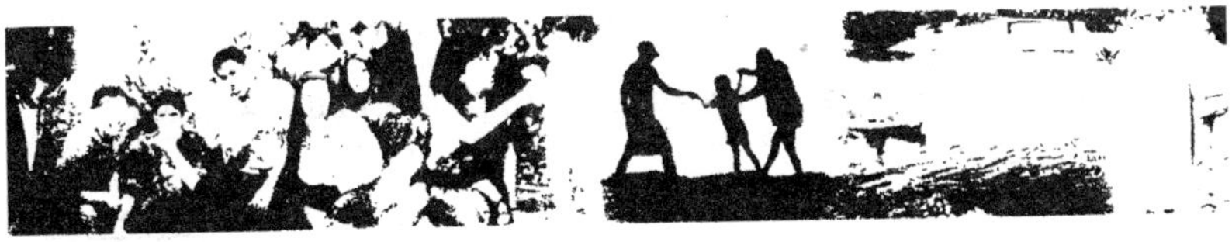

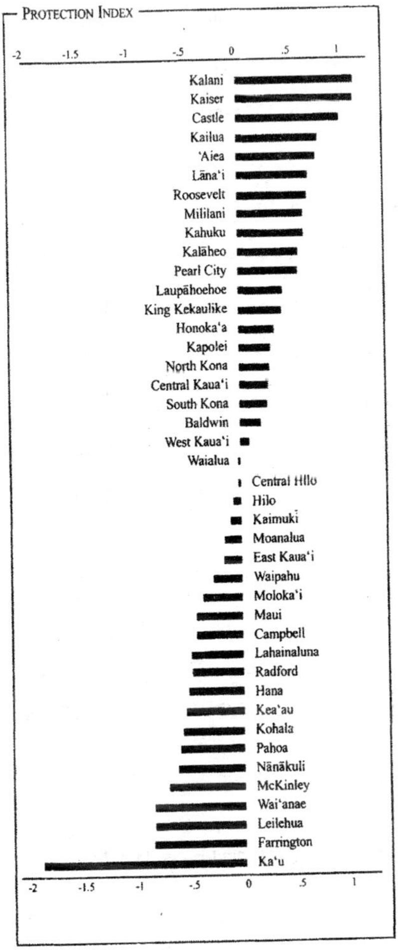

PROTECTION INDEX

There are various ways to assess the strength of a community. For this report, nine indicators of child, family, and community strengths were selected. Standard scores were derived for each of the nine indicators and summarized into a cumulative score for each of 42 school complex areas. A 43rd community, Ni'ihau, was omitted from the index because some data were unavailable. Those communities that scored highest on the protection index are more likely to have children who are nurtured and doing well in school, families that are healthy, and communities which are economically vital.

REFERENCES

Klingle, R.S. (2001). Ka leo o nā keiki: The 2000 Hawai'i student alcohol, tobacco, and other drug use study. Kapolei, HI: State of Hawai'i, Department of Health, Alcohol and Drug Abuse Division

State of Hawai'i, Department of Education, Planning and Evaluation Branch, Evaluation Section, (2001). School quality survey. (2001). School status and improvement reports. [Online:] http://arch.k12.hi.us/ (April 15, 2002).

_____. (2002). Senior exit plans survey. [Online:] http://arch.k12.hi.us/ (October 25, 2002).

State of Hawai'i, Department of Health, Dental Health Division. (2002). Statewide public school oral health assessment.

State of Hawai'i, Department of Human Services. (1999). TANF and food stamps data. Unpublished raw data.

State of Hawai'i, Department of Labor and Industrial Relations. (2001). Labor force and unemployment data. Unpublished raw data.

U.S. Census Bureau. (2000). Census 2000. [Online:] http:// www.census.gov/ census2000/ states/ hi.html (September 30, 2002).

Wood, D. William (2001). Hawai'i Covering Kids data project. Unpublished raw data.

CENTER ON THE FAMILY
COLLEGE OF TROPICAL AGRICULTURE & HUMAN RESOURCES
UNIVERSITY OF HAWAI'I
2515 CAMPUS ROAD, MILLER HALL 103
HONOLULU, HI 96822

PH: 808.956.4132 FX: 808.956.4147
VISIT OUR WEBSITE AT www.uhfamily.hawaii.edu

COF 2003

ALCOHOL AND DRUG ABUSE DIVISION – STATE FY 2004

OAHU – SUBSTANCE ABUSE PREVENTION – ALL FEDERAL FUNDS

AGENCY	SAPT FUNDS*	SIG FUNDS**
Boys & Girls Club (Waianae & Nanakuli	$ 132,000	$ ---
Ka'ala Farms (Waianae)	$ 80,000	$ ---
Waimanalo Health Center	$ 137,000	$ ---
Maui Center for Health Care	$ 70,000	$ ---
Coalition For A Drug-Free Hawaii – Ewa Beach	$ 130,037	$ ---
Waipahu Community Association	$ ---	$ 123,100
Boys & Girls Club – Nuuanu/Kalihi	$ ---	$ 140,000
Boys &Girls Club – Kaimuki/Palolo	$ ---	$ 140,000
YMCA of Honolulu – Waialua/Haleiwa	$ ---	$ 140,000
Coalition For A Drug-Free Hawaii – Kahuku/Laie	$ ---	$ 150,000
Coalition For A Drug-Free Hawaii – Ewa	$ ---	$ 150,000
Susannah Wesley Community Center – Kalihi	$ ---	$ 150,000
Parents and Children Together - Kaneohe	$ ---	$ 123,100
Waianae Coast Comprehensive Health Center	$ ---	$ 123,100
SUBTOTAL:	$ 549,037	$1,239,300

* SAPT Grant – Federal Substance Abuse Prevention & Treatment Block Grant
**SIG Grant – Federal State Incentive Grant

ALCOHOL AND DRUG ABUSE DIVISION – STATE FY 2004

MAUI – SUBSTANCE ABUSE PREVENTION - ALL FEDERAL FUNDS

AGENCY	SAPT FUNDS*	SIG FUNDS**
Alu Like – Hana	$ 75,000	$ ---
Aloha House - Maui	$ 75,000	$ ---
Maui Center for Health Care Education	$ 60,000	$ ---
Boys & Girls Club of Maui – Makawao	$ ---	$ 135,500
Maui Youth & Family Services – Wailuku	$ ---	$ 150,000
MOLOKAI:		
Alu Like – Molokai	$ 75,000	$ ---
Hawaii Conference of Seventh-day Adventists	$ ---	$ 123,100
LANAI:		
Lanai Youth Center	$ ---	$ 150,000
SUBTOTAL:	$ 285,000	$ 558,600

* SAPT Grant – Federal Substance Abuse Prevention & Treatment Block Grant
**SIG Grant – Federal State Incentive Grant

ALCOHOL AND DRUG ABUSE DIVISION – STATE FY 2004

HAWAII – SUBSTANCE ABUSE PREVENTION - ALL FEDERAL FUNDS

AGENCY	SAPT FUNDS*	SIG FUNDS**
YWCA of Hawaii – East Hawaii	$ 75,000	$ ---
Alu Like – West Hawaii	$ 75,000	$ ---
Family Support Services of West Hawaii – South Kona	$ ---	$ 110,000
Family Support Services of West Hawaii – Kohala	$ ---	$ 130,000
Laupahoehoe Train Museum		$ 123,100
SUBTOTAL:	$ 150,000	$ 363,100

* SAPT Grant – Federal Substance Abuse Prevention & Treatment Block Grant
**SIG Grant – Federal State Incentive Grant

ALCOHOL AND DRUG ABUSE DIVISION – STATE FY 2004

KAUAI – SUBSTANCE ABUSE PREVENTION - ALL FEDERAL FUNDS

AGENCY	SAPT FUNDS*	SIG FUNDS**
Alu Like	$ 70,000	$ ---
West Kauai Community Business & Professional Association – Waimea	$ ---	$ 69,000
Kauai Economic Opportunity – Central Kauai	$ ---	$ 150,000
Office of the Mayor	$ 5,000	$ ---
SUBTOTAL:	$ 75,000	$ 219, 000

* SAPT Grant – Federal Substance Abuse Prevention & Treatment Block Grant
**SIG Grant – Federal State Incentive Grant

ALCOHOL AND DRUG ABUSE DIVISION – STATE FY 2004

STATEWIDE SUBSTANCE ABUSE PREVENTION

AGENCY	SAPT FUNDS*	TOBACCO SETTLEMENT FUNDS
DOE - Parenting	$ 95,000	$ ---
MADD Youth In Action	$ 60,000	$ ---
Coalition For A Drug-Free Hawaii - RADAR	$ 176,000	$ ---
STATEWIDE SYSTEM SUPPORT:		
Starling Consulting -- MIS	$ 30,000	$ ---
UH Conf. Ctr. – Training	$ 70,000	$ ---
UH CRC – Synar	$ 68,989	$ ---
UH SSRI – Student Survey	$ 232,924	$ ---
UH SSRI – Evaluation	$ 130,033	$ ---
UH Center on Family	$ 100,000	$ ---
UH CRC (Enforcement)	$ ---	$ 206,325
Honolulu Police Dept.	$ ---	$ 24,576
Hawaii Police Dept.	$ ---	$ 12,912
Maui Police Dept.	$ ---	$ 11,216
Kauai Police Dept.	$ ---	$ 5,076
SUBTOTAL:	$ 962,946	$ 260,105

* SAPT Grant – Federal Substance Abuse Prevention & Treatment Block Grant

ALCOHOL AND DRUG ABUSE DIVISION – STATE FY 2004

SUBSTANCE ABUSE PREVENTION - ALL FEDERAL FUNDS

ENFORCING UNDERAGE DRINKING LAWS (OJJDP ** FEDERAL FUNDS)

AGENCY	FED. OJJDP	SAPT BLOCK GRANT	TOTAL
• MADD	$ 272,740	-0-	$272,740
• Honolulu Police Dept.	$ 49,000	-0-	$ 49,000
• Maui Police Dept.	$ 6,248	-0-	$ 6,248
• Kauai Police Dept.	$ 13,260	-0-	$ 13,260
• Hawaii Police Dept.	$ 20,000	-0-	$ 20,000
SUBTOTAL:	$ 361,248		$361,248

* SAPT Grant - Federal Substance Abuse Prevention & Treatment Block Grant
** OJJDP - Federal Office of Juvenile Justice & Delinquency Prevention

PREVENTING UNDERAGE DRINKING
DEPARTMENT OF TRANSPORTATION (DOT) FEDERAL FUNDS

AGENCY	FEDERAL DOT	TOTAL
Coalition for a Drug Free Hawaii	$100,000	$100,000

ALCOHOL AND DRUG ABUSE DIVISION – STATE FY 2004

OAHU – ADULT SUBSTANCE ABUSE TREATMENT

	General Funds	Federal Funds	Total
GENERAL TREATMENT:			
* Salvation Army ATS	$ 812,426	$ 198,585	$1,011,011
* Hawaii Alcoholism Foundation	$ 64,264	$ 115,736	$ 180,000
* Ho'omau Ke Ola	$150,000	$ 238,329	$ 388,329
* Hina Mauka (ARSH)	$ 118,938	$ 255,250	$ 374,188
. Queen's Medical Center	$ 50,000	-0-	$ 50,000
. Salvation Army ATS (ex-offenders)	-0-	$ 63,153	$ 63,153
. Salvation Army ATS (**DDRA funds**)	$ 50,000	-0-	$ 50,000
NON-MEDICAL RESIDENTIAL DETOX:			
. Salvation Army ATS	$100,000	$ 269,340	$ 369,340
SPECIALIZED TREATMENT FOR THE HOMELESS:			
. Hina Mauka (ARSH) at Institute for Human Services	-0-	$ 42,000	$ 42,000
SPECIALIZED TREATMENT FOR INJECTION DRUG USERS-METHADONE/LAAM			
. Drug Addiction Services of Hawaii	$ 166,316	$ 119,934	$ 286,250
SPECIALIZED TREATMENT FOR DUAL DIAGNOSIS:			
* Po'ailani	$ 158,500	$ 10,000	$ 168,500
. Queens Medical Center	$ 97,591	$ 10,000	$ 107,591
SPECIALIZED TREATMENT FOR PREGNANT & PARENTING WOMEN & CHILDREN:			
* Salvation Army FTS	$ 862,150	$ 620,119	$1,482,269
. Family Court – First Circuit	-0-	$ 250,000	$ 250,000
SUBTOTAL:	$2,630,185	$2,192,446	$4,822,631

* Provider has a residential treatment program that can admit clients from any island.

ALCOHOL AND DRUG ABUSE DIVISION – STATE FY 2004

MAUI --ADULT SUBSTANCE ABUSE TREATMENT

	General Funds	Federal Funds	Total
GENERAL TREATMENT:			
* Aloha House	$ 152,065	$ 140,543	$ 292,608
SPECIALIZED TREATMENT FOR PREGNANT & PARENTING WOMEN & CHILDREN			
. Malama Na Makua A Keiki	$ 200,000	-0-	$ 200,000

MOLOKAI--ADULT SUBSTANCE ABUSE TREATMENT

GENERAL TREATMENT:			
. Hale Ho'okupa'a	$ 54,547	$ 90,453	$ 145,000

LANAI -- ADULT SUBTANCE ABUSE TREATMENT

NO ADULT SUBSTANCE ABUSE TREATMENT FUNDS

SUBTOTAL:	$ 406,612	$ 230,996	$ 637,608

* Provider has a residential treatment program that can admit clients from any island.

ALCOHOL AND DRUG ABUSE DIVISION – STATE FY 2004

KAUAI -- ADULT SUBSTANCE ABUSE TREATMENT

	General Funds	Federal Funds	Total
GENERAL TREATMENT:			
. Hina Mauka	$ 150,278	$ 16,160	$ 166,438
SPECIALIZED TREATMENT FOR PREGNANT & PARENTING WOMEN & CHIDLREN			
. Child and Family Services	-0-	$ 140,524	$ 140,524
SUBTOTAL:	$ 150,278	$ 156,684	$ 306,962

ALCOHOL AND DRUG ABUSE DIVISION – STATE FY 2004

HAWAII – ADULT SUBSTANCE ABUSE TREATMENT

	General Funds	Federal Funds	Total
GENERAL TREATMENT:			
. Big Island Substance Abuse Council (BISAC) – East Hi	$ 174,695	$ 224,303	$ 398,998
. Big Island Substance Abuse Council (BISAC)-West Hi	$ 59,620	$ 67,133	$ 126,753
. Big Island Substance Abuse Council (BISAC) (West Hawaii-TLP)	$ 300,000	-0-	**$ 300,000(GIA)**
. Bridge House – West Hi	$ 66,380	$ 104,717	$ 171,097
. Drug Addiction Services of Hawaii (DASH) – Puna	$ 150,000	-0-	$ 150,000
. Big Island Substance Abuse Council (BISAC) - East Hi (TLP)	-0-	$ 175,000	$ 175,000
SPECIALIZED TREATMENT FOR INJECTION DRUG USERS-METHADONE/LAAM:			
. Drug Addiction Services of Hawaii (DASH) East and West Hawaii	$ 110,750	$ 79,000	$ 189,750
SUBTOTAL:	$ 861,445	$ 650,153	$1,511,598

ALCOHOL AND DRUG ABUSE DIVISION – STATE FY 2004

ADULT TREATMENT SYSTEM SUPPORT SERVICES

	General Fund	Federal Funds	Total
. Drug Addiction Services of Hawaii (DASH) – Early Intervention Services (HIV/AIDS, TB, Hepatitis) (Oahu & Big Island)	-0-	$360,071	$360,071
. Legal Action Center – 24 hour legal advise on substance abuse issues and legal matters	-0-	$ 2,050	$ 2,050
. Independent Peer Review	-0-	$ 5,000	$ 5,000
. Oxford House – loans for independent private group homes for adults in recovery	-0-	$ 68,000	$ 68,000
. ICRC	-0-	$ 1,057	$ 1,057
. Board of Examiners	-0-	$ 12,350	$ 12,350
. Castle Assessment Exam	-0-	$ 5,660	$ 5,660
. NASADAD Dues	-0-	$ 7,400	$ 7,400
. Criminal Justice Technical Assistance	-0-	$ 78,241	$ 78,241
SUBTOTAL:		$539,829	$539,829

ALCOHOL AND DRUG ABUSE DIVISION – STATE FY 2004

ADOLESCENT SUBSTANCE ABUSE TREATMENT

	General Funds	Federal Funds	Total
I. SCHOOL-BASED TREATMENT:			
OAHU:			
. YMCA	$ 588,577	$ 387,260	$ 975,837
. Hina Mauka (ARSH)	$ 601,079	$ 142,120	$ 743,199
. Hina Mauka (ARSH) – Radford H.S.	$ 90,000**		$90,000
**Rainy Day Funds			
MAUI			
. Aloha House	$ 76,223	$ 23,777	$ 100,000
. Maui Youth and Family Services	$ 76,223	$ 58,777	$ 135,000
KAUAI			
. Hina Mauka (ARSH)	$ 113,927	$ 36,073	$ 150,000
HAWAII:			
. Big island Substance Abuse Council (BISAC) – East Hi	$ 80,494	$ 39,094	$ 119,588
. Big Island Substance Abuse Council (BISAC) – West Hi	$ 65,860	$ 31,986	$ 97,846
LANAI:	See Maui Youth and Family Services		
MOLOKAI:	No Dedicated Funds		
II. RESIDENTIAL SUBSTANCE ABUSE TREATMENT			
OAHU:			
* Bobby Benson Center	$ 145,000	$ 100,000	$ 245,000
MAUI:			
* Maui Youth & Family Services	$ 144,997	$100,000	$ 244,997
SUBTOTAL:	$1,982,380	$ 919,087	$2,901,467

*Provider has a residential treatment program that can admit clients from any island.

ALCOHOL AND DRUG ABUSE DIVISION – STATE FY 2004

INTEGRATED CASE MANAGEMENT/SUBSTANCE ABUSE TREATMENT FOR THE CRIMINAL JUSTICE POPULATION

	General Funds	Federal Funds	Total
• CARE Hawaii, Inc. (Overall Case Management)	$ 780,000	-0-	$ 780,000
• Salvation Army ATS (Oahu)	$ 515,000	-0-	$ 515,000
• Hina Mauka (Oahu)	$ 255,000	-0-	$ 255,000
• Hina Mauka (Kauai)	$ 68,000	-0-	$ 68,000
• Hina Mauka (Maui)	$ 92,000	-0-	$ 92,000
• Aloha House (Maui)	$ 210,000	-0-	$ 210,000
• Queen's Medical Center (Oahu)	$ 50,000	-0-	$ 50,000
• Big Island Substance Abuse Council (Hawaii)	$ 230,000	-0-	$ 230,000
		TOTAL:	**$2,200,000**

JOINT HOUSE-SENATE COMMITTEE ON ICE AND DRUG ABATEMENT

FOCUS– ADOLESCENTS

HANDOUT

Elaine Wilson, ACSW, LSW, MPH
Chief, Alcohol and Drug Abuse Division
Hawaii Department of Health
September 8, 2003

2002 HAWAII STUDENT ALCOHOL, TOBACCO AND OTHER DRUG USE STUDY

EXECUTIVE SUMMARY (66 PAGES)

http://www.state.hi.us/doh/resource/adad/report2002/index.html

2002 HAWAII STUDENT ALCOHOL, TOBACCO AND OTHER DRUG USE STUDY

"ICE" PREVALENCE

LIFETIME PREVALENCE ("ICE")

GRADE	1989	1991	1993	1996	1998	2000	2002	2000-2002
6th	1.4%	1.0%	1.3%	1.4%	1.8%	0.5%	0.4%	-0.1%
8th	6.1%	4.3%	4.9%	4.4%	4.6%	2.3%	2.0%	-0.3%
10th	9.9%	7.0%	7.8%	5.9%	6.7%	4.5%	4.2%	-0.3%
12th	11.7%	8.9%	8.4%	7.5%	7.7%	5.8%	5.3%	-0.5%

MONTHLY PREVALENCE ("ICE")

GRADE	1989	1991	1993	1996	1998	2000	2002	2000-2002
6th	0.4%	0.2%	0.3%	1.0%	1.0%	0.3%	0.2%	-0.1%
8th	2.7%	1.6%	1.9%	3.0%	3.1%	1.1%	1.2%	+0.1%
10th	4.8%	2.9%	3.2%	2.8%	3.0%	1.6%	1.8%	+0.2%
12th	5.5%	3.4%	3.1%	2.8%	2.3%	1.6%	1.8%	-0.1%

DAILY PREVALENCE ("ICE")

GRADE	1996	1998	2000	2002	2000-2002
6th	0.2%	0.1%	0.0%	0.1%	+0.1%
8th	0.9%	0.5%	0.1%	0.1%	0.0%
10th	0.8%	0.6%	0.3%	0.2%	-0.1%
12th	0.6%	0.4%	0.3%	0.3%	0.0%

/

2002 HAWAII STUDENT ALCOHOL, TOBACCO AND OTHER DRUG USE STUDY

ALCOHOL PREVALENCE

LIFETIME PREVALENCE (ALCOHOL USE BY PERCENTAGE)

GRADE	1987	1989	1991	1993	1996	1998	2000	2002	2000-2002
6th	47.6	34.6	31.1	34.9	29.8	31.6	24.2	20.0	-4.2
8th	64.7	57.3	55.8	57.4	54.0	52.6	49.2	42.5	-6.7
10th	76.1	71.1	72.9	73.3	73.4	72.3	67.1	64.7	-2.4
12th	85.9	80.5	79.8	79.2	79.7	81.2	77.2	75.4	-1.8

MONTHLY PREVALENCE (ALCOHOL USE BY PERCENTAGE)

GRADE	1987	1989	1991	1993	1996	1998	2000	2002	2000-2002
6TH	3.2	3.1	2.8	2.5	14.4	12.0	9.1	7.8	-1.3
8TH	14.0	13.2	14.0	15.2	30.2	25.3	22.1	20.4	-1.7
10TH	28.0	27.1	28.3	28.8	41.2	37.6	32.5	33.9	+1.4
12TH	42.7	37.8	38.6	35.4	46.3	45.0	43.2	43.0	-0.2

DAILY PREVALENCE (ALCOHOL USE BY PERCENTAGE)

GRADE	1996	1998	2000	2002	2000-2002
6TH	0.9	0.9	0.7	0.5	-0.2
8TH	3.1	2.8	1.6	1.8	+0.2
10TH	3.8	3.8	2.4	2.5	+0.1
12TH	4.7	3.2	3.5	3.3	-0.2

2002 HAWAII STUDENT ALCOHOL, TOBACCO AND OTHER DRUG USE STUDY

MARIJUANA PREVALENCE

LIFETIME PREVALENCE (MARIJUANA USE IN PERCENTAGE)

GRADE	1987	1989	1991	1993	1996	1998	2000	2002	2000-2002
6TH	10.6	8.7	7.2	9.4	9.7	10.1	5.3	5.6	+0.3
8TH	14.9	13.0	12.7	16.6	15.2	12.5	9.9	9.1	-O.8
10TH	13.4	12.8	14.2	15.6	11.2	10.2	7.0	8.4	+1.4
12TH	11.5	11.2	10.2	12.0	7.9	8.1	5.7	7.3	+1.6

MONTHLY PREVALENCE (MARIJUANA USE BY PERCENTAGE)

GRADE	1987	1989	1991	1993	1996	1998	2000	2002	2000-2002
6TH	0.4	0.6	0.4	0.5	3.4	2.6	1.3	1.3	0.0
8TH	5.2	4.9	4.9	7.5	14.8	11.8	8.9	9.1	+0.2
10TH	12.4	11.1	12.7	16.0	21.2	22.3	17.2	18.4	+1.2
12TH	17.2	13.9	14.6	17.9	25.0	23.0	22.7	21.1	-1.6

DAILY PREVALENCE (MARIJUANA USE BY PERCENTAGE)

GRADE	1996	1998	2000	2002	2000-2002
6TH	0.7	0.4	0.2	0.2	0.0
8TH	3.1	2.4	1.5	1.6	+0.1
10TH	4.2	4.7	3.4	4.4	+1.0
12TH	6.4	5.2	4.6	4.8	+0.2

2002 HAWAII STUDENT ALCOHOL, TOBACCO AND OTHER DRUG USE STUDY

ECSTASY PREVALENCE

LIFETIME PREVALANCE TREND (ECSTASY)

GRADE	HAWAII 1998	HAWAII 2000	HAWAII 2002	NATION 2002
6TH	1%	0%	0%	-
8TH	3%	2%	3%	4%
10TH	4%	5%	7%	7%
12TH	5%	8%	11%	11%

MONTHLY PREVALENCE TREND (ECSTASY)

GRADE	HAWAII 1998	HAWAII 2000	HAWAII 2002	NATION 2002
6TH	.7%	.1%	.1%	-
8TH	2.0%	1.3%	1.7%	1.4%
10TH	1.9%	2.9%	2.3%	1.8%
12TH	1.7%	3.9%	2.5%	2.4%

HAWAII 2002 STUDENT PERCEPTION THAT ECSTASY IS HARMFUL:

67% of 8th graders; 73% of 10th graders; and 77% of 12th graders think ecstasy use is harmful. Fewer students perceive ecstasy use as harmful compared to hallucinogens, methamphetamine and cocaine.

HAWAII 2002 STUDENT PERCEPTION OF AVAILABILITY OF ECSTASY

GRADE	HAWAII 2002	NATION 2002
6th	5%	-
8th	15%	23%
10th	34%	41%
12th	44%	59%

HAWAII AVAILABILTY TREND (ECSTASY)

GRADE	HAWAII 1998	HAWAII 2000	HAWAII 2002
6TH	3%	4%	5%
8TH	6%	10%	15%
10TH	15%	26%	34%
12TH	22%	39%	44%

Reported availability perceptions of ecstasy have been increasing at all grade levels and are up 2 to 8 percentage points in 2002.

HAWAII YOUTH SUBSTANCE ABUSE PREVENTION STRATEGY

GOALS OF THE STRATEGY:

- To combat the use of alcohol and other drugs among Hawaii's youth by coordinating, leveraging, and/or redirecting substance abuse prevention resources in order to identify gaps in services to communities and to fill those gaps with science-based "Best Practices" prevention programs

- To prevent youth alcohol and other drug use by reducing those factors that may put youth at higher risk and increase those factors that buffer or protect them from risky behaviors.

ALIGNING STATE PREVENTION EFFORTS AROUND SIX PLANNING PRINCIPLES:

- FORMING PARTNERSHIPS AMONG STATE AGENCIES
- SUPPORTING AND SUSTAINING COMMUNITY-BASED PARTNERSHIPS
- USING RISK AND PROTECTIVE FACTORS AS A FRAMEWORK FOR PLANNING
- SUPPORTING EFFECTIVE, SCIENCE-BASED PREVENTION PROGRAMS ("BEST PRACTICES")
- ACHIEVING MEASURABLE OUTCOMES AND RESULTS
- SUPPORTING PROGRAMS THAT ARE EFFECTIVE AND REFLECTIVE OF HAWAII'S CULTURAL DIVERSITY

ADAD, August 2003

Risk and Protective Factors for Prevention Planning

1. Risk Factors

Risk factors are characteristics of people or their family, school, and community environments that are associated with increases in alcohol, tobacco, marijuana, and other drug use. Seventeen factors have been identified that increase the likelihood that children and youth will develop problem behaviors such as substance abuse.

2. Protective Factors

Factors associated with reduced potential for drug are called protective factors. Protective factors encompass psychological, behavioral, family, and characteristics that can insulate children and yout the effects of risk factors that are present in his/he environment.

Risk and Protective Factors Related to Substance Use

	Risk Factors	Protective Factors
COMMUNITY	➢ Alcohol and other drugs readily available ➢ Laws and ordinances are unclear or inconsistently enforced. Norms are unclear or encourage use ➢ Residents feel little sense of "connection" to community and communities are disorganized ➢ Neighborhoods have high transitions and residents are very mobile ➢ Communities have extreme poverty	➢ Opportunities exist for community involvement ➢ Laws and ordinances are consistently enforced ➢ Policies and norms encourage non-use ➢ Community service opportunities are available for youth ➢ Resources (housing, healthcare, childcare, jobs, recreation, etc.) are available
FAMILY	➢ Family member with history of alcohol or other drug abuse ➢ Parents have trouble keeping track of their teens and do not have clear rules and consequences regarding alcohol and other drug use ➢ Parents use drugs, involve youth in their use ("get me a beer, would you?") or tolerate use by youth ➢ Family members have many conflicts	➢ Close family relationships ➢ Education is valued and encouraged, and parents are actively involved ➢ Copes with stress in a positive way ➢ Clear expectations and limits regarding alcohol and other drug use ➢ Encourages supportive relationships with caring adults beyond the immediate family ➢ Shares family responsibilities, including chores and decision-making ➢ Family members are nurturing and support each other
SCHOOL	➢ Students lack commitment or sense of belonging at school ➢ High number of students fail academically at school ➢ Students exhibit persistent problem behaviors in school	➢ Communicates high academic and behavioral expectations ➢ Encourages goal-setting, academic achievement, and positive social development ➢ Provides leadership and decision-making opportunities for students ➢ Fosters active involvement of students, parents and community members ➢ Sponsors substance-free events
INDIVIDUAL	➢ Youth associates with friends who use ➢ Has attitude that alcohol and drug use is "cool" ➢ Begins using at a young age ➢ Has certain physical, emotional or personality traits ➢ Feels alienated and/or are rebellious	➢ Involved in alcohol and other drug-free activities ➢ Views parents, teachers, doctors, law enforcement officers and other adults as allies ➢ Has positive future plans ➢ Has friends who disapprove of alcohol and other drug use

Risk and Protective Factor Definitions
Continued

SCHOOL	**Risk Factors**	
	Low School Commitment	Defined as the student's inability to see the role of a student as a viable one. Factors such as disliking school and perceiving the course work as irrelevant are positively related to drug use.
	Poor Academic Performance	Defined as poor performance in school. Beginning in the late elementary grades (grades 4-6), academic failure increases the risk of drug abuse and delinquency.
	Protective Factors	
	School Opportunities for Positive Involvement	Defined as opportunities to become involved in school activities. When young people are given more opportunities to participate meaningfully in important activities at school, they are less likely to engage in drug use or problem behaviors.
	School Rewards for Positive Involvement	Defined as positive feedback by school personnel for student achievement. When young people are recognized and rewarded for their contributions at school, they are less likely to be involved in substance use and other problem behaviors.
PEER-INDIVIDUAL	**Risk Factors**	
	Early Initiation of Problem Behaviors	Defined as early substance use and early onset of problem behaviors. The earlier the onset of any drug use, the greater the involvement in other drug use. Onset of drug use prior to the age of 15 is a consistent predictor of drug abuse; later age of onset of drug use has been shown to predict lower drug involvement and a greater probability of discontinuation of use.
	Favorable Attitudes Toward ATOD Use	Defined as perceptions that it is not wrong for young people to engage in ATOD use. Initiation of use of any substance is preceded by values favorable to its use. During the elementary school years, most children express anti-drug, anti-crime, and prosocial attitudes and have difficulty imagining why people use drugs. However, in middle school, as more youths are exposed to others who use drugs, their attitudes often shift toward greater acceptance of these behaviors. Youths who express positive attitudes toward drug use are at higher risk for subsequent drug use.
	Low Perceived Risk of ATOD Use	Defined as perceived harmfulness associated with ATOD use. Young people who do not perceive drug use to be risky are far more likely to engage in drug use.
	Antisocial Behaviors (ASBs)	Defined as engaging in problem behaviors such as violence and delinquency.
	Favorable Attitudes Toward ASB	Defined as a student's acceptance of drug use, criminal activity, violent behavior, or ignorance of rules. Young people who accept or condone antisocial behavior are more likely to engage in a variety of problem behaviors, including drug use.
	Friends' ATOD Use	Defined as having several close friends who engage in ATOD use. Peer drug use has consistently been found to be among the strongest predictors of substance use among youths – even when young people come from well-managed families and do not experience other risk factors.
	Interaction with Antisocial Peers	Defined as having several close friends who engage in problem behaviors. Young people who associate with peers who engage in problem behaviors are at higher risk for engaging in antisocial behavior themselves.
	Rewards for Antisocial Involvement	Defined as having friends who approve of ATOD use and who are ignorant of laws and rules. Young people who receive rewards for their ASB are at higher risk for engaging further in ASB and ATOD use.
	Rebelliousness	Defined as not being bound by rules and taking an active rebellious stance toward society. Young people who do not feel like part of society, are not bound by rules, do not believe in trying to be successful or responsible, or who take an active rebellious stance toward society, are at higher risk of abusing drugs.
	Sensation Seeking	Defined as having a high need for sensation or arousal experiences. Young people with a high need for arousal have increased risk for participating in ATOD use and other problem behaviors.
	Gang Involvement	Defined as the degree of involvement in gangs or with gang members. Gang involvement often increases youth exposure to ATOD use and ASB, which puts them at greater risk for engaging in similar behaviors.
	Depression	Defined as signs of depression or lack of self-worth. Lack of self-worth is often associated with ATOD use.
	Protective Factors	
	Peer Disapproval of ATOD Use and Handguns	Defined as student perceptions that his or her close friends would disapprove of him or her using substances or carrying handguns. Peer pressure is a strong factor influencing adolescent behavior, and peer pressure not to use alcohol, tobacco, and other drugs is a very powerful deterrence.
	Religiosity	Defined as perceiving oneself to be religious and enjoying religious activities. Young people who regularly attend religious services are less likely to engage in problem behaviors.
	Belief in the Moral Order	Defined as beliefs that one is bound by societal rules. Young people who have a belief in what is "right" and "wrong" are less likely to use drugs.
	Educational Aspirations	Defined as aspirations for continuing on to and graduating from college. National surveys of high school seniors have shown that ATOD use is significantly lower among students who expect to attend and graduate from college than among those who do not.

Risk and Protective Factor Definitions
For the Community, Family, School, and Individual Domains

Domain	Factor	Definition
COMMUNITY	**Risk Factors**	
	Low Neighborhood Attachment	Defined as a lack of connection to the community. Low levels of bonding to the neighborhood are related to higher levels of juvenile crime and drug selling.
	Community Disorganization	Defined as the prevalence of crime, violence, and delinquency in the neighborhood. Research has shown tha neighborhoods with high population density, lack of public surveillance, physical deterioration, and high rates of adult crime also have higher rates of juvenile crime and drug selling.
	Transition & Mobility	Defined as amount of movement from one community or school to another. Neighborhoods with high rates of residential mobility have been shown to have higher rates of juvenile crime and drug selling, while childre who experience frequent residential moves and stressful life transitions have been shown to have higher risk for school failure, delinquency, and drug use.
	Exposure to Community Alcohol, Tobacco, and other Drug (ATOD) Use	Defined as frequent exposure to ATOD use by people in one's neighborhood or school. Frequent exposure t ATOD use influences normative beliefs and understanding of how to engage in the behavior and, thus, increases likelihood of ATOD use.
	Laws & Norms Favorable to Drug Use	Defined as the attitudes and policies a community holds about drug use and crime. Research has shown tha legal restrictions on alcohol and tobacco use, such as raising the legal drinking age, restricting smoking in public places, and increasing taxation have been followed by decreases in consumption. Moreover, national surveys of high school seniors have shown that shifts in normative attitudes toward drug use have preceded changes in prevalence or use.
	Perceived Availability of Drugs & Handguns	Defined as the perceived ease in obtaining drugs and firearms for adolescents. The availability of cigarettes alcohol, marijuana, and other illegal drugs has been related to the use of these substances by adolescents. Availability of handguns is also related to a higher risk of crime by adolescents.
	Ability to Purchase Alcohol or Tobacco	Defined as whether or not a student has been able to purchase alcohol and/or tobacco from a store employee, a bar, or a restaurant. Corresponding with perceived availability, opportunities to purchase alcoh and tobacco have been related to use of these substances by adolescents.
	Protective Factors	
	Community Opportunities for Positive Involvement	Defined as opportunities to engage in prosocial activities in the community such as sports or adult-supervis clubs. When opportunities are available in a community for positive participation, children are less likely to engage in substance use and other problem behaviors.
	Community Rewards for Positive Involvement	Defined as community encouragement for adolescents engaging in positive activities. Rewards for positive participation in activities help children bond to the community, thus lowering their risk for substance use.
FAMILY	**Risk Factors**	
	Poor Family Supervision	Defined as a lack of clear expectations for behavior and a failure of parents to monitor their children. Pare failure to provide clear expectations and to monitor their children's behavior makes it more likely that their children will engage in drug use whether or not there are family drug problems.
	Family Conflict	Defined as the degree to which family members fight or argue. Children raised in families high in conflict, whether or not the child is directly involved in the conflict, appear at risk for both delinquency and drug us
	Lack of Parental Sanctions for ATOD Use	Defined as a low probability that parents will sanction their children for ATOD use. Parents' failure to clea communicate to their children that their children would be in trouble if caught using alcohol, tobacco, or o drugs places children at higher risk for substance use.
	Parental Attitudes Favorable Toward ATOD Use	Defined as parental attitudes approving of young people's ATOD use. In families where parents are tolera of children's use, children are more likely to become drug abusers during adolescence.
	Exposure to Family ATOD Use	Defined as a high degree of exposure to parents' ATOD use. In families where parents use illegal drugs o are heavy users of alcohol, children are more likely to become drug abusers during adolescence. The risk further increased if parents involve children in their own substance-using behavior – for example, asking t child to light the parent's cigarette or to get the parent a beer from the refrigerator.
	Parental Attitudes Favorable Toward Anti-Social Behavior (ASB)	Defined as parental attitudes excusing children for breaking the laws. In families where parents are toler of antisocial behavior, children are more likely to engage in antisocial behavior.
	Family (Sibling) History of ASB	Defined as high ASB prevalence among brothers and sisters. When children are raised in a family with a history of problem behaviors, the children are more likely to engage in these behaviors.
	Protective Factors	
	Family Attachment	Defined as feeling connected to and loved by one's family. Young people who feel that they are a value of their family are less likely to engage in substance use and other problem behaviors.
	Family Opportunities for Positive Involvement	Defined as opportunities for positive social interaction with parents. Young people who are exposed to opportunities to participate meaningfully in the responsibilities and activities of the family are less likely engage in drug use and other problem behaviors.
	Family Rewards for Positive Involvement	Defined as positive experiences with parental figures. When family members praise, encourage, and at to their children's accomplishment, children are less likely to engage in substance use and ASB.

WHAT WOULD A COORDINATED PREVENTION SYSTEM LOOK LIKE?

An integrated prevention system for Hawaii could take many forms. A system based on the ideas in the Hawaii Youth Substance Abuse Prevention Strategy might look something like this.

- Prevention planning would be based in 42 local communities defined by the enrollment areas of the State's public High Schools.
- There would be some form of permanent Community Prevention Coalition in each of the 42 local communities. Local people and institutions would come together to assess their community needs, identify service gaps, plan, and operate prevention programs.
- State prevention agencies would develop and maintain a system to help organize, train, and provide technical assistance to local community coalitions.
- Communities would assess their prevention needs in terms of specific risk and protective factors and would implement science-based "Best Practice" prevention programs that had been proven to work.
- State agencies would adopt common outcomes for prevention in Hawaii and would make a long-term, common commitment to funding local community coalitions and local programs based on community assessments of local risk and protective factors and locally determined Best Practice prevention programs.
- State prevention agencies would develop and maintain a system to provide up to date information to community coalitions on risk and protective factors and other local community data. State agencies would work together to provide local communities with information, training, and technical assistance on Best Practices in prevention.
- State prevention agencies would work together to develop and support prevention programs responsive to Hawaii's unique cultural diversity and to develop a State level process to evaluate locally developed prevention approaches and certify them as Best Practices if they are effective.
- State agencies would collaborate to provide staff development for prevention workers, to develop common information systems and data resources, and to build other tools for a developing prevention system.
- State agencies would reach out to federal, county, and private funders to integrate their programs with State efforts to support local community prevention planning based on risk and protective factor analysis and using science-based, best practices in prevention.

Hawai`i State Incentive Grant

FACT SHEET

Hawai`i was awarded a three-year $8.4 million State Incentive Grant (SIG) from the Center for Substance Abuse Prevention (CSAP), Substance Abuse and Mental Health Services Administration.

The SIG has two major goals. The first is to reduce youth alcohol, tobacco, marijuana, and other drug use and abuse among Hawai`i's 12 to 17 year olds by building a statewide system of enduring substance abuse prevention partnerships. This will be accomplished by working at the state and community levels. The second goal is to coordinate, leverage, and redirect substance abuse prevention resources to communities, families, schools, and workplaces. At the community level, community people and organizations will partner to develop and implement effective locally focused prevention activities and programs that are founded on science-based research.

Approximately $2 million per year will be awarded to approximately 18 communities. Up to $150,000 will be awarded per community applicant, for each of the three years of funding. The State plans to publish a Request For Proposals in July 2001, and award contracts before December, 2001.

Communities applying for the SIG will be required, at a minimum, to:

- Demonstrate partnerships that will provide coordinated and collaborative substance abuse prevention efforts
- Identify a school/community complex geographic base in which the substance abuse prevention activities and program services will be provided
- Conduct a needs assessment of their community, including the risk and protective factors
- Identify available prevention resources and gaps in prevention services in their community
- Use a risk and protective factor framework to design prevention services to be implemented in their community
- Select and implement science-based prevention activities and programs
- Participate in evaluation process

Statewide community workshops and trainings will take place in June-July 2001 and will be open to all interested organizations and individuals.

Questions regarding the Hawaii SIG should be directed to Dr. Catherine Sorensen, SIG Program Manager at (808) 692-7530 or Raymond Gagner, SIG Program Coordinator at (808) 692-7531.

THE EIGHTEEN STATE INCENTIVE GRANT PARTNERSHIPS

LEAD ORGANIZATION	AREA	AWARD	BEST PRACTICE
Boys & Girls Club of Hawaii	Nuuanu/Makiki	$420,000	Smart Moves Smart Leaders FAN Club Mentoring
Boys & Girls Club of Hawaii	Kaimuki/Palolo	$420,000	Smart Moves Smart Leaders FAN Club
YMCA of Honolulu	Waialua/Haleiwa	$420,000	Positive Action
Coalition for Drug-Free Hawaii	Kahuku/Laie	$450,000	Reconnecting Youth ATLAS
Coalition for Drug-Free Hawaii	Ewa	$450,000	Reconnecting Youth Smart Moves Smart Leaders
Susannah Wesley Community Center	Kalihi	$450,000	Parenting Adolescents Wisely
Lanai Youth Center	Lanai	$450,000	Creating Lasting Family Connections Smart Leaders/FAN Club Mentoring
Family Support Services of West Hawaii	South Kona	$ 330,000	Across Ages
Family Support Service of West Hawaii	Kohala	$390,000	Project Venture
Boys & Girls Club of Maui	Makawao	$405,500	Smart Moves Smart Leaders FAN Club
Maui Youth & Family Services	Wailuku	$450,000	Project Venture Solutions For Families Mentoring
West Kauai Community Business & Professional Association	Waimea	$207,000	Smart Moves Smart Leaders
Kauai Economic Opportunity, Inc.	Central Kauai	$450,000	Life Skills Training
Laupahoehoe Train Museum	Honokaa	$369,300	Communities That Care
Hawaii Conference of Seventh-day Adventists	Molokai	$369,300	Communities That Care
Waianae Coast Comprehensive Health Center	Waianae	$369,300	Communities That Care
Parents and Children Together	Kaneohe	$369,300	Communities That Care
Waipahu Community Association	Waipahu	$369,300	Communities That Care

ALCOHOL AND DRUG ABUSE DIVISION – STATE FY 2004

OAHU – SUBSTANCE ABUSE PREVENTION – ALL FEDERAL FUNDS

AGENCY	SAPT FUNDS*	SIG FUNDS**
Boys & Girls Club (Waianae & Nanakuli	$ 132,000	$ ---
Ka'ala Farms (Waianae)	$ 80,000	$ ---
Waimanalo Health Center	$ 137,000	$ ---
Maui Center for Health Care	$ 70,000	$ ---
Coalition For A Drug-Free Hawaii – Ewa Beach	$ 130,037	$ ---
Waipahu Community Association	$ ---	$ 123,100
Boys & Girls Club – Nuuanu/Kalihi	$ ---	$ 140,000
Boys &Girls Club – Kaimuki/Palolo	$ ---	$ 140,000
YMCA of Honolulu – Waialua/Haleiwa	$ ---	$ 140,000
Coalition For A Drug-Free Hawaii – Kahuku/Laie	$ ---	$ 150,000
Coalition For A Drug-Free Hawaii – Ewa	$ ---	$ 150,000
Susannah Wesley Community Center – Kalihi	$ ---	$ 150,000
Parents and Children Together - Kaneohe	$ ---	$ 123,100
Waianae Coast Comprehensive Health Center	$ ---	$ 123,100
SUBTOTAL:	$ 549,037	$1,239,300

* SAPT Grant – Federal Substance Abuse Prevention & Treatment Block Grant
**SIG Grant – Federal State Incentive Grant

ALCOHOL AND DRUG ABUSE DIVISION – STATE FY 2004

MAUI – SUBSTANCE ABUSE PREVENTION - ALL FEDERAL FUNDS

AGENCY	SAPT FUNDS*	SIG FUNDS**
Alu Like – Hana	$ 75,000	$ —
Aloha House - Maui	$ 75,000	$ —
Maui Center for Health Care Education	$ 60,000	$ —
Boys & Girls Club of Maui – Makawao	$ ---	$ 135,500
Maui Youth & Family Services – Wailuku	$ ---	$ 150,000
MOLOKAI:		
Alu Like – Molokai	$ 75,000	$ —
Hawaii Conference of Seventh-day Adventists	$ ---	$ 123,100
LANAI:		
Lanai Youth Center	$ ---	$ 150,000
SUBTOTAL:	$ 285,000	$ 558,600

* SAPT Grant – Federal Substance Abuse Prevention & Treatment Block Grant
**SIG Grant – Federal State Incentive Grant

ALCOHOL AND DRUG ABUSE DIVISION – STATE FY 2004

HAWAII – SUBSTANCE ABUSE PREVENTION - ALL FEDERAL FUNDS

AGENCY	**SAPT FUNDS***	**SIG FUNDS****
YWCA of Hawaii – East Hawaii	$ 75,000	$ ---
Alu Like – West Hawaii	$ 75,000	$ ---
Family Support Services of West Hawaii – South Kona	$ ---	$ 110,000
Family Support Services of West Hawaii – Kohala	$ ---	$ 130,000
Laupahoehoe Train Museum		$ 123,100
SUBTOTAL:	$ 150,000	$ 363,100

* SAPT Grant – Federal Substance Abuse Prevention & Treatment Block Grant
**SIG Grant – Federal State Incentive Grant

ALCOHOL AND DRUG ABUSE DIVISION – STATE FY 2004

KAUAI – SUBSTANCE ABUSE PREVENTION - ALL FEDERAL FUNDS

AGENCY	**SAPT FUNDS***	**SIG FUNDS****
Alu Like	$ 70,000	$ ---
West Kauai Community Business & Professional Association – Waimea	$ ---	$ 69,000
Kauai Economic Opportunity – Central Kauai	$ ---	$ 150,000
Office of the Mayor	$ 5,000	$ ---
SUBTOTAL:	$ 75,000	$ 219, 000

* SAPT Grant – Federal Substance Abuse Prevention & Treatment Block Grant
**SIG Grant – Federal State Incentive Grant

ALCOHOL AND DRUG ABUSE DIVISION – STATE FY 2004

STATEWIDE SUBSTANCE ABUSE PREVENTION

AGENCY	SAPT FUNDS*	TOBACCO SETTLEMENT FUNDS
DOE - Parenting	$ 95,000	$ ---
MADD Youth In Action	$ 60,000	$ ---
Coalition For A Drug-Free Hawaii - RADAR	$ 176,000	$ ---
STATEWIDE SYSTEM SUPPORT:		
Starling Consulting -- MIS	$ 30,000	$ ---
UH Conf. Ctr. – Training	$ 70,000	$ ---
UH CRC – Synar	$ 68,989	$ ---
UH SSRI – Student Survey	$ 222,924	$ ---
UH SSRI – Evaluation	$ 130,033	$ ---
UH Center on Family	$ 100,000	$ ---
UH CRC (Enforcement)	$ ---	$ 206,325
Honolulu Police Dept.	$ ---	$ 24,576
Hawaii Police Dept.	$ ---	$ 12,912
Maui Police Dept.	$ ---	$ 11,216
Kauai Police Dept.	$ ---	$ 5,076
SUBTOTAL:	$ 952,946	$ 260,105

* SAPT Grant – Federal Substance Abuse Prevention & Treatment Block Grant

OFFICE OF JUVENILE JUSTICE AND DELINQUENCY PREVENTION ENFORCING UNDERAGE DRINKING LAWS

Title of the Grant: "Enforcing the Underage Drinking Laws Program," Supported under the Juvenile Justice and Delinquency Prevention Act of 1974, as amended.

Amount of the Grant: $360,000 for FY 2003

Purpose of the Grant:

To reduce underage drinking by expanding the number of communities taking a comprehensive approach to the problem, with a special emphasis on increasing law enforcement activities with regard to the sale of alcohol to minors by increasing State-level planning and program activities, preventing the purchase or consumption of alcoholic beverages by minors under the age of twenty-one and changing community norms and attitudes regarding underage drinking.

How the grant is being used:

- Collaboration with each county police department and liquor commission to implement and document a statewide system of compliance checks to enforce underage drinking laws.
- Maintaining contacts with appropriate liquor commission staff regarding administrative hearings in cases of alcohol sales to minors resulting from the inspections, and with the appropriate County Prosecutor's Office regarding criminal proceedings, and ensuring that participating minors are available as witnesses in administrative and criminal proceedings.
- Coordinating the Statewide Advisory Council and updating the Council's Strategic Plan.
- Developing and implementing an annual media strategy which includes media coverage of penalties associated with breaking underage drinking laws, increasing merchant education of the penalties of selling to minors and gives a message educating parents and minors on the harm and consequences of underage drinking.
- Attending the required annual OJJDP conference.

ALCOHOL AND DRUG ABUSE DIVISION – STATE FY 2004

SUBSTANCE ABUSE PREVENTION - ALL FEDERAL FUNDS

ENFORCING UNDERAGE DRINKING LAWS (OJJDP ** FEDERAL FUNDS)

AGENCY	FED. OJJDP	SAPT BLOCK GRANT	TOTAL
• MADD	$ 272,740	$ 60,000	$332,750
• Honolulu Police Dept.	$ 49,000	-0-	$ 49,000
• Maui Police Dept.	$ 6,248	-0-	$ 6,248
• Kauai Police Dept.	$ 13,260	-0-	$ 13,260
• Hawaii Police Dept.	$ 20,000	-0-	$ 20,000
SUBTOTAL:	$ 361,248		$421,259

* SAPT Grant - Federal Substance Abuse Prevention & Treatment Block Grant
** OJJDP - Federal Office of Juvenile Justice & Delinquency Prevention

PREVENTION RESEARCH PRINCIPLES FOR CHILDREN AND ADOLESCENTS

- Prevention programs should be designed to enhance "protective factors" and move toward reversing or reducing "risk factors".
- Prevention programs should target all forms of drug abuse, including the use of tobacco, alcohol, marijuana and inhalants.
- Prevention programs should include skill to resist drugs when offered, strengthen personal commitments against drug use, and increase social competency (e.g., in communications, peer relationship, self-efficacy, and assertiveness), in conjunction with reinforcement of attitudes against drug use.
- Prevention programs for adolescents should include interactive methods, such as peer discussion groups, rather than didactic etching techniques alone.
- Prevention programs should include a parent's or caregiver's component that reinforces what the children are learning – such as facts about drugs and their harmful effects – and that opens opportunities for family discussions about use of legal and illegal substance and family policies and their use.
- Prevention programs should be long-term, over the school career with repeat interventions to reinforce the original prevention goals. For example, school-based efforts directed at elementary and middle school students should include booster sessions to help with critical transitions from middle to high school.
- Family-focused prevention efforts have a greater impact than strategies that focus on parents only or children only.
- Community programs that include media campaigns and policy changes, such as new regulations that restrict access to alcohol, tobacco, or other drugs, are more effective when they are accompanied by school and family interventions.
- Community programs need to strengthen norms against drug use in all drug abuse prevention settings, including the family, the school, and the community.
- Schools offer opportunities to reach all populations and also serve as important settings for specific subpopulations at risk for drug abuse, such as children with behavior problems or learning disabilities and those who are potential droopiest.
- Prevention programming should be adapted to address the specific nature of the drug abuse problem in the local community.
- The higher the level of risk of the target population, the more intensive the prevention effort must be and the earlier it must begin.
- Prevention programs should be age-specific, developmentally appropriate, and culturally sensitive.
- Effective prevention programs are most effective. For every dollar spent on drug use prevention, communities can save $4 to $5 in costs for drug treatment and counseling.

Source: Preventing Drug Use Among Children and Adolescents: A Research Bases Guide, National Institute on Drug Abuse, National Institutes of Health

SUBSTANCE ABUSE PREVENTION RECOMMENDATIONS

- **Make substance abuse prevention a priority in every community.**
  - Involving community
  - Using protective factors important
  - Community efforts to reduce availability through merchant compliance, enforcement of laws
  - Restricting alcohol and smoking

- **Strengthen the family's roles and skills in substance abuse prevention efforts.**
  - Exposure puts youth at risk
  - Parents' expressed disapproval is a powerful deterrent
  - Parents talking an active role in child's life
  - Talk about dangers; monitor activities; communicating; family time

- **Ensure that every adolescent who has substance abuse problems get treatment**
  - School-based treatment accessible
  - Make sure students know there is treatment

- **Increase mass media coverage on substance abuse prevention & treatment**
  - Alter the myth that everyone is using
  - Educate parents about their critical role
  - Increase public awareness of prevention and treatment programs
  - Printed material in workplace, physicians' office

- **Increase community awareness of the serious consequences of underage drinking**
  - Limit alcohol
  - Enforce laws

- **Strengthen substance abuse prevention programs in the school and community.**
  - Begin no later than 4th grade and continue through high school
  - Community approaches also
  - Address risk and protective factors
  - Use "Best Practices"

ADAD, August 2003

2002 Hawaii Statewide Treatment for Students in Grades 6 Through 12

COUNTY/DISTRICT INFORMATION		Alcohol Abuse *Only* Treatment Needs		Drug Abuse *Only* Treatment Needs		*Both* Alcohol and Drug Abuse Treatment Needs		ANY SUBSTANCE ABUSE TREATMENT NEEDS		*Any* Alcohol Abuse Treatment Needs		*Any* Drug Abuse Treatment Needs	
	Total N	%	n	%	n	%	n	%	n	%	n		
City & County of Honolulu	58,645	2.3%	1,355	2.8%	1,621	4.3%	2,490	9.3%	5,458	6.5%	3,785	6.1%	3,591
Honolulu District	16,517	2.2%	356	2.3%	373	3.9%	636	8.3%	1,364	5.9%	980	5.1%	840
Central District	15,714	2.0%	318	2.3%	361	3.8%	597	8.1%	1,277	5.8%	903	5.5%	862
Leeward District	17,841	2.5%	444	2.5%	450	4.0%	705	8.9%	1,593	6.3%	1,129	5.7%	1,020
Windward District	8,573	2.8%	237	5.1%	437	6.4%	552	14.3%	1,224	9.0%	773	10.1%	869
Hawaii County/District	13,077	4.2%	545	3.8%	491	5.8%	756	13.7%	1,787	9.8%	1,284	8.8%	1,150
Kauai County/District	5,268	2.9%	151	4.4%	233	5.5%	288	12.7%	671	8.2%	430	9.0%	476
Maui County/District	10,813	2.8%	304	4.2%	457	7.4%	796	14.4%	1,558	10.0%	1,082	10.3%	1,115
All Public Schools	87,803	2.7%	2,355	3.2%	2,802	4.9%	4,330	10.8%	9,474	7.5%	6,581	7.2%	6,332
Private Schools	19,058	2.9%	561	2.2%	413	4.6%	872	9.7%	1,845	7.5%	1,423	6.2%	1,187
TOTAL STATEWIDE	106,861	2.7%	2,916	3.0%	3,215	4.9%	5,202	10.6%	11,319	7.5%	8,004	7.0%	7,519

ADDICTION

- **Bio-psycho-social disease**
- **Requires ongoing treatment and intervention, not just episodic or acute care**
- **Addictive disorder cannot be addressed in isolation from biological, psychological or social needs**

FACTS ABOUT TREATMENT

- **Drug addiction is a preventable disease**
- **Drug addiction is a treatable disease**
- **Prolonged drug use changes the brain in fundamental and long lasting ways**
- **Addiction is a brain disease expressed as compulsive behavior**
- **The brains of addicts are different from the brains of non-addicts**
- **Those differences are an essential element of addiction**
- **A major task for treatment is changing the brain back**
- **The most effective treatment strategies will address all aspects of addiction: medical, psychological, social, vocational, and legal problems**

MOTIVATION TO ENTER TREATMENT

- **Effective treatment need not be voluntary**
- **Sanctions/enticements (family, employer, criminal justice system) can increase treatment entry/retention**
- **Treatment outcomes are similar for those who enter treatment under legal pressure vs voluntary**

EFFECTIVENESS OF TREATMENT

- **Addiction can be treated as readily as hypertension, diabetes and asthma**
- **The goal of treatment is to return to productive functioning**
- **Treatment reduces drug use by 40%-60%**
- **Treatment reduces crime by 40%-60%**
- **Treatment increases employment prospects by 40%**
- **Treatment is less expensive than not treating or incarceration**
- **Every $1 invested in treatment yields up to $7 in reduced crime-related costs**
- **Savings can exceed costs by 12:1 when health care costs are included**
- **Reduced interpersonal conflicts**
- **Improved workplace productivity**
- **Fewer drug-related accidents**

FOR TREATMENT TO BE EFFECTIVE

- **Duration for at least 3 months to one year**
- **Intensive, comprehensive and highly structured**
- **Focus on all aspects of patient's life - medical, psychological, social, vocational, educational and legal**
- **Support groups - most treatment programs encourage participation during/after treatment**

ADAD, August 2003

ADOLESCENT DRUG ABUSE DIAGNOSIS

A diagnostic instrument used to:

- Assess substance use and other life problems
- Assist with individualized treatment planning
- Assess changes in life problem areas and severity over time.

The instrument provides a comprehensive, relevant, and dynamic picture of the problems currently impacting on a troubled adolescent.

It is a structured interview designed to address nine potential problem areas in substance usii adolescents:

- Medical status
- School
- Employment
- Social
- Family
- Psychological
- Delinquent behavior
- Drug
- Alcohol

ADAD, August 2003

TREATMENT ADMISSIONS FROM ALCOHOL AND DRUG ABUSE DIVISION

TREATMENT EPISODE SYSTEM (TEDS)

Treatment Admissions - By any drug/alcohol 1998-2002

	1998	1999	2000	2001	2002
Adults	5,518	5,745	6,500	6,454	6,369
Adolescents	1,821	1,525	1,633	1,641	1,552
TOTAL	7,339	7,270	8,133	8,095	7,921

A. Treatment Admissions - Primary substance of abuse – Methamphetamine

	1998	1999	2000	2001	2002
Adults	1,423	1,517	2,136	2,332	2,730
Adolescents	189	126	143	150	158
TOTAL	1,612	1,643	2,279	2,482	2,888

B. Treatment Admissions - Primary substance of abuse - Alcohol

	1998	1999	2000	2001	2002
Adults	2,231	2,337	2,469	2,435	2,051
Adolescents	429	379	432	442	378
TOTAL	2,660	2,716	2,901	2,877	2,429

C. Treatment Admissions - Primary substance of abuse - Marijuana

	1998	1999	2000	2001	2002
Adults	343	404	495	552	558
Adolescents	1,158	961	956	979	949
TOTAL	1,501	1,365	1,451	1,531	1,507

Source: Hawaii DOH, Alcohol and Drug Abuse Division (August 2003)

KEY ELEMENTS OF EFFECTIVENESS FOR ADOLESCENT SUBSTANCE ABUSE TREATMENT

- ASSESSMENT AND TREATMENT MATCHING
  - Use standardized screening instruments
  - In-depth assessment including medical, psychiatric and family
  - Use ASAM Patient Placement Criteria
- COMPREHENSIVE, INTEGRATED TREAMENT APPROACH
  - Address co-occurring mental disorders, juvenile justice problems; STD problems; school failure; health; etc.
- FAMILY INVOLVEMENT IN TREATMENT
- DEVELOPMENTALLY APPROPRIATE PROGRAM
  - Can't just be adult programs modified for adolescents
- ENGAGE AND RETAIN TEENS IN TREATMENT
  - Creative techniques to engage and retain teens in treatment
  - Often referred or coerced by parents, school, juvenile justice systems
  - Teens view treatment as curtailing their independence
  - Climate of trust and acceptance is vitally important
- QUALIFIED STAFF
  - Knowledge and experience in treating youth
  - Clinical supervision
- GENDER AND CULTURAL COMPETENCE
  - Many girls report having been sexually/physically abused
  - Depression and trauma in girls often precedes drug use
  - Girls reluctant to talk freely in front of boys about some of their experiences.
  - Retention rates higher when culturally appropriate
- CONTINUING CARE
  - Gains made in treatment need to be supported
  - Relapse prevention
- TREATMENT OUTCOMES
  - Routinely measure progress
  - Check school performance, disruptive behavior, family problems

Source: "Treating Teens: A Guide To Adolescent Drug Programs"

ADAD, August 2003

TEN IMPORTANT QUESTIONS TO ASK AN ADOLESCENT TREATMENT PROGRAM

1) How does your program address the needs of adolescents?

2) What kind of assessment does the program conduct of the adolescent's problems?

3) How often does the program review and update the treatment plan in light of the adolescent's progress?

4) How is the family involved in the treatment process?

5) How do you engage adolescents so that they stay in treatment?

6) What are the qualifications of program staff and what kind of clinical supervision is provided?

7) Does the program separate single sex groups as well as male and female counselors for girls and boys?

8) How does the program follow up with the adolescent and provide continuing care after treatment is completed?

9) What evidence do you have that your program is effective?

10) What is the cost of your program?

Source: "Treating Teens: A Guide to Adolescent Drug Programs"

ADAD, August 2003

SCHOOL-BASED SUBSTANCE ABUSE TREATMENT

THE NEED:

Results of the "2002 Hawaii Student Alcohol, Tobacco and Drug Use Survey," were extrapolated to provide a projection of the number of youths ages 12-17 in need of substance abuse treatment. The findings indicate the following:

- 2,916 youths statewide need treatment for alcohol abuse while an additional 3,215 need treatment for drug abuse. Additionally, 5,202 require treatment for both alcohol and drug abuse, leading to a combined total of 11,319 students or 10.6% who have either an alcohol abuse problem or both.

THE GOAL OF SCHOOL-BASED SUBSTANCE ABUSE TREATMENT:

- To ensure that substance abuse treatment is available to youth statewide at public middle and high schools to reduce the severity and disabling effects related to alcohol and other drug abuse.
- Measurable outcomes:
  - Improved school attendance, tardiness and/or grades
  - No new drug-related or any other arrests
  - Alcohol and/or drug abstinence or at least reduction in use
  - Tobacco abstinence or at lest reduction in use
  - Reduction of school alcohol and drug abuse
  - Improved social relations (reduction in conflicts with families, peers and teachers)
  - Lower rates of emotional, physical and sexual abuse
  - Successful completion of treatment
  - Lower rates of sexually transmitted disease

DESCRIPTION OF SCHOOL-BASED SUBSTANCE ABUSE TREATMENT:

The programs provide treatment, intervention and counseling services and include outreach; crisis intervention; individual, group and family sessions for education and counseling; peer and adult role modeling; and clean and sober recreational activities. The combination of individual and group sessions is supplemented by family education and counseling.

In addition, school-based programs provide education and consultation to school faculty in identifying and referring students. On campus programs have proven to provide consistency, visibility, accessibility and support for both school staff and students alike. Successful results are changes in personal attitudes, behavior and lifestyle, as well as reduced use and abstinence.

THE ESTIMATED BUDGET PER SCHOOL FOR TREATMENT:

The cost for two counselors at each site and related operational and administrative expenses is $90,000 per school per year.

ADAD, August 2003

2003-2004
HAWAII PUBLIC HIGH SCHOOLS (Grades 9-12)

School District	SCHOOL	ADAD Treatment*
Honolulu District (Oahu)	ANUENUE	
	FARRINGTON	X
	KAIMUKI	X
	KAISER	
	KALANI	X
	MCKINLEY	
	ROOSEVELT	X
Central District (Oahu)	AIEA	X
	LEILEHUA	X
	MILILANI	X
	MOANALUA	X
	RADFORD	
	WAIALUA	X
Leeward District (Oahu)	CAMPBELL	X
	KAPOLEI	
	NANAKULI	X
	PEARL CITY	X
	WAIANAE	X
	WAIPAHU	X
Windward District (Oahu)	CASTLE	X
	KAHUKU	X
	KAILUA	X
	KALAHEO	X
	OLOMANA	X
Hawaii District	HILO	X*
	HONOKAA	X*
	KONAWAENA	X
	KAU	X
	KEAAU	
	KEALAKEHE	X*
	KOHALA	
	LAUPAHOEHOE	X*
	PAHOA	X
	WAIAKEA	X
Maui District (Maui, Lanai, Molokai)	BALDWIN	X
	HANA	
	King KEKAULIKE	X
	LAHAINALUNA	X
	MAUI	X
	LANAI	X
	MOLOKAI	
Kauai District (Kauai, Niihau)	KAPAA	X
	KAUAI	
	WAIMEA	X
	NIIHAU	

X School-based treatment programs funded by ADAD.
X* School-based treatment programs funded by SAMHSA.
Of the 45 high schools, 29 have ADAD-funded treatment and 16 do not. 28

2003-2004
HAWAII PUBLIC MIDDLE SCHOOLS (Grades 7 & 8)

School District	SCHOOL	ADAD Treatment*
Honolulu District (Oahu)	ANUENUE	
	CENTRAL	
	DOLE	
	JARRETT	
	KAIMUKI	
	KALAKAUA	
	KAWANANAKOA	
	NIU VALLEY	
	STEVENSON	
	WASHINGTON	
Central District (Oahu)	AIEA	
	ALIAMANU	
	MILILANI	
	MOANALUA	
	WAHIAWA	
	WAIALUA	
	WHEELER	
Leeward District (Oahu)	HIGHLANDS	
	KAPOLEI	
	NANAKULI	
	WAIANAE	
	WAIPAHU	
	ILIMA	
Windward District (Oahu)	KAHUKU	
	KAILUA	
	KING	X
	WAIMANALO	
	OLOMANA	
Hawaii District	HILO	
	HONAUNAU	
	HONOKAA	
	HOOKENA	
	KALANIANAOLE	
	KAU / PAHALA	
	KEAAU	
	KOHALA	
	KONAWAENA	
	LAUPAHOEHOE	
	NAALEHU	
	PAAUILO	
	PAHOA	
	WAIAKEA	
	WAIMEA	
	KEALAKEHE	
Maui District (Maui, Lanai, Molokai)	HANA	
	IAO	
	LAHAINA	
	SAMUEL E. KALAMA	X
	MAUI-WAENA	
	LOKELANI	
	LANAI	
	MOLOKAI	
Kauai District (Kauai, Niihau)	KAPAA	X
	KAUAI	
	KAMAKAHELEI CHIEFESS	
	WAIMEA CANYON	
	NIIHAU	

Of the 57 middle schools, 3 have ADAD-funded treatment, 54 do not.
Note: Enrollment counts include regular and special education students.

STATE OF HAWAII
DEPARTMENT OF HEALTH
ALCOHOL AND DRUG ABUSE DIVISION
ADOLESCENT SCHOOL-BASED SUBSTANCE ABUSE TREATMENT SERVICES
STATE FY 2004

ISLAND	AGENCY	SCHOOLS	BUDGET/ year
Oahu	Hina Mauka	Kalani High School Kalaheo High School Castle High School Pearl City High School Olomana Youth Center Mililani High School Kahuku High School King Int. & High School	$743,199
	YMCA of Honolulu	Leilehua High School Roosevelt High School Farrington High School Moanalua High School Aiea High School Waipahu High School Campbell High School Kailua High School Kaimuki High School Waialua Int & High School Waianae High School Nanakuli Int & High School	$975,837
Hawaii	BISAC	Waiakea High School Pahoa High School Konawaena High School Ka`u High School	$217,434
Kauai	Hina Mauka	Kapaa Intermediate School Kapaa High School Waimea High School	$150,000
Maui	Aloha House	Baldwin High School Maui High School	$100,000
	MYFS	King Kekaulike High School Lahainaluna High School	$135,000
Lanai	MYFS	Lanai Elementary, Int & High School	

TREATMENT PROGRAM PERFORMANCE RESULTS

During the state Fiscal Year 2002 (July 1, 2001 to June 30, 2002), six-month follow-ups were completed for a sample of 901 adolescents. Listed below are the outcomes for this sample:

ADOLESCENT SUBSTANCE ABUSE TREATMENT-FY 2002	
MEASURE	PERFORMANCE OUTCOME ACHIEVED SIX-MONTHS AFTER DISCHARGE
Employment/School/Vocational Training	95.2%
No Arrests Since Discharge	87.3%
No Substance Use 30 Days Prior to Follow Up	44.4%
No New Substance Abuse Treatment	79.2%
No Hospitalizations	95.4%
No Emergency Room Visits	93.1%
No Psychological Distress Since Discharge	78.8%
Stable Living Arrangements	94.8%

ADAD, August 2003

JOINT HOUSE-SENATE COMMITTEE ON ICE AND DRUG ABATEMENT

FOCUS – ADULTS

HANDOUT

Elaine Wilson, ACSW, LSW, MPH
Chief, Alcohol and Drug Abuse Division
Hawaii Department of Health
August 27, 2003

A COMPREHENSIVE APPROACH TO REDUCE SUBSTANCE ABUSE

- LOWER PEOPLE'S VULNERABILITY
- PREVENT INITIAL USE
- PREVENT VOLUNTARY USERS FROM PROGRESSING TO ADDICTION
- TREAT ADDICTS
- REDUCE ACCESS TO DRUGS AND THE DRUG MARKETING AND DISTRIBUTION SYSTEM

ADDICTION

- Bio-psycho-social disease
- Requires ongoing treatment and intervention, not just episodic or acute care
- Addictive disorder cannot be addressed in isolation from biological, psychological or social needs

FACTS ABOUT TREATMENT

- Drug addiction is a preventable disease
- Drug addiction is a treatable disease
- Prolonged drug use changes the brain in fundamental and long lasting ways
- Addiction is a brain disease expressed as compulsive behavior
- The brains of addicts are different from the brains of non-addicts
- Those differences are an essential element of addiction
- A major task for treatment is changing the brain back
- The most effective treatment strategies will address all aspects of addiction: medical, psychological, social, vocational, and legal problems

MOTIVATION TO ENTER TREATMENT

- Effective treatment need not be voluntary
- Sanctions/enticements (family, employer, criminal justice system) can increase treatment entry/retention
- Treatment outcomes are similar for those who enter treatment under legal pressure vs voluntary

EFFECTIVENESS OF TREATMENT

- Addiction can be treated as readily as hypertension, diabetes and asthma
- The goal of treatment is to return to productive functioning
- Treatment reduces drug use by 40%-60%
- Treatment reduces crime by 40%-60%
- Treatment increases employment prospects by 40%
- Treatment is less expensive than not treating or incarceration
- Every $1 invested in treatment yields up to $7 in reduced crime-related costs
- Savings can exceed costs by 12:1 when health care costs are included
- Reduced interpersonal conflicts
- Improved workplace productivity
- Fewer drug-related accidents

FOR TREATMENT TO BE EFFECTIVE

- Duration for at least 3 months to one year
- Intensive, comprehensive and highly structured
- Focus on all aspects of patient's life - medical, psychological, social, vocational, educational and legal
- Support groups - most treatment programs encourage participation during/after treatment

ADAD, August 2003

ADDICTION DIAGNOSIS
BASED ON THE DIAGNOSTIC AND STATISTICAL MANUAL – IV (DSM-IV)

Addiction is manifested by 3 or more of the following, occurring at any time in the same 12-month period:

- **Substance is taken in larger amounts or over longer period than intended**
- **Persistent desire or unsuccessful efforts to cut down or control substance**
- **Great deal of time is spent in activities necessary to obtain the substance (e.g., visiting multiple doctors, driving long distances), use the substance, or recover from its effects**
- **Important social, occupational, or recreational activities given up or reduced because of substance abuse**
- **Continued substance use despite know of having a persistent or recurrent psychological or physical problem that is caused or exacerbated by use of the substance**
- **Tolerance of the substance, as defined by either: need for markedly increased amounts of the substance in order to achieve intoxication or desired effect; or markedly diminished effect with continued use of the same amount**
- **Withdrawal, as manifested by either: characteristic withdrawal syndrome for the substance; or the same (or closely related) substance is taken to relieve or avoid withdrawal symptoms.**

ADDICTION SEVERITY INDEX (ASI)

Semistructured interview designed to address seven potential problem areas in substance abusing patients:

- **Medical status**
- **Employment and support**
- **Drug Use**
- **Alcohol use**
- **Legal status**
- **Family/social status**
- **Psychiatric**

The ASI is used for treatment planning and outcome evaluation.

ADAD. August 2003

ADDICTION DIAGNOSIS
BASED ON THE DIAGNOSTIC AND STATISTICAL MANUAL – IV (DSM-IV)

Addiction is manifested by 3 or more of the following, occurring at any time in the same 12-month period:

- **Substance is taken in larger amounts or over longer period than intended**
- **Persistent desire or unsuccessful efforts to cut down or control substance**
- **Great deal of time is spent in activities necessary to obtain the substance (e.g., visiting multiple doctors, driving long distances), use the substance, or recover from its effects**
- **Important social, occupational, or recreational activities given up or reduced because of substance abuse**
- **Continued substance use despite know of having a persistent or recurrent psychological or physical problem that is caused or exacerbated by use of the substance**
- **Tolerance of the substance, as defined by either: need for markedly increased amounts of the substance in order to achieve intoxication or desired effect; or markedly diminished effect with continued use of the same amount**
- **Withdrawal, as manifested by either: characteristic withdrawal syndrome for the substance; or the same (or closely related) substance is taken to relieve or avoid withdrawal symptoms.**

ADDICTION SEVERITY INDEX (ASI)

Semistructured interview designed to address seven potential problem areas in substance abusing patients:

- **Medical status**
- **Employment and support**
- **Drug Use**
- **Alcohol use**
- **Legal status**
- **Family/social status**
- **Psychiatric**

The ASI is used for treatment planning and outcome evaluation.

ADAD. August 2003

AMERICAN SOCIETY OF ADDICTION MEDICINE (ASAM) PATIENT PLACEMENT CRITERIA FOR THE TREATMENT OF SUBSTANCE-RELATED DISORDERS

- **Clinical guide used in matching patients with the appropriate level of treatment.**

- **Patient matched to services based on clinical severity and level of functioning.**

- **A mutildimensional assessment addressing 6 primary problem areas (or dimensions) in order to be able to make patient placement decisions and to formulate an individual treatment plan. The six dimensions addressed are:**

  1. **Acute intoxication and/or withdrawal potential**

  2. **Biomedical conditions and complications**

  3. **Emotional/behavioral conditions and complications (e.g., psychiatric conditions, psychological or emotional/behavioral complications of known or unknown origin, poor impulse control, changes in mental status, or transient neuropsychiatric complications)**

  4. **Treatment acceptance/resistance**

  5. **Relapse/continued use potential**

  6. **Recovery/living environment**

- **Once the severity assessment has been completed, the client is placed in a level of care that most efficiently and effectively can provide the specific modalities and services required.**

- **The overall structure of the levels of care and services are as follows:**

  - **Early Intervention Service (Level 0.5)**
  - **Opiate Maintenance Therapy**
  - **Detoxification Service**
  - **Level I Outpatient Services**
  - **Level II Intensive Outpatient/Partial Hospitalization Services**
  - **Level III Residential/Inpatient Services**
  - **Level IV Medically-Managed Intensive Inpatient Services**

ADAD, August 2003

WHAT IS SUBSTANCE ABUSE TREATMENT?

- **BROAD RANGE OF SERVICES, INCLUDING:**
  - **IDENTIFICATION**
  - **ASSESSMENT**
  - **DIAGNOSIS**
  - **COUNSELING**
  - **MEDICAL SERVICES**
  - **PSYCHIATRIC SERVICES**
  - **PSYCHOLOGICAL SERVICES**
  - **SOCIAL SERVICES**
  - **FOLLOW-UP (CONTINUING CARE)**

- **OVERALL GOAL OF TREATMENT:**
  - **REDUCE OR ELIMINATE THE USE OF ALCOHOL AND/OR DRUGS AS A CONTRIBUTING FACTOR TO PHYSICAL, PSYCHOLOGICAL, AND SOCIAL DYSFUNCTION**
  - **REVERSE PROGRESS OF ANY ASSOCIATED PROBLEMS**

ADAD, August 2003

ADULT SUBSTANCE ABUSE TREATMENT NEEDS

- The 1998 Hawaii Adult Household Survey indicates there are 82,880 adults in need of treatment (about 9% of the adult population). Approximately 19,062 adults will need publicly funded treatment. Of the 19,062 adults, 50% or 9,531 would enter treatment if treatment were available. There are public resources to provide treatment to approximately 6,369 adults, leaving a gap of 3,162 adults untreated.

- Child Protective Services (CPS) has about 6,261 active family cases (as of July 2003). It is estimated that between 80% and 90% of CPS clients need substance abuse treatment.

- The 1996 DOH "Blind Study of Substance Abuse and Need for Treatment Among Women of Child-Bearing Age in Hawaii" revealed that 15.7% of non-pregnant women in prenatal clinics tested positive for use within the last 48 hours of one or more illegal drugs, while 12.7% of the clinics' pregnant women tested positive for one or more illegal drugs. Based on 18,552 births (1995), 2,356 infants would be born exposed to illegal drugs prenatally.

- It is estimated that over 80% of the adult criminal justice population is in need of substance abuse treatment. Diverting offenders who are at risk of being incarcerated or re-incarcerated can reduce dependence and rescue criminality.

- 2002 Hawaii Student Alcohol, Tobacco and Other Drug Use Survey indicates that approximately 11,319 (10.6%) of students in grades 6 through 12 meet the criteria for needing substance abuse treatment.

- Wait list for publicly funded adult substance abuse treatment - between 150 and 300 clients per day.

PRIVATE INSURANCE AND QUEST TREATMENT BENEFIT

- Chapter 431M, HRS mandates a substance abuse benefit for people working 20 or more hours per week. The covered benefit includes not less than 30 days of in-hospital services per year which can be exchanged for 2 days of non-hospital residential or 2 days of day treatment or partial hospitalization, or 2 days of outpatient treatment. The total covered benefit for outpatient treatment is not less than 12 visits per year. For the substance abuse benefit, the insurer may limit the number of treatment episodes to 2 treatment episodes per lifetime.

- QUEST eligible clients can access treatment based on medical necessity determined by each QUEST health plan. Length of treatment reimbursed varies greatly with 4-8 weeks of intensive outpatient appearing like the maximum length of stay. Clients entering treatment without QUEST can face a 30-day wait once they are approved for QUEST, before they can access the substance abuse treatment benefit.

ADAD, August 2003

LICENSED ADULT RESIDENTIAL SUBSTANCE ABUSE TREATMENT FACILITIES (Short and long term programs)

OAHU:
- **Salvation Army Family Treatment Services - 41 beds**
- **Salvation Army Addiction Treatment Services - 45 beds/20 detox**
- **Hina Mauka - 45 beds**
- **Hawaii Alcoholism Foundation (Sand Island) - 53 beds**
- **Ho'omau Ke Ola - 14 beds**
- **Po'ailani - 16 beds**
- **Habilitat - 150 beds**

MAUI:
- **Aloha House - 26 beds/6 detox**

MOLOKAI:
- **There are no adult residential treatment facilities on Molokai**

LANAI:
- **There are no adult residential treatment facilities on Lanai**

KAUAI:
- **There are no adult residential treatment facilities on Kauai**

BIG ISLAND:
- **There are no adult residential treatment facilities on the Big Island**
- **Big Island Substance Abuse Council (BISAC) operates 24 hour therapeutic homes.**
- **Bridge House operates 24 hour therapeutic homes**

Total licensed adult residential treatment beds = 390
Total licensed adult detoxification beds = 26
NOTE: ADAD has sufficient resources to pay for approximately 85 beds.

Except for Ho'omau Ke Ola and Habilitat, all licensed adult residential treatment facilities are also accredited by the National Commission on Accreditation of Rehabilitation Facilities (CARF).

ADAD, August 2003

TREATMENTS FOR METHAMPHETAMINE

- Cognitive behavior approach - based on the theory that learning processes play a critical role in the development of maladaptive behavior patterns. The interventions help modify a patient's thinking and harmful behaviors through teaching more effective coping skills.

- Withdrawal from "ice" is typically characterized by drug craving, depressed mood, disturbed sleep patterns, and increased appetite. Antidepressant medications can help the depressive symptoms associated with withdrawal.

- Ice is often used in dangerous combinations with other substances, including cocaine/crack, marijuana, heroin and alcohol.

- Contingency Management - behavioral intervention that is designed to increase or decrease desired behaviors by providing immediate reinforcing or punishing consequences when the target behavior occurs. It sets short-term and long-term goals and emphasizes positive behavioral changes. Reliance should be on positive reinforcing approaches, not punitive consequences, because punitive consequences can promote treatment dropout.

- MATRIX Model - an outpatient approach which integrates treatment elements from a number of specific strategies, including relapse prevention, motivational interviewing, psychoeducation, family therapy and 12-Step program involvement. (St. Francis WATCH program replicated this model in Hawaii.)

- New Medications (in development)

- Self-help groups as support for treatment

ALL TREATMENT FOR "ICE" ADDICTION NEEDS A LENGTH OF STAY OF 90 DAYS OR MORE, WITH FOLLOW-UP FOR AT LEAST ONE YEAR.

ADAD, August 2003

PREREQUISITES FOR APPROPRIATE TREATMENT

- **Adequate resources**
- **Effective service systems**
- **Higher standards of treatment**

ADEQUATE RESOURCES (Invest for Results):

- **Close serious gap in treatment capacity**
- **Align financing and reimbursement mechanisms to ensure the most effective and efficient use of available resources**
- **Establish standard insurance benefits for both public and private insurance that provide coverage for substance abuse and dependence equivalent to other medical conditions and that include a full array of appropriate treatment and continuing care (parity).**
- **Set reimbursement rates and funding level to cover reasonable costs of providing care, including evidence-based practice improvements, capitol improvements ad reinvestment; workforce recruitment, retention and development; and care for persons without public or private insurance.**

EFFECTIVE SERVICE SYSTEMS ("No Wrong Door")– ensure that an individual needing treatment will be identified and assessed and will receive treatment, either directly or through appropriate referral, no matter where he or she enters the realm of services.

- **Require appropriate assessment, referral, and treatment in all systems service people with substance abuse and dependency problems.**
- **Ensure that in all systems individuals enter and become engaged in the most appropriate type and level of substance abuse treatment and that they receive continuing services at the level needed.**
- **Apply a commonly accepted, evidence-based model for the continuum of services and care for substance abuse and dependence across health, human services, and justice systems as well as in the substance abuse specialty sector.**

HIGHER STANDARDS OF TREATMENT (A Commitment to Quality) - effective treatment and the wise use of resources depend upon ongoing improvement in the quality of care.

- **Establish a system that more effectively connects services and research, with the goal of providing treatment based on the best scientific evidence.**
  - **The system should specifically:**
    - **a) promote consistent communication and collaboration among service providers, academic institutions, researchers, and other relevant stakeholders; and**
    - **b) establish incentives and assistance for programs and staff in applying the new standards and treatment methods.**
- **Utilizing the connecting services and research principle, develop commonly accepted standards for the treatment field.**
  - **Specifically:**
    - **a) define evidence-based standards for quality of care and practices that apply to all systems and payors;**
    - **b) derive or achieve consensus on critical elements to measure quality of care and treatment outcomes for payors and providers;**
    - **c) establish standards for education, training and credentialing of alcohol and drug treatment professionals and for other health and human service providers; and**
    - **d) adopt best business practices for program management and operations.**
- **Attract, support, and maintain a high quality, diverse workforce, responsive to the client population.**

Source: "Changing the Conversation" – The National Treatment Plan Initiative, November 200, U.S DHHS, Substance Abuse and Mental Health Services Administration, Center for Substance Abuse Treatment (www.samhsa.gov)

ADAD August 2003

TREATMENT ADMISSIONS FROM ALCOHOL AND DRUG ABUSE DIVISION

TREATMENT EPISODE SYSTEM (TEDS)

Treatment Admissions - By any drug/alcohol 1998-2002

	1998	1999	2000	2001	2002
Adults	5,518	5,745	6,500	6,454	6,369
Adolescents	1,821	1,525	1,633	1,641	1,552
TOTAL	7,339	7,270	8,133	8,095	7,921

A. Treatment Admissions - Primary substance of abuse – Methamphetamine

	1998	1999	2000	2001	2002
Adults	1,423	1,517	2,136	2,332	2,730
Adolescents	189	126	143	150	158
TOTAL	1,612	1,643	2,279	2,482	2,888

B. Treatment Admissions - Primary substance of abuse - Alcohol

	1998	1999	2000	2001	2002
Adults	2,231	2,337	2,469	2,435	2,051
Adolescents	429	379	432	442	378
TOTAL	2,660	2,716	2,901	2,877	2,429

C. Treatment Admissions - Primary substance of abuse - Marijuana

	1998	1999	2000	2001	2002
Adults	343	404	495	552	558
Adolescents	1,158	961	956	979	949
TOTAL	1,501	1,365	1,451	1,531	1,507

Source: Hawaii DOH, Alcohol and Drug Abuse Division (August 2003)

ALCOHOL AND DRUG ABUSE DIVISION

FUNDING FOR SUBSTANCE ABUSE TREATMENT AND PREVENTION FOR ADULTS AND ADOLESCENTS

STATE FISCAL YEAR	GENERAL FUNDS FOR POS TREATMENT CONTRACTS (Expenditures)	FEDERAL SUBSTANCE ABUSE PREVENTION & TREATMENT BLOCK GRANT (20% IS PREVENTION)
1992	$5,104,244	$6,078,000
1993	$5,651,197	$6,279,545
1994	$6,106,186	$5,323,812
1995	$5,923,860	$5,810,235
1996	$5,019,979	$5,690,381
1997	$5,319,979	$5,867,429
1998	$5,796,711	$6,382,425
1999	$5,654,887	$6,382,425
2000	$5,633,837	$6,810,019
2001	$5,666,740	$6,983,864
2002	$5,779,949*	$7,070,824
2003	$7,783,598**	$7,164,579
2004	$7,790,900***	$7,164,579****

* Includes $192,692 ICM funds
** Includes $2,192,698 ICM funds
***Includes $2,200,000 ICM funds
****Federal award not received yet.

ADAD, August 2003

ADULT TREATMENT
PROGRAM PERFORMANCE RESULTS

In the state Fiscal Year 2002 (July 1, 2001 to June 30, 2002), six-month follow-ups were completed for a sample of 1,558 adults. Listed below are the outcomes for this sample:

ADULT SUBSTANCE ABUSE TREATMENT-FY 2002	
MEASURE	**PERFORMANCE OUTCOME ACHIEVED SIX-MONTH**
Employed/School/Vocational Training	**50.2%**
No Arrests Since Discharge	**85.6%**
No Substance Use 30 Days Prior to Follow Up	**67.9%**
No New Substance Abuse Treatment	**81.5%**
No Hospitalizations	**90.4%**
No Emergency Room Visits	**89.8%**
Participated in Self-Help Group (NA, AA, Etc.)	**41.7%**
No Psychological Distress Since Discharge	**81.8%**
Stable Living Arrangements	**83.7%**

PRINCIPLES OF EFFECTIVE TREATMENT

1. No single treatment is appropriate for all individuals
2. Treatment needs to be readily available
3. Effective treatment attends to multiple needs of the individual, not just his or her drug use.
4. An individual's treatment and services plan must be assessed continually and modified as necessary to ensure that the plan meets the person's changing needs.
5. Remaining in treatment for an adequate period of time is critical for treatment effectiveness.
6. Counseling (individual and/or group) and other behavioral therapies are critical components of effective treatment for addiction.
7. Medications are an important element of treatment for many patients, especially when combined with counseling and other behavioral therapies.
8. Addicted or drug-abusing individuals with coexisting mental disorders should have both disorders treated in an integrated way.
9. Medical detoxification is only the first stage of addiction treatment and by itself does little to change long-term drug use.
10. Treatment does not need to be voluntary to be effective.
11. Possible drug use during treatment must be monitored continuously.
12. Treatment programs should provide assessment for HIV/AIDS, hepatitis B and C, tuberculosis, and other infectious diseases, and counseling to help individuals modify or change behaviors that place themselves or others at risk of infection.
13. Recovery from drug addiction can be a long-term process and frequently requires multiple episodes of treatment.

National Institute on Drug Abuse, *Principles of Drug Addiction Treatment*, 1999

PREVENTION PLANNING PRINCIPLES

- FORM PARTNERSHIP AMONG STATE AGENCIES FOR STATE-LEVEL PREVENTION SYSTEM CHANGES AND DEVELOP PARTNERSHIPS AT THE COMMUNITY LEVEL FOR SUBSTANCE ABUSE PREVENTION
- SUPPORT AND SUSTAIN COMMUNITY PARTNERSHIPS
- USE THE RISK AND PROTECTIVE FACTORS AS A FRAMEWORK FOR PREVENTION
- SUPPORT EFFECTIVE, SCIENCE-BASED PROGRAMS
- ACHIEVE MEASURABLE OUTCOMES AND RESULTS
- SUPPORT PROGRAMS THAT ARE EFFECTIVE AND REFLECTIVE OF HAWAII'S CULTURAL DIVERSITY

What we will do without a law!

Internal Controls

- Properly check in deliveries.
- Lock up all inventory to reduce theft of product.
- Place all products in a highly visible location.
- Place company imposed limits on sale of product.
- Post signs advising customers of the challenge.
- Train employees on how to report suspicious transactions and actions.

Public Relations

- Promote Meth Watch Program.
- Support education of consumers on what to look for and how to report.
- Promote the registration of all retailers selling psuedophederine products to allow government to create a database on locations.
- Promote the reporting of wholesale sales to government to allow for a baseline on sales by stores via store size.

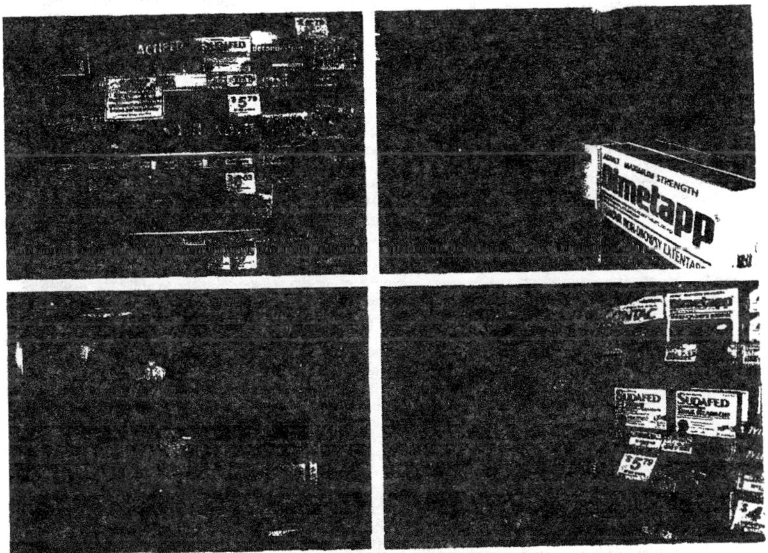

HAWAII FOOD INDUSTRY ASSOCIATION
677 Ala Moana Blvd., Suite 815
Honolulu, HI 96813
www.hawaiifood.com / Phone 808-533-1292 / Fax 808-599-2606

CHPA® FOUNDED 1881
Consumer Healthcare Products Association

Methamphetamine/ CHPA Meth Watch Program

Background on methamphetamine:

Communities across America plagued by the proliferation of methamphetamine are looking for effective and innovative ways to combat this emergent trend. The most significant problem for state and local law enforcement, especially in rural communities, is the manufacturing of methamphetamine in what have become known as small, home-made labs. These labs often use pseudoephedrine, a safe and effective ingredient found in many over-the-counter cough/cold products, in the illegal manufacture of methamphetamine. These labs have a devastating effect on the environment, communities, and the children who are often times present, and for these reasons are referred to as small toxic labs by law enforcement officials.

What is Meth Watch?

"Meth Watch" is a program designed to help curtail suspicious sales and theft of pseudoephedrine and other precursor products used in the illicit manufacturing of methamphetamine. Meth Watch was started in Kansas as a public-private partnership between the Kansas Department of Health and Environment, the Kansas Bureau of Investigation, the Kansas Methamphetamine Prevention Project (part of the non-profit statewide drug prevention system), and Kansas retailers. As news spread of its success, several states have begun to adopt the Kansas model, including Washington, Oregon, and South Dakota. Many more have expressed interest, but have been deterred by lack of resources and know-how.

How does Meth Watch work?

Meth Watch is a voluntary program that involves a variety of people at the community and state level, although retail involvement is the cornerstone of this program. Participating retailers place the precursor products where they can be easily monitored, and strategically post Meth Watch signs and tags on their doors and windows, around their cash registers and on the shelves where precursor products are located. They may impose purchase limits to prevent high volume sales. They train their employees to recognize, but not to confront, suspicious customers and to contact law enforcement with as much identifying information as possible.

Participants in the Meth Watch program report safer stores, better customer relations, increased employee awareness, and improved communications with law enforcement. In areas that have been hard hit by the meth scourge, Meth Watch partners are helping to unify their communities against drug abuse. The Meth Watch program in Kansas is a proven and replicable program which has significantly affected meth lab seizures.

How can individual states become involved?

The Consumer Healthcare Products Association (CHPA) has developed a uniform Meth Watch model that serves as an online resource center for interested states (www.methwatch.com). This site provides a one-stop shop to help states implement Meth Watch in their communities. CHPA will provide direct resources to states for the implementation of Meth Watch, including training, technical assistance, and retail support and education.

What does the future hold for Meth Watch?

Law enforcement officials and anti-drug abuse coalitions across the country are seeing a dramatic increase in meth abuse. As other states begin to benefit from the Meth Watch program, CHPA anticipates a greater need for funding a comprehensive methamphetamine prevention program and will join with those states most affected by this problem to call on Congress to authorize a permanent grant program for states that can demonstrate a need.

74-5035 Queen Ka'ahumanu Hwy, 3B
P.O. Box 4698
Kailua-Kona, Hawai'i 96745
(808) 327-9755 fax (808) 331-1454
Kawika-ka2020@verizon.net

Kealakehe Ahupua'a 2020, Inc.

To:	Representative Ed Case	Fax:	808-538-0233
From:	David Marquez, Executive Director	Date:	8/1/2004
Re:	Drug policy comments, Big Island Meeting	Pages:	9
CC:			

☒ Urgent For Review ☐ Please Comment ☒ Please Reply ☐ Please Recycle

Honolulu office at)

Aloha kakou.

There has been much written and talked about in addressing our growing substance abuse problem. Ice is NOT new. For ten years, the "Ice Epidemic" has been upon us. During this time, the 'experts' in treatment have been doing business as usual. Hawai'i island is still woefully lacking in effective treatment facilities, and few go beyond the initial cessation of illicit drug use and often transfer dependencies to pharmaceutical drugs. That is not drug rehab. Providing more treatment slots for that kind of treatment will not turn this epidemic. And there will always be another 'epidemic' around the corner. Getting people off drugs is a start; it's what's done next that will spell the success of failure of the individual to assume a responsible, self-reliant role in society.

Law enforcement has escalated, and there have been more arrests, but what then? Ultimately, offenders will be released from jail or prison, and little if any effective work will have been done to change their destructive behavior.

Prevention that only addresses the deleterious impact of drugs is not effective; prevention must address positive life skills and activities. Given the state of our schools, it is doubtful that there is much attention to other than passing standardized academic testing .

What is truly needed is an approach which will actively prevent participation in substance abuse and will help to restructure the lives that have been impaired through substance abuse. Kealakehe Ahupua'a 2020, a non-profit community development organization, has embraced the concept of a Local Conservation Corps, to conserve our most precious resources, including our people. The Corps' program envisioned for Hawai'i is attached.

We most respectfully request your support and assistance in finding funding to bring this program into full operation. Help us by becoming an advocate for real change, help us find funding through congressional programs, help us by working with us to develop private resources. Help us by not simply having more meetings. We are ready to get busy changing lives. Are you?

Thank you for your kind attention.

David "Kawika" Marquez
Executive Director
Kealakehe Ahupua'a 2020
808-327-9755, or 987-9101

745035 Queen Kahumanu Hwy, 3-B
P.O. Box 4698
Kailua-Kona, Hawai'i 96745
(808) 327-9755 fax (808) 331-145
Kawika-ka2020@verizon.net

KEALAKEHE AHUPUA'A 2020, Inc.

'OHANA AHUPUA'A LOCAL CONSERVATION CORPS 2004 Program narrative

The 'Ohana Ahupua'a Local Conservation Corps ('OALCC) has been formed to fulfill primary purposes: (1) to provide service to the Island of Hawai'i (Hawai'i County) community by performing work on community facilities, performing work on restoring forest, watershed, native plants, and reefs, and all its habitants, and providing assistance to vulnerable populations such as the elderly and the disabled; and , (2) to provide individuals between the ages of 16 and 60, with work and knowledge of Western and Hawai'ian traditional practices and other skills needed to become self-sufficient. It is expected that the majority – approximately 80% of the intergenerational participates enrolled in the 'OALCC will be economically, social and/or educationally challenged

An overarching principal of the Ohana Ahupua'a Local Conservation Corps is building of a community that will not tolerate or accept abuse and crime, and that seeks to mitigate the personal and societal consequences of the abuse of alcohol other drugs.

Work performed by the 'Ohana Ahupua'a Local Conservation Corps will be conducted on behalf of private not-for-profit organizations, and federal, state and local public agencies. For these agencies, 'OALCC crews of up to 10 corps members will engage in a variety of work projects that will include: (1) activities that involve physical improvements, such public park facilities, fresh water pond and other wetland restoration, native plant and tree restoration, beach and reef restoration and maintenance, and maintenance and renovation to low-income or substandard housing, and improvements to neighborhood centers, settlements houses, senior centers, and shelters to serve the homeless; and, (2) activities that services to the elderly, disabled, and the other challenged populations.

Activities for program participants/corps members will consist of the following

- ✓ A one-week residential/non-residential training program in which corps members are prepared for the full 'OALCC program through team building and other personal development.
- ✓ Physical training each morning.
- ✓ Work, as part of a crew of ten corps members, for 35 hours of each week. Through work participants learn valuable western and Hawai'ian traditional job skills as dependability (e.g. punctuality, and good attendance); good worksite relations (e.g. constructive criticism, working cooperatively with other corps members and staff); on some projects corps members will learn Hawai'ian traditional practices job-specific skills.
- ✓ Education, for eight hours of each week, in which corps members will work on such goals as: genealogy, Hawai'ian language

A COMMUNITY PARTNERSHIP

and traditional practices, reading, math, and communication skills, English language proficiency, and GED/college preparation. In addition, participants will receive instruction in life skills, conflict resolution, job search and employment retention, personnel money management, goal setting and decision making.

After completion of the program, 'OALCC staff will work with participants to find specific employment opportunities and /or continuation of their education.

'OALCC recognizes that the abuse of alcohol and other drugs, just like other abuses and social ills, is not a problem for law enforcement, jails, probation/parole officers, or schools or any single segment alone to solve. Indeed, we view this partnership as a process, one that encourages Hawai'ians to take responsibility for creating a healthy future for all people and neighborhoods. To this extent that we have focused on the problem of substance abuse, we have, in the past, come up with solutions in the form of programs targeted to the symptoms. We now recognize that programs do not, by themselves, create change. Change will occur only if the individual programs are planned and implemented in the context of changes in the larger community and a holistic approach to community wellness.

'OALCC expects to be fully operational by spring of 2005, when the first group of thirty corps members- three crews- will be enrolled. Efforts are currently underway to develop job description for recruiting and hiring key program staff, staff positions include work project coordinator, corps members development coordinator, Hawai'ian traditional practices coordinator, recruiter/job developer and crew leaders.

Site location and lease negotiations, space planning for 'OALCC offices are in the planning stages.

74-5035 Queen Ka'ahumanu Hwy, 3B
P.O. Box 4698
Kailua-Kona, Hawai'i 96745
(808) 327-9755 fax (808) 331-1454
kawika-ka2020@verizon.net

KEALAKEHE AHUPUA'A 2020

Island of Hawai'i

'Ohana Ahupua'a Conservation Corps

(Space to grow, place to learn)

Local Conservation Corps is not a new concept: other states, counties, and cities have different names for their organizations. The goals and strategies are the similar, which are developing a program that is consistent and effective that reflect the highest standards of conduct, integrity and excellence, through education, career development, leadership, enriching ones culture, caring for the land, trees, plants and water, and all its habitants. What is unique about the 'Ohana Ahupua'a Conservation Corps is that normal corps efforts will be expanded to help restore active use of Hawaiian traditional practices that are essential to fostering a recognition of the interdependence between nature and the 'Ohana (the Hawaiian family system) and the community. The Island of Hawaii through this unique blend of Hawaiian and western practices would receive a measurable ecological, educational, social and/or economic benefit from a high quality organization such as the 'Ohana Ahupua'a Conservation Corps.

BACKGROUND

The islands of Hawaii pose challenges and opportunities not as clearly observed in other locations in the Unites States of America. As islands, the resources needed for life are limited to what is <u>on</u> the island. While this is true in all geographic settings, it was perhaps better recognized here; getting resources from afar could take months to years, if at all. Under traditional Hawaiian practices, the conservation of the people and natural resources to provide for life-sustenance was a principal role of the leadership of the Ahupua'a communities. There was a depth of knowledge regarding the lifecycles of edible marine and plant life, and restrictions were placed on collection of specific resources during certain times, to allow for population growth or colony repair or to prevent collection during toxic periods. Over-collection and waste were severe crimes in Hawaiian practices, as damaging to the whole ecosystem, including the people. People were considered a part of the whole ecosystem, and respect for and preservation of the land and sea were dominant themes in the Ahupua'a system. A very responsible system of resource conservation was developed: the Ahupua'a system. An Ahupua'a was usually a triangular piece of land like a slice of pie, the narrow point in mountain uplands and extending and widening to the sea. This land division included the high forests, the agriculturally rich mid-elevations, and the shoreline and coastal reefs. There was an appreciation that what was done in the mountains had an impact on all lower elevations, including the sea. Water, soils, etc., were thus recognized as critical elements.

Land in the Ahupua'a system was or supervised by a Konohiki (landlord), who was entrusted by the Chief of the Ahupua'a, who was responsible for the people and resources within the Ahupua'a. With the introduction of Western/European land ownership concepts, the Ahupua'a system was abandoned and replaced by rectangular land divisions were defined and sold. This broke down the ecosystem management, and with the loss of the full range of land for community sustenance, it broke as well the collective social responsibility that was integrated in the Ahupua'a system.

Just prior to the arrival of the Western religious missionaries, there was an abandonment of the traditional Hawaiian "kapu" system, a system of rules and prohibitions, which constituted the moral and social codes of the Hawaiian people. While introduction of Christianity, and later religions of other immigrant groups, filled a moral void in Hawaiian society, the devaluing of the traditional practices of the host culture resulted in the loss of very valuable tools in guiding ecosystem and social interaction.

Among a broad range of ethnic groups on the island, the native Hawaiian population, while possessing a rich background, suffer from deteriorating social and economic conditions not uncommon in colonized communities: high rates of alcohol and substance abuse, high rates of child abuse and other domestic abuse, high rates of teen pregnancies, disproportionate rate of adjudicated youth, disproportionate rates of incarceration among youth and adults, high rates of school drop out, and inadequate reading and math skills among high school graduates. These indicators produce low self-esteem and desperation.

At present there is higher than the national average unemployment, with an economy based on tourism and, recently, new construction development and emerging high-tech company expansion. There are too few skilled workers to meet the increasing demand. Often, Hawaii Island residents have two or more part-time or lower paying jobs to make enough to support family needs. This detracts from the quality of family life and spins into a continually deteriorating condition. Many of the unemployed and under-employed population live in very small communities or in rural areas, far from the centers of business, tourism, construction and high tech development. There is not adequate public transportation to serve rural employees getting to job sites. There are inadequate training and employment opportunities in these areas.

Despite a recent surge in development of new housing and vacation accommodations, local infrastructure is inadequate and deteriorating from excessive use. Likewise, more forest and other wild natural land is being built over.

PROGRAM PROPOSAL

The ʻOhana Ahupua'a Conservation Corps proposes to create programs that could develop work and service projects that are of value to the community and to Corps members, which integrate best practices from Western science and relevant traditional practices from the host culture, native Hawaiian. Those service projects are those which:

- Fill an unmet, but valued, community need
- Are visible, tangible, meaningful and achievable
- Have educational dimension
- Provide introductory skills training
- Would be conducted according to accepted safety and design principles
- Provide long-term benefits to the community
- Will be environmentally sound, and respecting the traditional ecosystem principles of the Ahupua'a system.
- Lend themselves to group effort and close supervision
- Involve youth, young adults, adults and elders in both skills development and community enhancement
- Teach traditional Hawaiian values and employ traditional Hawaiian methods of rehabilitation.

The ʻOhana Ahupua'a Conservation Corps will be subject to a well defined monitoring and evaluation process, consistent with needs of funding sources and to maintain good standing within the National Association of Service Conservation Corps.

ʻOhana Ahupua'a Conservation Corps Members Development

ʻOhana Ahupua'a Conservation Corps will develop programs that provide Corps members with **structured opportunities to learn** academic, Western scientific and traditional Hawaiian practical skills, genealogy awareness, spiritual enhancement, and other skills which will meet the individual needs of each participant. The individual programs for Corps members will include case-management and collaboration with relevant treatment providers for substance abuse and health issues.

Corps members - focused education:

- Occupies a substantial and consistent place on the Corps schedule
- Is based upon individual assessment of Corps members needs
- Is carried out by Corps staff or under written contract
- Builds upon and embraces work and service project experiences
- Involves goal setting and rewards for accomplishments

The 'Ohaha Ahupa'a Conservation Corps will develop programs that would provide **life skills** that prepare Corps members for a successful life. This is especially important for Corps members who are recovering from substance abuse.

Life skills training:

- Occupies a substantial and consistent place on the Corps schedule
- Effectively address topics critical to young adults, adults and elders
- Makes use of and trains Corps members in the use of common resources
- Provide leadership opportunities and develops group skills
- Encourages community service within the Corps members experience
- Is linked to basic education through reading, writing and discussion
- Encourages career planning and development and ties into post-Corps job and education placement
- Encourages a sense of 'Ohana within the Corps
- Helps youth and young adults, adults and elders to see themselves as resources
- Encourages youth, young adults, adults and elders to value differences
- Builds a sense of pride and connection to traditional Hawaiian practices

The 'Ohana Ahupua'a Conservation Corps will develop programs that would provide Corps members with a **disciplined, positive and supportive experience**. Such an experience results from:

- The payment of stipends or wages (and benefits) tied to work
- Clearly stated rules and procedures
- Initial orientation and on-going training
- High standards of attendance and strong retention efforts
- The provision of needed support and/or remediation services directly, or through case management and referral to specific service providers
- Effective deployment of Corps members using the crew structure

The 'Ohana Ahupua'a Conservation Corps will develop programs that will work to achieve the goal of **diversity**...an understanding and appreciation of people with different backgrounds, experiences and ideas, at all levels of the organization, while enhancing respect for and understanding of the traditional host culture. To achieve the goal of diversity, Corps programs will:

- Ensure to the greatest extent possible and appropriate that their governing bodies, staff and participants reflect the pluralism of the community which they serve
- Design work projects, collaborative exchanges with other community service programs and educational components to ensure that the Corps members are exposed to a broad range of experiences that help overcome stereotypical attitudes and behavior
- Develop mission statements that define diversity within the content of each programs and community, as well as written plans for moving toward that diversity
- Consistently make use of uniforms, insignia and other markings
- Respond to community needs, including the need to bridge ethnic and socioeconomic gaps

The 'Ohana Ahupua'a Conservation Corps will develop programs that **employ sound management and administration practices**. Such sound practices are those which:

- Ensure that the sizes of the crews and the ratio of the crew supervisors to Corps members in a crew allow for work projects to be conducted with safety, efficiency and opportunities for learning

- Utilize a governing or advisory board representative of the community
- Maintain thorough record keeping and reporting systems regarding participants, work accomplishments and finances
- Establish and adhere to clear criteria and processes for the selection of work projects
- Enlist a wide range of community partnerships to ensure recruitment funding stability and visibility, as well as non-duplication of services
- Maintain administrative and financial systems that allow for continued growth and complexity of programming
- Assure ongoing staff training and development at all levels in the organization
- Conduct strategic planning

The 'Ohana Ahupua'a Conservation Corps will develop programs to cultivate such relationships throughout the broader community. To cultivate such relationships, Corps programs:

- Adopt a collaborative spirit toward community, and its citizens, the "Aloha Spirit"
- Interact regularly in the community
- Constructively approach perceived problems and issues
- Avoid duplication of effort and competition for local funding
- Seek to build the capacity of the entire 'Ohana Ahupua'a Conservation Corps by sharing best practices and special organizational and program strengths with the community.

FACILITIES PLAN

The 'Ohana Ahupua'a Conservation Corps is in discussion with a few major landholders for facilities to lease which will initially facilitate non-residential training and service projects. It is hoped that in the future the Corps will be able to expand to include a residential component to meet higher service needs or corps members.

It is expected that Corps members will rehabilitate or construct any properties that we seek to occupy as part of their practical experience, under the tutelage and guidance of professionals.

BUDGET

We speculate a budget of approximately $800,000 the first year to develop facilities, equip facilities and work projects and to serve initial Corp members. The second year the anticipated budget will be $500,000, and the third year and subsequent years, we anticipate an operating budget of approximately $300,000.

FUNDING PERIOD

From start-up, through operation and graduation of a first class of Corps members into employment and tracking for maintained employment, we anticipate minimally 3 years funding.

PROGRAM MANAGEMENT

The 'Ohana Ahupua'a Conservation Corps is incorporated as a non-profit corporation in the State of Hawaii and will operate under the umbrella of Kealakehe Ahupua'a 2020, a non-profit corporation in the State of Hawaii recognized by the IRS under code sections 501 c-3 and 509.

The 'Ohana Ahupua'a Conservation Corps will become a member of the National Association of Service Conservation Corps, for support in curriculum development, program design, and guidance and consulting as needed from successful Corps elsewhere.

The Chief Executive Officer will be David Marquez. Mr. Marquez has significant experience in managing and operation employment development and rehabilitation programs, as evidence by his attached resume. He has operated secure residential half-way houses for corrections departments, and has operated job preparation and placement programs for hard to employ populations. Perhaps most notable is his depth of experience in collaborative projects, engaging a variety of community interests and parties to work toward common goals.

A Chief Fiscal Officer is being recruited. That person will be a Certified Public Accountant, with background in community service projects.

Key personnel will include specialists in land conservation, forestry practices, marine biology, traditional Hawaiian practices, as well as teachers for all necessary skill and educational development, and crew managers.

lcc/concept.doc

R4-04-0030/ UGA3D
Seizure of Approximately 5 pounds of Crystal Methamphetamine/Arrest of 3 Subjects

On January 22, 2004, the Hawaii Airport Task Force ("HATF") seized approximately 3 pounds of crystal methamphetamine from within a suspicious FedEx parcel pursuant to a federal search warrant. A controlled delivery was then conducted which resulted in the arrest of Jaime AGTANG, Felipe DOMANGUERA, and Dan TAUYAN. A consent search was conducted of the delivery address and another FedEx box similar to the first was discovered; this box contained another 2 pounds of crystal methamphetamine. AGTANG cooperated and stated that his source of supply was Antonio LNU from California, who uses telephone number (808) 341-3782 (Antonio lived in Hawaii for approximately 6 months and still uses a Hawaii cellular number). The Hawaii owner of the crystal methamphetamine is a Filipino male named Dan LNU, who uses the following telephone numbers (all area code 808): 224-4759, 341-1450, 222-5568, 630-7551, 341-1450, and 630-6311. AGTANG stated that over the past 6 months, he has received at least 5 other parcels similar to those seized on this date. The arrests in this investigation will disrupted a mid-level crystal methamphetamine trafficking organization operating in Honolulu.

R4-04-0044/UGA3I
Seizure of Approximately 20 pounds of Crystal Methamphetamine and Arrest of Three Defendants

On March 14, 2004, CBP (Customs) Inspectors at the FedEx hub in Memphis, TN discovered methamphetamine concealed inside 4 aluminum 6' pipes sent from Mexico to Honolulu, HI. The pipes were forwarded to the Honolulu ICE (Customs) office, where a joint investigation was initiated with the Hawaii Airport Task Force (HATF). A controlled delivery was made on March 16, 2004. 7 days later, the pipes were opened and 3 defendants were arrested and $200,000.00 in U.S. currency was seized from a residence. Debriefings revealed that the true sender of the parcel was arrested in a DEA Honolulu case 6 years ago; this avenue of investigation is ongoing. The cooperators were turned over to the long term investigation group, which has identified the source of supply and is actively seeking his arrest.

R4-04-0022 / UGA3D
Seizure of Approximately 1698 grams of Crystal Methamphetamine/arrest of Gavien DANIEL and Dwayne GOUVEIA.

On January 5, 2004, members of the Riverside District Office informed the Hawaii Airport Task Force that the FedEx Delivery Station in 1111 Bird Center Drive, Palm Springs, CA, had opened a parcel containing suspected methamphetamine destined to Hawaii from California. On January 7, 2004, HATF received the parcel which contained approximately 1698 grams of methamphetamine. A controlled delivery was conducted to 74-5156 Haleolono Place, Kailua-Kona, Hawaii, and subsequently, Dwayne GOUVEIA and Gavien DANIEL were arrested. Both declined to cooperate with law enforcement. Federal search warrants were executed on both of their residences resulting in the seizure of various documents and two Harley Davidson Motorcycles which were identified as purchased with drug proceeds. Both subjects will be charged in Federal court. Incident to GOUVEIA and DANIEL's arrest and execution of search warrants, six cellular telephones were seized.

The Riverside District Office, Hilo Post of Duty and HDO will continue to coordinate identified leads in this investigation.

IMPACT STATEMENT:

This investigation was initiated on January 5, 2004. This organization receives and distributes approximately 3 to 5 pounds of methamphetamine every month on the island of Hawaii. In this investigation, a mid to high level dealer of this organization, along with an associate, was arrested. 1698 grams of methamphetamine was removed from the drug trafficking element in the community of west Hawaii.

SIGNIFICANT ACTIVITY REPORT

EVENT: R4-04-0093 / UGA3D
Seizure of Approximately 1416.0 grams of Crystal Methamphetamine and $103,200.00 in U.S. Currency.

DATE OF EVENT: July 21-22, 2004

HOW REPORTED: Firebird

WHEN REPORTED: July 22, 2004

DETAILS: On July 21, 2004, the Hawaii Airport Task Force (HATF) conducted a controlled delivery of 1973.0 grams of methamphetamine to Jorge Ormeno at 3281 Kehau Place, Honolulu. Federal search warrants were obtained and additional 1416.0 grams of methamphetamine and $63,500 in U.S. Currency was recovered from the backpack of Carlos Becerrada. A search warrant was obtained for Becerrada's vehicle, 1998 Ford F150, documents and $1,000.00 was seized along with the vehicle. Another Federal Search Warrant was obtained for the residence of Becerrada at 91-1005 Kaope Street, Ewa Beach, HI. A small safe was found and $38,700 in U.S. Currency was seized from it.

On July 22, 2004, two federal search warrants were obtained for the address, 94-111 Pupuole Street, Apartment 17, Waipahu, HI. Documents were recovered from this address. The other search warrant was served on seven boxes that Becerrada had addressed to himself at 91-1005 Kaope Street and mailed from California. The seven boxes contained only household goods and clothing.

Total amount of methamphetamine seized from 3281 Kehau Place was 3389.0 grams and the amount of U.S. Currency seized from three locations was $103,200.00.

Carlos BECERRADA (FBI#433648EA5) was arrested without incident.

IMPACT STATEMENT:

This investigation was initiated on July 21, 2004. BECERRADA receives and distributes an unknown large quantity of methamphetamine on the island of Oahu. In this investigation a high level dealer, for an island such as Oahu, was arrested and 3389.0 grams of methamphetamine was removed from the drug trafficking element in the community Honolulu, which is a metropolitan community in the center area of Oahu. A kilo of methamphetamine in Hawaii is valued at $50,000 to $70,000 wholesale; 3389.0 grams would retail for $1,016,700.00.

Critical Event/ WSIN Database Activity Report:
State of Hawaii
January through June 2004

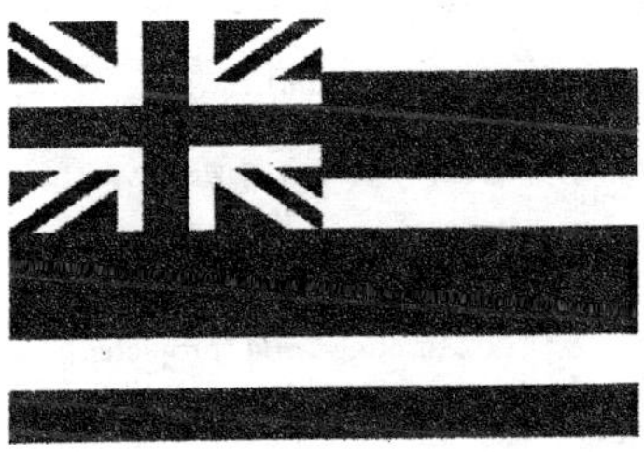

Published/Prepared By:
Western States Information Network
Sacramento, CA
7/23/04

Table of Contents

Critical Event Overview

Law enforcement agencies from the state of Hawaii have actively submitted operations (e.g. undercover buys, search warrants, etc) to the Western States Information Network's Watch Center since May 2002. This is accomplished by contacting the Watch Center located in Sacramento, California via phone or fax. The operation information is entered into the Critical Event application.

The Critical Event application is designed to electronically monitor law enforcement activities. This process increases officer safety by plotting event locations on island maps that identify and portray conflicting operations. Typically, conflicts occur when operations are located within two thousand yards of another. Conflicts can also occur when the focus is on a similar subject, moniker, vehicle, phone number, organization, and drug commodity/dollar amount. When a conflict is identified, Watch Center staff notifies the appropriate agencies.

Any type of law enforcement activity can be reported for deconfliction purposes. Agencies or officers posting operations into the Critical Event application are not required to be WSIN members. Conflicts between member and non-member agencies are releasable. However, only essential information about the conflict will be released for officer safety purposes.

Critical event information is also searched in the WSIN database. These searches often provide valuable intelligence. The critical event information can be stored into the WSIN database if it is related to a criminal activity. However, an agency must be a member in order to store the information into the WSIN database. An officer has to have a WSIN Security Control Card on file in order to receive any intelligence data from the WSIN database.

Total Critical Event (Operation) Submissions
January 1st through June 30th 2004

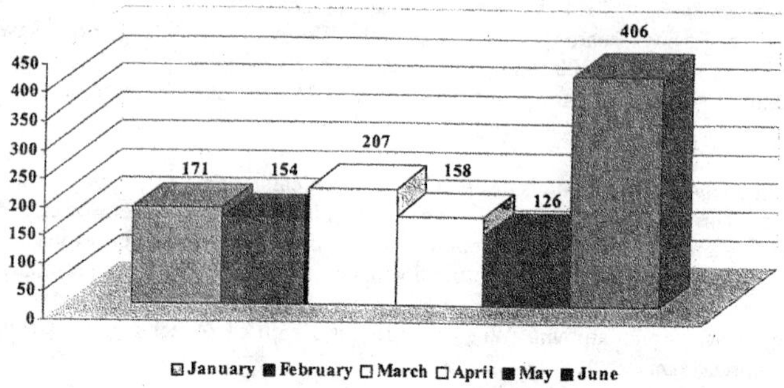

WSIN posted a total of 1,222 law enforcement critical events (operations) for deconfliction purposes in the state of Hawaii during the first six months of 2004. Monthly critical event submissions increased significantly from last year. As of the end of June, the average amount of operations submitted per month in 2004 is 203. This number is about twice as higher than the average from 2003 (111 per month).

There was a dramatic increase from May to June. A large part of this involved Honolulu Police Department's increased reporting on "knock and talk" related operations.

DECONFLICTION RATES

The WSIN Watch Center reported 44 location conflicts were resolved January 1st through June 30th 2004. During this time, approximately four percent of all operations received a conflict. Out of those 44 locations that received conflicts, 8 of those conflicted with operations submitted by another agency. These numbers are based on manual counts from the Watch Center staff.

Critical Event Submissions by Agencies
January 1st through June 30th 2004

	January	February	March	April	May	June	Total
Hawaii County PD, Hilo	8	6	25	11	15	9	**74**
Hawaii County PD, Kona	11	9	4	7	4	8	**43**
Honolulu PD	95	88	128	97	76	301	**785**
Kauai PD	1	15	11	11	8	8	**54**
Maui PD	8	8	12	6	6	8	**48**
US Customs and Border Protection	0	0	1	0	0	2	**3**
US Drug Enforcement Administration	2	9	7	12	11	14	**55**
US Federal Bureau of Investigations	18	12	1	1	1	3	**36**
US Marshals Service	16	5	17	13	5	52	**108**
US Naval Criminal Investigative Service	1	2	1	0	0	0	**4**
US Postal Inspection Service	11	0	0	0	0	1	**12**
Total	**171**	**154**	**207**	**158**	**126**	**406**	**1222**

The counts for critical events are based on the agency that submitted the operation to the Watch Center.

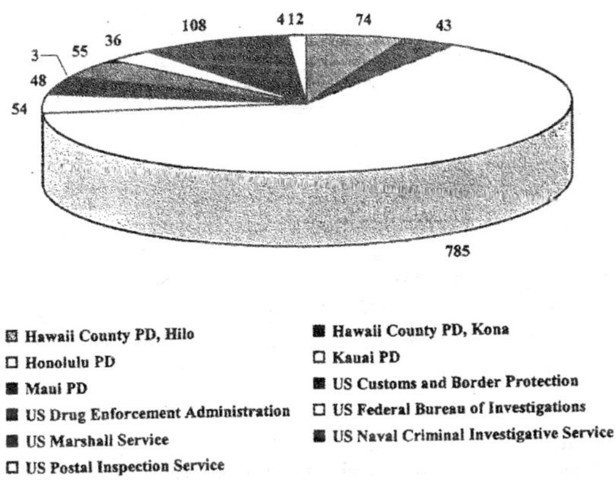

Honolulu Police Department submitted approximately 65 percent of all critical events reported January through June 2004. US Marshals Service and Hawaii County Police Department (Kona and Hilo) were the next largest contributors. Honolulu Police Department operations were significantly higher in June due to an increase in the number of "knock and talks" being reported (173 total in June).

Critical Event Submissions by Month (Average)
May 1st 2002 through June 30th 2004

	2002	2003	Jan – Jun 2004	Percentage Increase/Decrease 2003 to 2004
Hawaii County Police Dept, Hilo	5.63	5	12.33	**147%**
Hawaii County Police Dept, Kona	2	5.33	7.17	**35%**
Honolulu Police Dept	21.13	63.25	130.83	**107%**
Kauai Police Dept	1.5	1.83	9	**392%**
Maui Police Dept	5.88	5.42	8	**48%**
US Customs and Border Protection	0.13	0.42	0.5	**19%**
US Drug Enforcement Administration	10.75	5.5	9.17	**67%**
US Federal Bureau of Investigations	8.63	9.67	6	**-38%**
US Immigration and Customs Enforcement	0	0.17	0	**-100%**
US Immigration and Naturalization Service	0	0.08	0	**-100%**
US Internal Revenue Service	0	0.42	0	**-100%**
US Marshals Service	0	14.75	18	**22%**
US Naval Criminal Investigative Service	0	0.5	0.67	**34%**
US Postal Inspection Service	0.5	0	2	**0%**
Hawaii St Dept of Public Safety	0.13	0	0	**0%**
Average	56.25	111.08	203.67	**83%**

Yearly Averages are rounded to the nearest one hundredth. Percentage Increase/Decrease rounded to nearest whole number.

The above table represents the average number of monthly operations submitted to the WSIN Watch Center for deconfliction purposes and the percentage change from 2002 through June 2004. There were major increases from all of the top 8 submitting agencies*. The largest increases in operations have come from Hawaii County Police Department (Hilo and Kona), Honolulu Police Department and Kauai Police Department.

* Honolulu Police Department, US Marshals Service, Hawaii County Police Department, US Federal Bureau of Investigations, US Drug Enforcement Administration, and Maui Police Department, Kauai Police Department

Critical Event Submissions by Event Category
January 1st through June 30th 2004

	Drug Related	Non-Drug Related	Unknown
Hawaii County Police Dept, Hilo	73	1	0
Hawaii County Police Dept, Kona	43	0	0
Honolulu Police Dept	689	88	8
Kauai Police Dept	52	2	0
Maui Police Dept	48	0	0
US Customs and Border Protection	3	0	0
US Drug Enforcement Administration	54	1	0
US Federal Bureau of Investigations	36	0	0
US Marshals Service	67	37	4
US Naval Criminal Investigative Service	4	0	0
US Postal Inspection Service	12	0	0
Total	**1081**	**129**	**12**

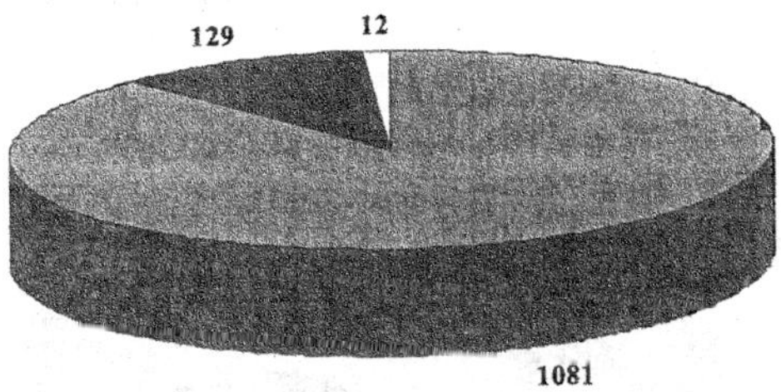

The primary event category was used to determine if a critical event was drug related or not. Though there is a possibility many of the critical events were both drug and non-drug related, only the primary event category was available. Based on that information, drug related operations represented approximately 88 percent of all activity while non-drug related operations represented slightly over 10 percent. These numbers are virtually the same as 2003.

Critical Event Submissions by Drug Types
January 1st through June 30th 2004

	Meth	Cocaine	Marijuana	Heroin	Other*	Not Specified
Hawaii County Police Dept, Hilo	56	4	9	0	3	1
Hawaii County Police Dept, Kona	37	0	5	0	0	1
Honolulu Police Dept	589	17	6	5	1	71
Kauai Police Dept	44	3	3	1	0	1
Maui Police Dept	41	0	4	0	2	1
US Customs and Border Protection	3	0	0	0	0	0
US Drug Enforcement Administration	35	4	2	0	4	9
US Federal Bureau of Investigations	33	2	0	0	0	1
US Marshals Service	33	1	2	1	0	30
US Naval Criminal Investigative Service	4	0	0	0	0	0
US Postal Inspection Service	12	0	0	0	0	0
Total	**887**	**31**	**31**	**7**	**10**	**115**

** Represents other drugs and activities such as: unknown precursors, hallucinogens, steroids, stimulants, depressants, narcotic equipment and currency*

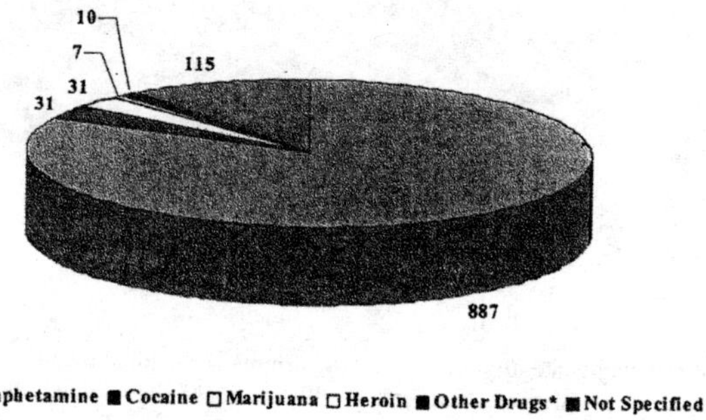

Though operations could involve multiple drug types, only the primary drug was captured. Methamphetamine (including amphetamines and crystal meth) accounted for approximately 73 percent of drug related critical event activity reported in Hawaii for 2003. Cocaine (including rock/crack cocaine) and marijuana accounted for approximately 2 1/2 percent each. Drugs not specified represented approximately 9 percent. The sharpest decrease from 2002 through June 2004 was shown in cocaine related events, dropping approximately 50 percent each year. Methamphetamine events percentages remained steady within that same time frame.

Critical Event Submissions by Non-Drug Types
January 1st through June 30th 2004

Criminal Event (General)	Honolulu Police Dept	US Marshals Service	Other Agencies*	Total
Assault	0	1	0	1
Burglary	0	1	0	1
Commercial Sex	22	0	0	22
Crimes Against Person	0	0	1	1
Criminal Gang	1	0	0	1
Flight	0	16	0	16
Fraud	0	2	1	3
Gambling	29	0	2	31
Money Laundering	1	0	0	1
Obstruct	0	4	0	4
Public Peace	8	0	0	8
Robbery	1	3	0	4
Sex Assault	1	0	0	1
Sex Offense	16	1	0	17
Smuggling	1	0	0	1
Stolen Property	1	3	0	4
Stolen Vehicle	6	1	0	7
Traffic Offense	1	4	0	5
Weapon Offense	0	1	0	1
Total	88	37	4	129

* *Other agencies: Hawaii County Police Department (Hilo), Kauai Police Department, US Drug Enforcement Administration*

Honolulu Police Department and the US Marshals Service were the only significant contributors of non-drug related critical events. A majority of Honolulu Police Department's non-drug operations were from gambling and sex related offenses; about half of the US Marshals Service's non-drug operations were flight (fugitive) related offenses.

Critical Event Submissions by Operation Types
January 1st through June 30th 2004

	Arrest and Probation/ Parole Search	Knock and Talk	Surveillance	Search Warrant	U/C Buy and Meeting*	Other**
Hawaii County Police Dept, Hilo	2	0	2	52	17	1
Hawaii County Police Dept, Kona	1	0	4	33	5	0
Honolulu Police Dept	5	218	43	54	398	67
Kauai Police Dept	1	0	2	12	38	1
Maui Police Dept	1	1	1	33	12	0
US Customs and Border Protection	0	2	0	0	1	0
US Drug Enforcement Administration	8	0	4	8	35	0
US Federal Bureau of Investigations	16	0	0	2	18	0
US Marshals Service	92	4	4	2	2	4
US Naval Criminal Investigative Service	0	0	0	0	4	0
US Postal Inspection Service	0	0	0	12	0	0
Total	**126**	**225**	**60**	**208**	**530**	**73**

**Undercover buys include buy/walks, buy/busts, informant buys, and stings*
*** e.g. unknown operations, etc*

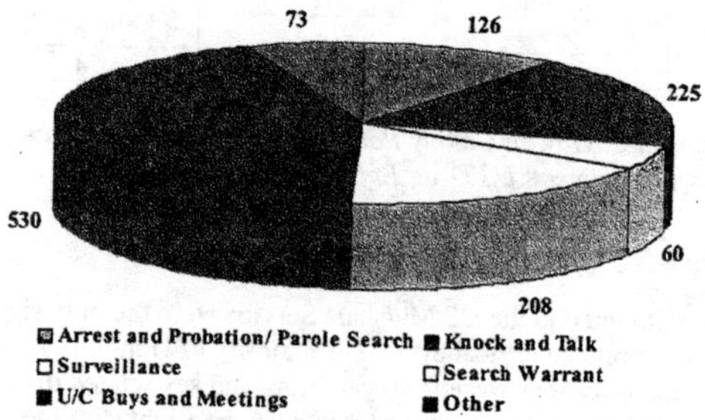

Undercover buys and meetings accounted for approximately 45 percent of all operations submitted in Hawaii. Other operations such as knock and talks represented about 18 percent of the operations, search warrants 17 percent, arrests/probation/parole searches 10 percent, surveillances 5 percent, and other operations 6 percent.

Critical Event Submissions by City/County
January 1st through June 30th 2004

HONOLULU (COUNTY)		
CITY	*ZIP*	*#**
Aiea	96701	51
Ewa Beach	96706	18
Kapolei	96707	3
Haleiwa	96712	11
Hauula	96717	4
Kaaawa	96730	1
Kailua	96734	37
Kaneohe	96744	19
Laie	96762	3
Pearl City	96782	40
Wahiawa	96786	66
Mililani Town	96789	17
Waialua	96791	15
Waianae	96792	23
Waimanalo	96795	26
Waipahu	96797	52
Honolulu	96813	17
Honolulu	96814	39
Honolulu	96815	15
Honolulu	96816	36
Honolulu	96817	125
Honolulu	96818	31
Honolulu	96819	250
Honolulu	96821	2
Honolulu	96822	36
Honolulu	96825	4
Honolulu	96826	13
Ewa Beach/ Barbers Point	96862	1
TOTAL		**955**

MAUI (COUNTY)		
CITY	*ZIP*	*#**
Kahului	96732	14
Kaunakakai	96748	1
Kihei	96753	5
Lahaina	96761	8
Makawao	96768	2
Maunaloa/ Kephui	96770	1
Paia	96779	3
Wailuku	96793	14
TOTAL		**48**
HAWAII (COUNTY)		
CITY	*ZIP*	*#**
Captain Cook	96704	6
Hilo	96720	55
Holualoa	96725	4
Honomu	96728	1
Kailua Kona	96740	24
Kamuela/Waikoloa Village	96743	14
Keaau	96749	12
Kurtistown	96760	2
Mountain View	96771	11
Pahoa	96778	29
Pepeekeo	96783	2
TOTAL		**160**
KAUAI (COUNTY)		
CITY	*ZIP*	*#**
Eleele	96705	3
Princeville	96722	5
Kapaa	96746	18
Kaumakani	96747	1
Koloa	96756	8
Lihue	96766	24
TOTAL		**59**

* *Number of Critical Event submissions*

Zip codes are generated by the Critical Event application after a location has been posted for deconfliction. The above listed cities are based according to the zip code.

Critical Event Submissions by Zip Codes (Map - Oahu)
January 1st through June 30th 2004

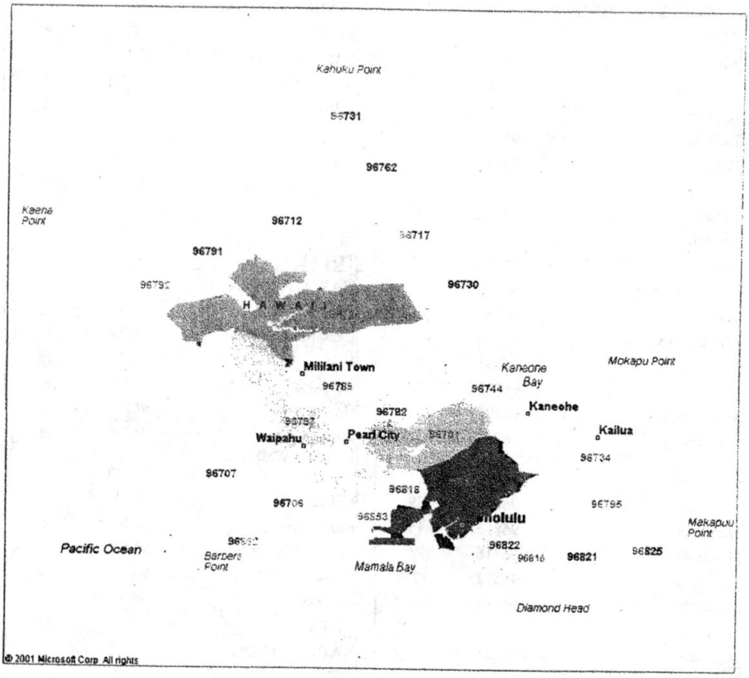

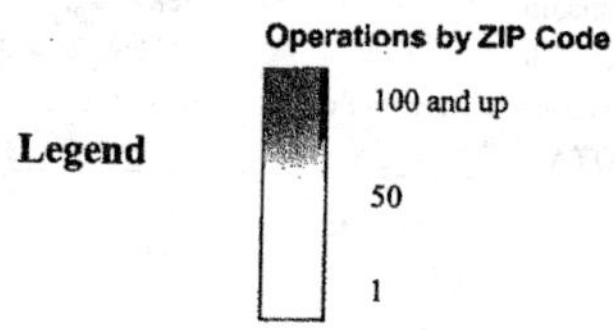

WSIN Database Overview

The WSIN Watch Center maintains and operates an automated criminal intelligence sharing database using the SINS network capable of controlled input; rapid retrieval and dissemination; and systematic updating of information. It also offers flexible search criteria and allows for close monitoring of narcotics subjects. WSIN operates this database to provide member agencies with quick access to accurate and current narcotics intelligence. The Watch Center operates 24 hours a day, 7 days a week.

Information entered into the WSIN database is submitted by member agencies though inquiries or critical events (operations) by contacting the Watch Center via phone or fax, remote access via the secure riss.net Intranet or on forms provided by WSIN. The following forms are available for use: Subject Card, Clandestine Laboratory Seizure Report, Unreliable Informant, Outlaw Motorcycle Gang Subject Card, Aircraft/Pilot Intelligence Report, Vessel Intelligence Report, Seizure Information Report.

The database may be searched by one or more of the following fields: name (or partial name), alias, moniker, associates, address, telephone number, vehicle description, licenses, organizations, infiltrated businesses and weapons. Information is stored in the database for either six months or five years with one of the following dissemination criteria: release information, release only submitting agency/officer's name or no release.

Security of the WSIN database intelligence is of paramount importance. Only those officers designated by their agency as Primary Liaison Officers (PLO) or Alternate Liaison Officers (ALO) may inquire. Each PLO and ALO provides WSIN with a personal data card. Information on the personal data card is used to verify the officer's identity when an inquiry is made. As an extra precaution, information is released on a call back basis only. Database access is also limited to specified WSIN personnel. Remote access is controlled by the respective member agency's security officer.

WSIN Database Activity Totals by Agencies
January 1st through June 30th 2004

	Hits	Inquiries	Entries
Hawaii Attorney General	0 (0)	7 (7)	0 (0)
Hawaii Co Police Dept, Hilo	58 (11)	265 (121)	217 (60)
Hawaii Co Police Dept, Kona	29 (5)	356 (250)	228 (120)
Hawaii St Dept Public Safety	2 (0)	33 (28)	30 (25)
Honolulu Police Dept	1269 (549)	4859 (3487)	3759 (2722)
Honolulu US ATF	1	3	2
Honolulu US Customs and Border Protection	6 (5)	42 (37)	6 (4)
Honolulu US DEA	138 (45)	521 (305)	210 (14)
Honolulu US FBI	96 (41)	618 (495)	404 (301)
Honolulu US Marshals Service	103 (1)	259 (1)	223 (0)
Honolulu US Postal Inspection Service	17	19	18
Kauai Police Dept	52 (4)	134 (17)	126 (11)
Maui Police Dept	60 (11)	293 (72)	222 (3)
Maui Prosecutors Office	8 (8)	7 (7)	0 (0)
Pearl Harbor US Navy NCIS	0 (0)	7 (1)	6 (0)
Schofield Barracks US Army CID	8 (1)	297 (271)	230 (205)
Remote Totals (Hawaii)	681	5099	3465
WSIN Watch Center	1166	2621	2216
TOTALS	**1847**	**7720**	**5681**

(Numbers in parentheses are from remote sites)

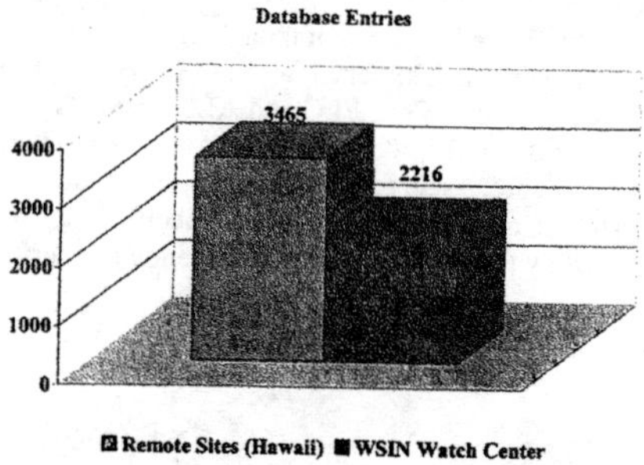

Approximately 60 percent of Hawaiian agencies' entries were submitted remotely into the WSIN database January 1st through June 30th 2004. In 2003, remote entries represented 75 percent. The number has declined primarily because of increased critical event submissions from Hawaiian agencies directly through the Watch Center. Most critical event information is submitted into the WSIN database.

From January 1st through June 30th 2004, 2229 WSIN database submittals were entered by Hawaiian agencies. There was an average of about 2.5 entries per submittal.

WSIN Database Activity by Agencies
2002 through 2004* (projected)

	2002			2003			2004*		
	Hits	Inq	Entries	Hits	Inq	Entries	Hits	Inq	Entries
Hawaii Attorney General	0	19	0	1	18	0	0	14	0
Hawaii Co Police Dept, Hilo	33	288	246	49	274	188	116	530	434
Hawaii Co Police Dept, Kona	16	219	241	55	515	434	58	712	456
Hawaii Co Prosecutors Office	5	30	0	1	18	0	0	0	0
Hawaii St Dept Public Safety	14	245	351	11	160	208	4	66	60
Honolulu Police Dept	728	3273	2741	1654	6892	6184	2538	9718	7518
Honolulu Prosecutors Office	0	0	0	0	2	3	0	0	0
Honolulu US ATF	0	0	0	88	438	420	2	8	4
Honolulu US Customs and Border Protection	0	0	0	27	88	39	12	84	12
Honolulu US Immigration and Customs Enf.	0	0	0	2	11	9	0	0	0
Honolulu US Customs C.E.T.	0	8	0	1	1	0	0	0	0
Honolulu US Customs Service**	16	123	53	22	99	55	0	0	0
Honolulu US DEA	182	613	376	149	460	272	276	1042	420
Honolulu US FBI	169	564	345	178	775	507	192	1236	808
Honolulu US INS	3	93	2	0	5	0	0	0	0
Honolulu US IRS	4	14	9	0	7	5	0	0	0
Honolulu US Marshals Service	0	1	0	104	325	254	206	518	446
Honolulu US Navy NCIC	0	0	0	3	44	6	0	0	0
Honolulu US Postal Inspection Service	2	8	4	5	11	0	34	38	36
Kauai Police Dept	10	64	59	28	106	96	104	268	252
Maui Police Dept	64	300	223	44	164	110	120	586	444
Maui Prosecutors Office	0	5	0	0	1	0	16	14	0
Pearl Harbor US Navy NCIS	0	0	0	6	8	7	0	14	12
Schofield Barracks US Army CID	11	477	599	36	458	587	16	594	460
Remote Totals (Hawaii)	715	5021	4080	986	7374	7187	1362	10198	6930
WSIN Watch Center	542	1323	1169	1478	3506	2206	2332	5242	4432
TOTALS	**1257**	**6344**	**5249**	**2464**	**10880**	**9393**	**3694**	**15440**	**11362**

**2004 statistics projected (as of 7/1/2004)*

*** US Customs split into two separate WSIN agencies May 2003 - US Customs and Border Protection and Honolulu US Immigration and Customs Enforcement*

A majority of Hawaii agencies are on pace this year to equal or significantly exceed the number of inquiries from each of the last two years. Honolulu Police Department continues to be the significant contributor for the entire state.

WSIN Database Entries and Hit Rates
2001 through 2004 (projected)*

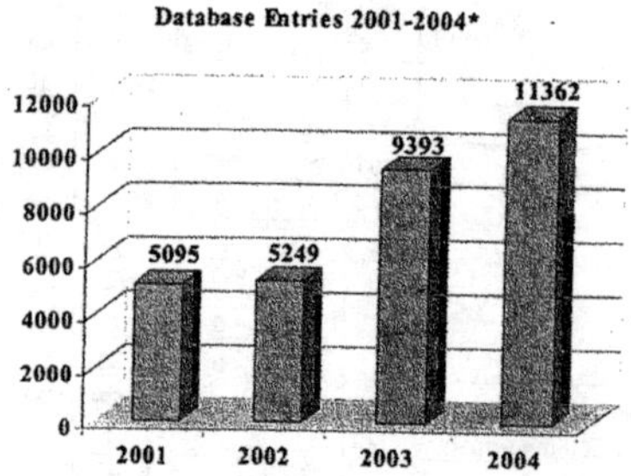

**2004 statistics projected (as of 7/1/2004)*

WSIN database entries remained consistent from 2001 through 2002. However, from 2002 through 2003 the number of entries dramatically increased by approximately 79 percent. According to 2004 projections, WSIN database entries will increase another 21 percent.

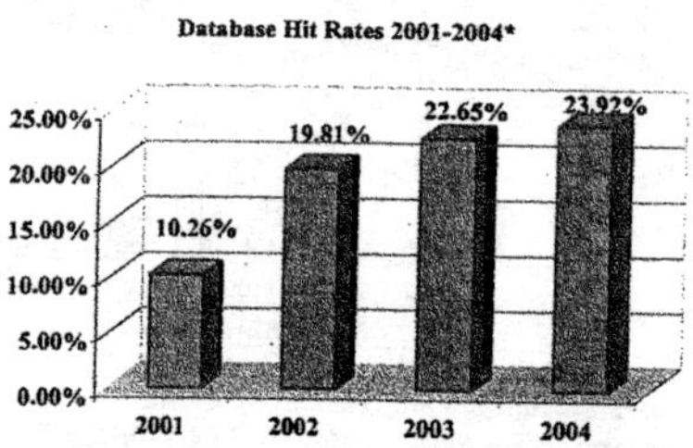

**2004 statistics projected (as of 7/1/2004)*

According to 2004 projections, WSIN database hit rates will remain consistent compared to the two previous years. There was approximately a 10 percent increase in hit rates from 2001 to 2002. This could have resulted from the increasing number of entities from Hawaiian agencies being entered into the WSIN database, thus improving the odds of a hit.

WSIN Database Drug/Non-Drug Frequency by Agencies
January 1st through June 30th 2004

	Drug Related Events	Non Drug Related Events	Total
Hawaii Attorney General	0	0	0
Hawaii Co Police Dept, Hilo	101	1	102
Hawaii Co Police Dept, Kona	95	0	95
Hawaii St Dept Public Safety	11	2	13
Honolulu Police Dept	846	880	1726
Honolulu US ATF	0	1	1
Honolulu US Customs and Border Protection	4	0	4
Honolulu US DEA	81	2	83
Honolulu US FBI	62	0	62
Honolulu US Marshals Service	63	35	98
Honolulu US Postal Inspection Service	1	0	1
Kauai Police Dept	57	0	57
Maui Police Dept	45	52	97
Maui Prosecutors Office	0	0	0
Pearl Harbor US Navy NCIS	3	0	3
Schofield Barracks US Army CID	125	0	125
Total	**1495**	**973**	**2467**

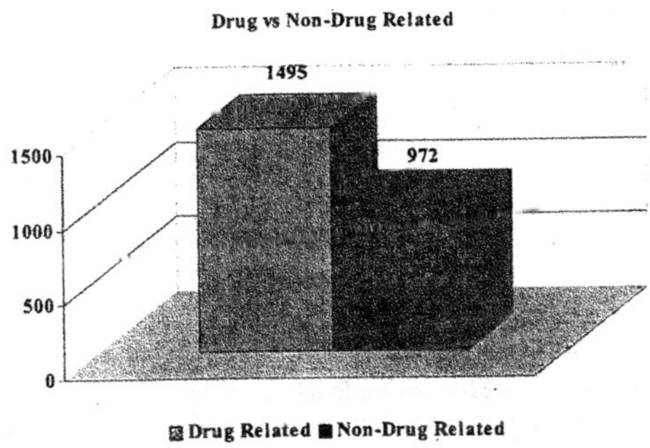

These numbers represent the frequency drug and non-drug related events appear in the above agencies' WSIN database submittals from January 1st through June 30th 2004. WSIN database submittals can contain more than one criminal event – a total of 2229 submittals were created with 2467 criminal events/predicates. Drug related events represented approximately 60 percent of the submittals and non-drug 40 percent. The only agencies to contribute a significant number of non-drug related events were Honolulu Police Department, Maui Police Department and US Marshals Service.

WSIN Database Drug Event Category Frequency for Hawaii
January 1st 2000 through June 30th 2004

	2000	2001	2002	2003	Jan - June 2004*
Methamphetamine	617 (41.19%)	495 (29.13%)	602 (41.18%)	1219 (47.45%)	917 (62.51%)
Cocaine	273 (18.22%)	219 (12.89%)	171 (11.70%)	260 (10.12%)	102 (6.95%)
Dangerous Drugs (other / not specified)	275 (18.36%)	583 (34.31%)	216 (14.77%)	628 (24.25%)	285 (19.43%)
Hallucinogens	8 (0.53%)	24 (1.41%)	34 (2.33%)	50 (1.95%)	6 (0.41%)
Heroin	81 (5.41%)	100 (5.89%)	41 (2.80%)	49 (1.91%)	10 (0.68)
Marijuana	244 (16.29%)	278 (16.36%)	398 (27.22%)	363 (14.13%)	147 (10.02)
Total	**1498**	**1699**	**1462**	**2569**	**1467**

** Current 2004 database statistics as of 7/1/04*

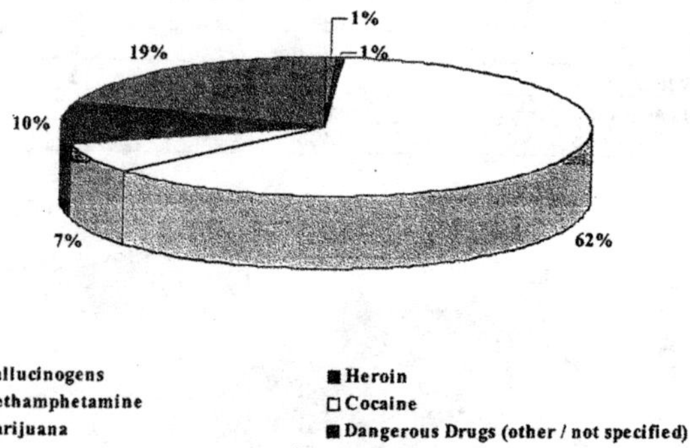

The table above reflects the number of times each drug has appeared as an event category for all submittals that were entered with an event location in Hawaii. Submittals from Hawaiian agencies that did not have an event location in Hawaii were not counted. Next to each number in the above table is the yearly percentage rounded to the nearest one hundredth. There has been a steady increase in the number of methamphetamine (with the exception of 2001) categories. The sharpest yearly decrease was shown in the cocaine categories, dropping approximately 60 percent from January 2000 to June 30th 2004.

WSIN Database Non Drug Event Category Frequency for Hawaii
January 1st through June 30th 2004

Criminal Event (General)			
Assault	105	Property Crimes	7
Burglary	62	Public Peace	7
Commercial Sex	42	Robbery	57
Criminal Gang	20	Sex Assault	52
Damage Property	18	Sex Offense	8
Flight	23	Stolen Property	21
Forgery	83	Stolen Vehicle	175
Fraud	20	Threat	75
Gambling	21	Traffic Offense	5
Homicide	32	Weapon Offense	27
Kidnapping	20	Other Crimes	19
Larceny	74	Total	**973**

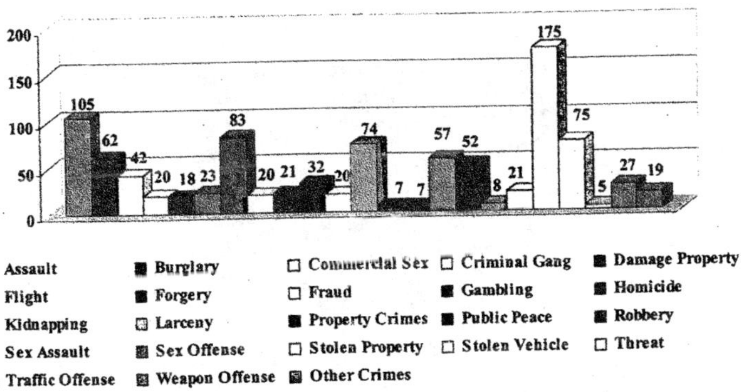

The table and chart above reflects the number of times each non-drug related has appeared as an event category for all submittals that were entered with an event location in Hawaii. Prior to 2003, crimes other than drugs to typically appear in the WSIN database from Hawaiian agencies involved either commercial sex (e.g. prostitution) or gambling related investigations.

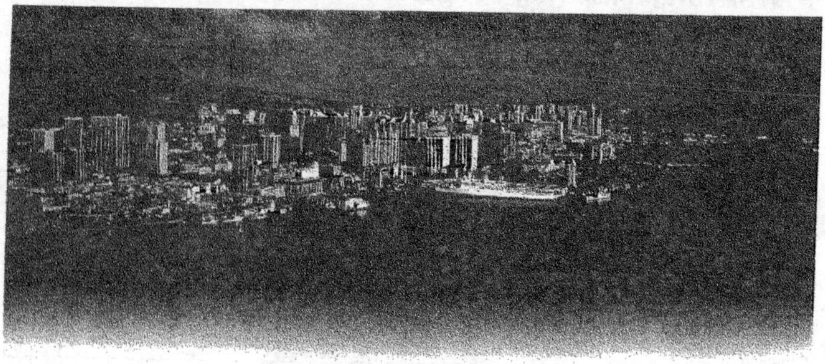

2005 STRATEGY

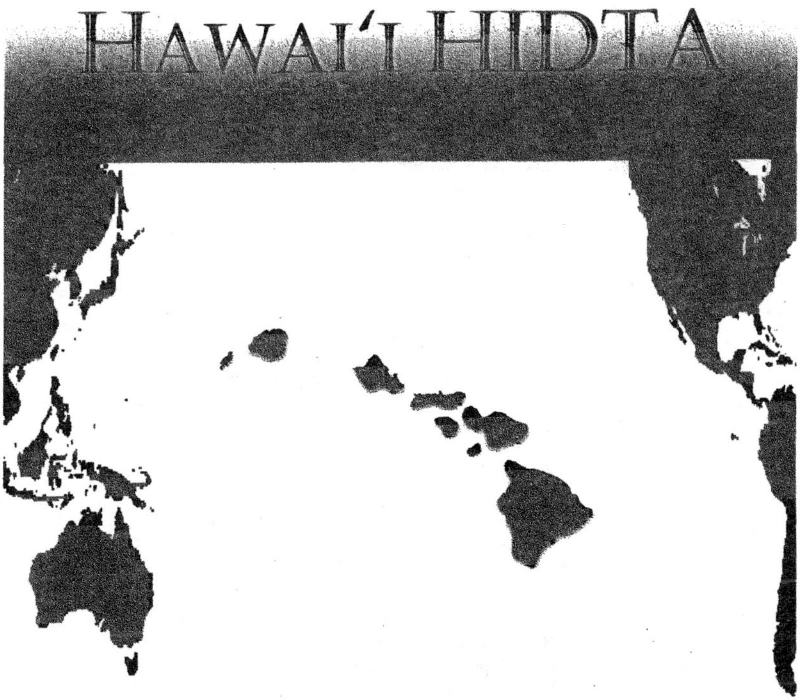

HAWAII HIDTA STRATEGY

This document and the information contained herein are unclassified.

TABLE OF CONTENTS

SECTION I.

EXECUTIVE SUMMARY

The Hawaii HIDTA Executive Board through its Oversight Committees has devised a clear, well planned, strategy to counter the drug threat facing Hawaii and the surrounding region.

> Hawaii, as in any populated area, faces a multitude of illicit drug abuse problems. Hawaii's drug trafficking and abuse can be categorized in three tiers. In the first tier are the two drugs causing the most serious problems—crystal methamphetamine and marijuana. Cocaine (usually crack cocaine) and heroin comprise the second tier; and drugs such as MDMA, GHB, steroids, and diverted pharmaceuticals make up the third tier. While it is imperative to continue combating all forms of drug abuse to prevent larger problems in the future, it is the trafficking and abuse of crystal methamphetamine as well as marijuana, cocaine, and heroin that currently pose the most viable drug threats to Hawaii. The magnitude of the crystal methamphetamine crisis in Hawaii—a far more socially disruptive problem—overshadows all other abuse threats.
>
> The crystal methamphetamine problem could not have reached such epidemic proportions if not for the constant pressure of drug traffickers. This constant pressure fuels a market that generates larceny, theft, burglary, homicides, abuse, and endangerment. Consequently, drug trafficking organizations (DTOs) — international and local — are a focus of law enforcement and pose a significant drug threat to Hawaii.

The process utilized by the Executive Board:

1) Identifies primary threats by geographic area;
2) Develops desired goals to counter the threats;
3) Assigns responsibility to accomplish the desired goals;
4) Evaluates effectiveness of the program's outcomes;
5) Provides oversight and implements changes as necessary.

This process is dynamic, ongoing, allowing for change and refinement.

The Hawaii HIDTA strategy has each subsystem, intelligence/operational initiative, task force, and support group target one or more of the identified threats and needs that are listed in the current Hawaii HIDTA Threat Assessment Matrix. For FY2005 law enforcement organizations will contribute a total of 311 (full and/or part time) law enforcement personnel and support staff, organized into 12 initiatives. Two additional far reaching initiatives will be implemented should supplemental funding become available.

- **HI-IMPACT** - the main investigative arm of the Hawaii HIDTA whose focus is on long term, complex, multi-jurisdictional case activity that disrupts and dismantles international, regional, and local drug trafficking organizations.

- **INTERDICTION** – intercepts illicit drugs destined for Hawaii, or transiting Hawaii's airports, harbors, and seaports, for the continental U.S. and other foreign destinations.

- **MONEY LAUNDERING/ASSET FORFEITURE** - dismantles and disrupts DTOs by seizing the money and assets used to operate illicit activities thereby impacting their ability to function.

- **CLANDESTINE LAB COORDINATION** - works with personnel throughout the State of Hawaii to provide oversight, consolidated training and coordination of first response to clandestine laboratories.

- **PROSECUTORIAL INITIATIVE** – supports investigation and prosecution activity in both State and Federal courts. Actively promotes model legislation to conform the state's laws to federal statute.

- **INTELLIGENCE SUBSYSTEM** - a main focus of the Hawaii HIDTA that provides a communication infrastructure to promote information sharing between participating law enforcement agencies. The analysis and deconfliction of strategic and operational intelligence is critical for effectively attacking drug traffickers and reducing drug availability. The Investigative Support Center is the main body of the intelligence subsystem and consists of the Investigative Support Group and the Strategic Intelligence Support Group. In addition, the Regional WSIN Coordinator and staff are housed under the intelligence subsystem umbrella.

- **MANAGEMENT AND COORDINATION** – facilitates efficient operation of initiatives by providing oversight, administrative, and budgetary support.

- **TRAINING** - provides on-site and coordinates off-site training including mainland travel. The main goal of the training initiative is to provide resources and improve the ability of investigative and analytical personnel to counter drug trafficking and related criminal activity.

Partial funding, full funding through baseline increase:

- **SAFE NEIGHBORHOODS** – removes guns from the street by targeting chronic violent drug offenders having significant impact on crime occurring in Hawaii. FY2003 seizure of 162 firearms.

Funded through baseline increase:

- **FUGITIVE** - assists other HIDTA initiatives in crippling the drug trade and related crime in Hawaii and throughout the Pacific region by bringing fugitives to justice.

- **MARIJUANA** – eradicates marijuana that can be abundantly grown in Hawaii's tropical climate, typically on public lands. FY2003 resulted in seizure of 392,276 plants (approximately 200 tons).

- **CIUs** – unites City/County intelligence units with the 24 Hawaii HIDTA participating federal, state and local law enforcement agencies.

Unfunded, full funding dependant on supplemental request:

- **WEED & SEED** – compliments Operation Weed & Seed by providing resources that are lacking under the larger umbrella program.

- **HI-PRIORITY - (PACIFIC RIM/BASIN)** – supports task force operations, provides funding for Title III's, and exploits regional intelligence linking Pacific Rim and Asian based traffickers to CPOT/RPOT investigations. A Pacific Rim/Basin intelligence component would also support this initiative and link to the Hawaii HIDTA Investigative Support Center.

Each HIDTA initiative develops a mission statement to focus their efforts on one or more of the National HIDTA Program's three goals, which are designed to reduce drug availability and its harmful consequences through a coordinated effort of federal, state, and local law enforcement agencies. The initiatives work to accomplish these goals through a clearly defined strategy fostered by examination of the region's threats and needs.

During CY2004 the Hawaii HIDTA began incorporating a new method of reporting and accountability as mandated by the Office of National Drug Control Policy (ONDCP) and developed through the National HIDTA Program Office (NHPO). This method, known as the Performance Management Process, is most obviously illustrated by the Performance Management Process Matrix. The Matrix is a tool designed to illustrate the Performance Management Process and keep it simple, direct and understandable. It serves as both a planning tool and an operational roadmap. The Matrix changes over time as the Hawaii HIDTA defines and redefines the threats and needs it faces. Based on this Matrix the Hawaii HIDTA Executive Board organized its task forces and initiatives into a carefully planned strategy to counter the drug threat facing Hawaii and the surrounding region.

SECTION II.

INTRODUCTION

By design, the Hawaii HIDTA provides a comprehensive response to illicit drug activity by fostering interagency cooperation, information sharing, collocating and commingling resources to create greater efficiency and effectiveness among participating agencies at the federal, state, and local level. Success of the HIDTA program is measured by its ability to achieve three goals established by ONDCP to achieve the HIDTA mission.

GOAL ONE. **REDUCE DRUG AVAILABILITY BY ELIMINATING OR DISRUPTING DRUG TRAFFICKING ORGANIZATIONS.**

The illegal drug market in the United States is one of the most profitable in the world. The prices in Hawaii and the Pacific Region are twice to four times as high as the continental U.S., which creates an attractive market for drug traffickers and organizations from both the continental U.S. and Asian countries.

GOAL TWO. **REDUCE THE HARMFUL CONSEQUENCES OF DRUG TRAFFICKING**

Drug trafficking causes various problems in the community and negatively impacts the quality and safety of life for citizens exposed to the dangers of the drug culture.

GOAL THREE. **IMPROVE THE EFFICIENCY AND EFFECTIVENESS OF LAW ENFORCEMENT ORGANIZATIONS.**

The guiding theme of the HIDTA Program is to attack drug trafficking from all angles, combining available resources from federal, state and local law enforcement organizations.

In order to achieve these goals, the Hawaii HIDTA promotes the team and task force concept that advances the National Drug Control Strategy and the National Gang Strategy by emphasizing multi-agency investigations and elevating cooperative efforts among HIDTA participants. These goals are supported by intelligence driven drug task forces aimed at eliminating or reducing domestic drug trafficking and its harmful consequences, through enhancement and coordination of drug trafficking control efforts among federal, state and local law enforcement agencies.

The Hawaii HIDTA strategy facilitates the relationship between the region's drug threat and the initiatives created to address it. It demonstrates how law enforcement agencies have shaped their drug control efforts to reduce drug trafficking, eliminate unnecessary duplicative efforts, maximize resources, and improve information and intelligence sharing under the coordinating umbrella of the HIDTA Program.

SECTION III.

HIDTA MATRIX

The National HIDTA Program Office (NHPO) is mandated by the Office of Management and Budget (OMB) to accurately account for the performance of the HIDTA program. In doing so, the NHPO has developed the Performance Management Process (PMP), which measures program efficiency and effectiveness. The cornerstone of this effort is the PMP Matrix, a tool designed to illustrate the performance process and keep it simple, direct and understandable. The Matrix is a grid system that:

1. Identifies primary threats by geographic area;
2. Develops desired goals to counter the threats;
3. Assigns responsibility to accomplish the desired goals;
4. Captures output measurements;
5. Illustrates the program's outcomes.

The left side of the Matrix contains a description of the primary threats and desired outputs (strategy) by geographic region. The right side of the Matrix lists the entities responsible for addressing the threats and outputs/outcomes.

The Hawaii HIDTA sits on the National HIDTA PMP Development Committee and is one of two HIDTAs using the PMP Matrix in the submission of its 2003 Annual Report, 2005 Threat Assessment, and the 2005 Strategy. We expect the PMP Matrix to be fully implemented by the end of CY2004.

A complete, fold-out, copy of the Hawaii HIDTA's matrix can be found in both the Annual Report and the Threat Assessment.

The 2005 Hawaii HIDTA Matrix was developed using information from the 2003 Annual Report, 2005 Threat Assessment, and FY2005 Initiative Submissions. The desired outcomes and responsibility sections are based on the expected outputs as indicated by each of the initiatives in their annual submission package.

The matrix based system establishes a mechanism that measures each HIDTA's performance and holds them accountable for what they do. Standardized outcome measurements have yet to be finalized by the NHPO and are not used in the development of the strategy. Therefore, they are not included in the matrix.

SECTION IV.

OVERVIEW OF HIDTA REGION

GEOGRAPHY

The State of Hawaii encompasses eight main islands and a 1,500-mile chain of islets covering more than 6,400 square miles in the north central Pacific Ocean. It is perhaps the most geographically isolated populated place in the world, situated approximately 2,500 miles from California, almost 4,000 miles from Guam and Japan, and more than 5,000 miles from Taiwan, Australia, the Philippines, and Hong Kong.[1] Hawaii's remote location, situated in the expanse of the Pacific Ocean, makes it an ideal transshipment point for illicit drugs to and from Asia and North America or to Pacific Basin locations, where profits two-four times higher are realized.

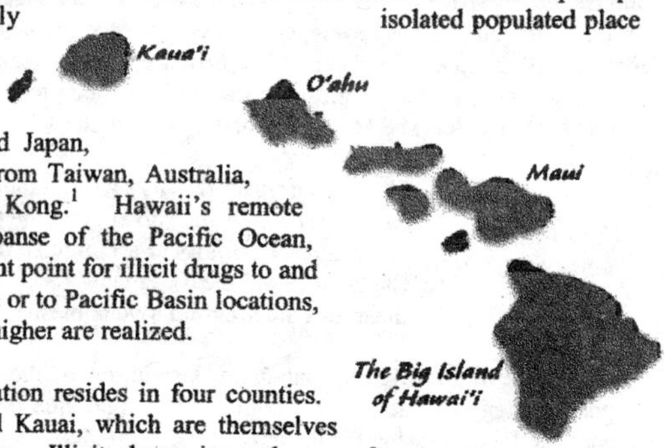

The State of Hawaii's population resides in four counties. Honolulu, Hawaii, Maui, and Kauai, which are themselves separated by miles of ocean. Illicit drugs in each are often controlled by DTOs that supply and distribute statewide. While Hawaii is a geographically expansive state, three-quarters of the population reside on the island of Oahu (Honolulu County), and, to a large extent, circumstances in the City and County of Honolulu drive the drug situation statewide.

DEMOGRAPHICS

Hawaii has the most racially diverse population of any state, with more than 1.2 million residents exposed to the influences of the illicit drug trade and the social costs associated with abuse. Asians account for 41.6 percent of the population, which includes Asian Indian (0.1), Chinese (4.7), Filipino (14.1), Japanese (16.7), Korean (1.9), Vietnamese (0.6), and other Asians (3.5). Caucasians represent 24.3 percent of the population, the lowest percentage of any state. Native Hawaiians account for 9.4 percent of the population, and African Americans account for 1.8 percent. Various mixed-racial groups account for most of the remaining 15.7 percent of the population[2]. A recent and significant change in Hawaii's population has been the increasing Mexican/Hispanic population, which now accounts for 7.2 percent of Hawaii's overall population. Mexican/Hispanic communities are primarily located on the islands of Maui and Hawaii and have strong links to Mexico and South America. Hawaii also has a large, possibility the largest per capita, transient population in the United States. When military personnel and visitors are factored in, daily population of the state grows by as much as 20 percent.

HIDTA REGION

The demand for illicit drugs in all counties is high, particularly in regards to crystal methamphetamine and marijuana. The drug threat includes the presence of international

DTOs, drug fugitives, armed violent drug offenders, smuggling/transportation and distribution of multi-pound quantities of illicit drugs, significant numbers of drug traffickers identified but not prosecuted, money laundering activity, use of public lands for cannabis cultivation, and the presence of weapons associated with drug trafficking.

Because of Hawaii's remote location in the Pacific Ocean, much of the Hawaii HIDTA's efforts focus on the transportation to, through, and from Hawaii of illicit drugs (at least one of which—marijuana—is produced in significant quantities in the state) and drug proceeds. As an interdiction and production HIDTA, the Hawaii HIDTA is not engaged in prevention or treatment initiatives; rather, it focuses on crippling the efforts of drug trafficking organizations smuggling illicit drugs into and out of the state.

ECONOMICS

Tourism, military, and agriculture are Hawaii's leading economic industries and play an important role in the State's drug threat. With over 6 million visitors arriving annually[3], the daily profusion of tourists can make it difficult for law enforcement to interdict drug couriers at Hawaii's airports.

Military personnel and their dependents contribute nearly 87,000 individuals to the State's population[4]. According to military law enforcement agencies, there has been an increase in the use of predatory drugs, such as MDMA and GHB among personnel. Because these drugs are not detectable in the body after a day or two, service members use the drugs over the weekend when they know they will not be tested.

Agriculture is Hawaii's third largest industry generating $1.07 billion to the State's economy each year[5]. Crops such as exotic fruits, coffee, macadamia nuts, flowers, and foliage not only provide products for Hawaii's markets but have become exports to destinations around the world. These products, especially flowers and foliage, may be used to conceal drug exports such as marijuana.

TRANSPORTATION

Hawaii's island makeup eliminates land-based border threats and allows law enforcement to concentrate on air and sea chokepoints. Airborne package delivery services and commercial aircraft are the most significant threats for transporting illicit drug to and from the State. In 2003, FedEx, UPS, and the U.S. Postal Service delivered over 28 million packages into the State. In addition, there were over one million takeoffs and landings at Hawaii's airports.

CLIMATE

Agricultural and weather conditions make Hawaii an optimal location to cultivate marijuana. Marijuana grown outdoors in Hawaii contains some of the highest THC levels in the nation. The windward side of each of the islands provides an optimal location for marijuana growth due to ample morning rain showers and afternoon sunlight. Marijuana cultivators often use public lands such as national forests and state parks. The majority of marijuana is cultivated at remote jungle locations in Hawaii County.

SECTION V.

SUMMARY OF THREAT & NEEDS ASSESSMENT

The CY2005 Hawaii HIDTA Threat Assessment contains a more comprehensive analysis of the illicit drug threat facing Hawaii. The information contained in this section is condensed and presented only as a limited overview for summary.

A multitude of illicit drugs are available to varying degrees in Hawaii, as in any populated area; however, these drugs can be categorized in three tiers based on the severity of the problems they pose to Hawaii's law enforcement and citizens.

Tier 1.
In the first tier are the two drugs causing the most serious problems—crystal methamphetamine and marijuana. Arrest and seizure data for both these drugs indicate that availability is high, while demand data suggest that use of both drugs, along with the consequences of that use, is high and increasing.

Nonetheless, the magnitude of the crystal methamphetamine problem in Hawaii—a far more socially disruptive problem—overshadows marijuana, which has seen an increase in associated violence, but not nearly to the same extent.

Tier 2.
The second-tier drugs are cocaine (usually crack cocaine) and heroin which, although they remain problems in Hawaii, appear to rank well behind crystal methamphetamine and marijuana in contributing to the state's drug troubles. Cocaine-related arrests and seizures are on an upswing, but demand data suggest declining prevalence and consequences of use. At the same time, heroin distribution and abuse appear to be diminishing in light of indicators suggesting declines in arrests, seizures, reported use, and treatment.

Tier 3.
In the third tier are drugs such as MDMA, GHB, steroids, and diverted pharmaceuticals, which are available and abused in Hawaii but to a much lesser extent. The focus of third tier drugs appears to be among young club goers and younger members of the military. While it is imperative to continue combating these drugs and thus preventing them from becoming a larger problem in the future, it is the trafficking and abuse of primarily crystal methamphetamine as well as marijuana, cocaine, and heroin that currently pose the most viable drug threats to Hawaii.

International and local DTOs have ample opportunity to traffic drugs to, through, and from the area because of Hawaii's high volume of international and domestic air and sea traffic including passengers, cargo, and mail. Hawaii is a destination for crystal methamphetamine, cocaine, and heroin supplied from the West Coast and Mexico by Mexican Consolidated Priority Organization Targets (CPOTs) and DTOs; for crystal methamphetamine and heroin transported from Asia, Canada, and the West Coast by Asian DTOs; and for marijuana transported from Canada and the Pacific Northwest by local DTOs. Hawaii is a trans-shipment point for methamphetamine transported from the West Coast to locations in the Pacific Basin, such as Guam, by local DTOs supplied by Mexican DTOs.[6] It also is a transshipment point for methamphetamine transported from the West Coast or Asia to locations in the Pacific Basin by Asian DTOs. Finally, Hawaii is the source of high potency marijuana transported to the U.S. mainland, Canada and, to a lesser extent, Mexico by local DTOs.

In addition to the threat posed by the presence of international and local DTOs, drug fugitives, armed violent drug offenders smuggling, money laundering, and the use of public lands for cannabis cultivation plague the counties. Because of the way Hawaii's drug laws are written, a significant number of drug traffickers are identified but not prosecuted.

Through its initiatives the Hawaii HIDTA and its participating agencies are disrupting and dismantling the DTOs responsible for trafficking illicit drugs in Hawaii through the interdiction of crystal methamphetamine, marijuana, cocaine, heroin, and other illicit drugs as they are transported throughout the state and region. The Hawaii HIDTA is also disrupting these DTOs by seizing the money they use to operate and the assets they acquire with illicit drug proceeds.

The Hawaii HIDTA and its federal and state/local law enforcement partners are removing weapons from the street and bringing drug offenders and fugitives to justice to in its efforts to cripple the drug trade and reduce drug-related crime in Hawaii. The future impact of Hawaii HIDTA initiatives will be measured in the continuing and increasing seizures of illicit drugs and proceeds as well as the arrests and successful prosecutions of those responsible for transporting drugs and drug proceeds through Hawaii's airports, parcel facilities, and ports.

SECTION VI.

VISION & MISSION STATEMENTS

HIDTA MISSION STATEMENT

The mission of the High Intensity Drug Trafficking Area (HIDTA) Program is to enhance and coordinate America's drug-control efforts among local, state and federal law enforcement agencies in order to eliminate or reduce drug trafficking and its harmful consequences in critical regions of the United States. The mission includes coordination efforts to reduce the production, manufacturing, distribution, transportation and chronic use of illegal drugs, as well as the attendant money laundering of drug proceeds.

HAWAII HIDTA VISION STATEMENT

The Hawaii HIDTA envisions a combined cultural and regional counterdrug effort that not only improves coordination and effectiveness among local, state and federal law enforcement agencies; but also embraces citizen stakeholders in education, prevention, health care, and public leadership, etc., in order to provide an inclusive community action plan and response to the harmful consequences of drug trafficking in our neighborhoods.

HAWAII HIDTA MISSION STATEMENT

As the crossroad of the Pacific and gateway into the continental United States, the Hawaii HIDTA's participating agencies work together through enhanced coordination and integrated initiatives to disrupt and dismantle illicit drug distribution, production, money laundering, transportation, and trafficking within the region.

This mission is consistent with (a) the goals of the National Drug Control Strategy and its comprehensive approach to counter the threat of illicit drugs, and (b) the overall mission of the HIDTA program-the enhancement and coordination of America's drug control efforts among federal, state, and local agencies in order to eliminate or reduce drug trafficking (including the production, manufacture, transportation, distribution, and chronic use of illegal drugs and money laundering) and its harmful consequences in critical areas of the United States.

SECTION VII.

CONCEPT OF STRATEGY

METHODOLOGY

Each year the Hawaii HIDTA conducts it Threat Assessment using information collected from its initiatives and other sources relevant to identifying and evaluating the region's drug threat. This provides the framework for HIDTA's strategy outlining the efforts needed to address the drug threat. The Hawaii HIDTA Executive Board evaluates the allocation of resources based on the Threat Assessment and makes changes to the program as needed to address the threat and achieve the program goals.

COMPOSITION

A. **Executive Board** – the role of the Executive Board is to provide direction and oversight in implementing the ONDCP/HIDTA concept and establishing the goals of the region. The Executive Board is comprised of eight federal and eight state/local law enforcement leaders (Agency Heads) in the Hawaii Region who make decisions together regarding the Hawaii HIDTA's strategy, initiatives/budget, and internal policies and procedures.

The board consists of the following member agencies:

Bureau of Alcohol, Tobacco and Firearms
City and County of Honolulu Prosecuting Attorney's Office
Drug Enforcement Administration
Federal Bureau of Investigation
Hawaii National Guard
Hawaii County Police Department
Hawaii State Department of Public Safety
Honolulu Police Department
Immigration and Customs Enforcement
Internal Revenue Service
Kauai Police Department
Maui Police Department
U. S. Attorney's Office
U. S. Marshal's Service
U. S. Postal Inspection Service
Western States Information Network
Bureau of Prisons*
U. S. Coast Guard*
Naval Criminal Investigative Service*
(* indicates non-voting Executive Board members.)

B. **Director's Office** – The Director reports to the Executive Board and is responsible for providing the day to day management of the Hawaii HIDTA. The Director is assisted by a staff consisting of a Fiscal Officer, Administrative Assistant, and Program Analyst. The Director and staff implements the policy established by the ONDCP/ NHPO and the Executive Board. They also implement an annual evaluation process of all initiatives to assess efficiency and effectiveness.

C. **Executive Board Subcommittees** – The Executive Board is divided into four subcommittees to facilitate efficiency in examining and implementing ONDCP/HIDTA policies and procedures:

a. **Intelligence** – provides oversight for the Intelligence Subsystem.

b. **Budget** – provides oversight for fiscal operations and approves operational budgets/funding for Initiatives and Task Forces.

c. **Administration** – sets policy & procedure and provides oversight to the Director and staff.

d. **Initiative Review** – conducts internal reviews and provides oversight for Initiatives and Task Forces.

D. **Participating Agencies**

AGENCY	TOTAL PARTICIPANTS (FULL-TIME PLUS PART-TIME)
Bureau of Alcohol, Tobacco and Firearms	9
Department of Public Safety	12
Drug Enforcement Administration	13
Federal Bureau of Investigation	15
Federal Bureau of Prisons	1
Fisheries Service	1
Hawaii County Police Department	38
Hawaii Department of Land & Natural Resources	17
Hawaii HIDTA Contract Personnel	8
Hawaii National Guard	21
Honolulu City & County Prosecutor's Office	5
Honolulu Police Department	73
Immigration and Customs Enforcement	24

Internal Revenue Service	5
Kauai Police Department	13
Maui County Prosecutor's Office	1
Maui Police Department	36
Naval Criminal Investigative Service	1
U.S. Attorney's Office	1
U.S. Coast Guard	1
U.S. Inspector General	1
U.S. Marshals Service	6
U.S. Postal Inspection Service	4
Western States Information Network	5
TOTALS	**311**

UNITY OF EFFORT

All components of the Hawaii HIDTA function in a unified effort under guidelines in the Hawaii HIDTA Policy and Procedures Manual. This manual establishes policy with regard to administrative, financial and organizational matters. These policies are included in signed Memorandums of Understanding (MOU) developed by each initiative with the participating law enforcement agencies governing operational policies and the assignment, supervision and responsibilities of those departments committing personnel to each initiative.

All initiatives meet the ONDCP requirements of multi-agency participation and collocation/commingling of personnel. Kauai which has no permanent federal presence is granted an exception to the collocation/commingling rule, via temporary assignment of federal personnel on an as-needed basis.

SECTION VIII.

GOAL 1

Reduce Drug Availability by Eliminating or Disrupting Drug Trafficking Organizations

The Hawaii HIDTA's primary goal is to dismantle, disrupt, arrest, and prosecute drug trafficking organizations (DTOs), drug gangs, and organized crime groups involved in drug distribution, drug manufacturing, money laundering, and other drug related crimes. This is accomplished through complex drug and money laundering investigations, an effective interdiction program targeting domestic and international drug traffickers, and reliable intelligence and analytical support. The following illustrates the combined Hawaii HIDTA strategy for accomplishing Goal 1:

COMBINED HAWAII HIDTA GOALS	Goal 1: Reduce Drug Availability by Eliminating or Disrupting DTOs
	TARGET AND DISMANTLE OR DISRUPT DRUG TRAFFICKING ORGANIZATIONS TO INCLUDE: INTERNATIONAL DTOs, CPOT LINKED DTOs, RPOT LINKED DTOs, AND LOCAL DTOs
	IDENTIFY LINKS TO CPOTS & RPOTS THROUGH INTELLIGENCE DRIVEN TASK FORCES
	APPREHEND DRUG FUGITIVES & ARMED VIOLENT DRUG OFFENDERS
	APPREHEND INDIVIDUALS WHO ATTEMPT TO SMUGGLE ILLICIT DRUGS THROUGH HAWAII'S AIRPORTS
	SEIZE ILLICIT DRUGS, FIREARMS, AND DRUG RELATED PROCEEDS
	SECURE FEDERAL INDICTMENTS AGAINST STATE/LOCAL DRUG TRAFFICKERS
	TARGET MONEY LAUNDERING ORGANIZATIONS
	ERADICATE MARIJUANA GROWN THROUGHOUT THE STATE

A. Investigative Subsystem

The Investigative and Interdiction Subsystems have primary responsibility for accomplishing Goal 1. The Investigative Subsystem consists of seven HI-IMPACT task force groups, the Hawaii Fugitive Task Force, the Safe Neighborhood Strike Force, and the Money Laundering/Asset Forfeiture Task Force. Accomplishing goal one is one of the primary responsibilities of the Investigative Subsystem. The investigative task forces are most closely aligned with law enforcement goals of impacting the crime rate through arrests and seizures, and thereby reducing drug availability.

1. HI-IMPACT

The HI-IMPACT initiative is the central investigative element of the Hawaii HIDTA whose focus is to disrupt and dismantle drug trafficking organizations (DTOs). HI-IMPACT utilizes state-of-the-art techniques to conduct complex multi-jurisdictional investigations.

2. Hawaii Fugitive Task Force

The Fugitive Task Force assists other HIDTA initiatives in crippling the drug trade and related crime in Hawaii and throughout the Pacific region by bringing fugitives to justice.

3. **Project Safe Neighborhoods Task Force (PSN)**
   By removing guns from the street, PSN targets chronic violent drug offenders who have a significant impact on the amount of crime occurring in Hawaii.

4. **Money Laundering/Asset Forfeiture Task Force**
   The Money Laundering initiative disrupts and dismantles DTOs by making an impact on their ability to function, through seizing the money they use to operate and the assets they acquire with illicit drug proceeds.

5. **Hawaii Weed & Seed Initiative (proposed - supplemental)**
   The Weed & Seed support initiative is a newly proposed initiative for FY2005, if supplemental funding becomes available. It is designed to compliment the operation "Weed & Seed" strategy within the U.S. Department of Justice and engages all member of the community in a balanced effort to attack drug trafficking in designated sites.

6. **Pacific Rim Task Force (proposed- supplemental)**
   Most federal law enforcement agencies in Hawaii are responsible for U.S. Territories in the Pacific. This initiative is an investigative element similar to HI-IMPACT that conducts complex multi-jurisdictional investigations focused on the transshipment of illicit drugs to and from Asia and North America or to Pacific Basin locations where drug profits are two to four times higher.

B. Interdiction Subsystem

The Interdiction Subsystem consists of the Hawaii Interdiction Task Force and includes a domestic interdiction group and a foreign interdiction group. Both groups are located at Honolulu International Airport, the state's hub for passenger transit and parcel shipments. Being located at the airport is the most efficient way to stop illicit drugs from entering Hawaii's market. The Interdiction Task Force focuses on chokepoints and is the region's first line of defense.

1. **Hawaii Interdiction Task Force**
   The domestic group is charged with stopping the transport of illicit drugs as they enter through Hawaii's airports and harbors from the continental U.S. Conversely, the foreign group targets illicit shipments that originate from international territories.

2. **Marijuana Initiative (proposed – base line)**
   The Marijuana interdiction Initiative is newly proposed for FY2005 and is designed to compliment DEA's Domestic Cannabis Eradication & Suppression Program by providing lacking resources to eradicate marijuana grown in Hawaii's tropical climate, typically on public lands and tough to penetrate jungle.

C. **Support Subsystem**

The support initiatives are broad based and provide services and support to other initiatives and HIDTA functions. Only the Prosecutor's Initiative under the Support Subsystem directly contributes to Goal 1.

1. **Prosecutor's Initiative**

The Prosecutorial Initiative works with the Investigation and Interdiction Subsystems to successfully prosecute those involved in illicit drug trafficking throughout the region. It has designated prosecutors collocated at the Hawaii HIDTA who may provide legal support for subpoenas, arrest and search warrants, electronic surveillance, undercover operations, and other issues related to Hawaii HIDTA initiatives .

D. **Intelligence Subsystem**

The Hawaii HIDTA Intelligence Subsystem provides tactical, operational, and strategic intelligence support to enforcement and interdiction initiatives in an effort to reduce drug trafficking in the State of Hawaii. It provides a communication infrastructure that promotes information sharing between participating law enforcement agencies. The analysis and deconfliction of strategic and operational intelligence is critical for effectively attacking drug traffickers and reducing drug availability.

1. **Investigative Support Center**

The main body of the Intelligence Subsystem is the Investigative Support Center (ISC). To facilitate the availability and exchange of information, the ISC is collocated with several HIDTA initiatives and links electronically to other initiatives through the Western States Information Network (WSIN). Operation of the ISC provides full support to all HIDTA task forces and other law enforcement within the HIDTA region to achieve an intelligence-based approach to all counterdrug operations.

2. **Combined Intelligence Unit (proposed – base line)**

The Hawaii HIDTA Combined Intelligence Unit initiative is comprised of sworn law enforcement personnel. One of its objectives is to help identify CPOT and RPOT linked drug trafficking organizations that operate within the Hawaii HIDTA region.

3. **Financial Intelligence Unit (proposed – base line)**

The Financial Intelligence Unit is a multi-agency initiative whose mission is detect and analyze money laundering trends, patterns, and activities in Hawaii in an effort to impair the ability of DTOs to operate.

4. **Pacific Rim Intelligence Unit (proposed - supplemental)**

The Pacific Rim Intelligence Unit facilitates the exchange of information to and between the ISC and law enforcement task forces in Guam, Saipan, and the U.S. Territories in the Pacific. It is the intelligence arm of the Pacific Rim Task Force.

SECTION IX.

GOAL 2

Reduce the Harmful Consequences of Drug Trafficking

Drug trafficking causes various problems in Hawaii's communities and negatively impacts the quality of life. The Hawaii HIDTA began funding two initiatives in FY2004 whose mission is to attack the elements that adversely affect public safety. In addition, the Hawaii Weed & Seed Initiative has been proposed for FY2005 to further combat these problems. Indicated below is the Hawaii HIDTA strategy for addressing Goal 2:

COMBINED HAWAII HIDTA GOALS	Goal 2 Reduce the Harmful Consequences of Drug Trafficking
	SEIZE FIREARMS FROM VIOLENT DRUG TRAFFICKERS
	APPREHEND DRUG FUGITIVES
	PROPOSE MODEL LEGISLATION TO INCREASE INVESTIGATIVE METHODS
	DEVELOP AND MAINTAIN RELATIONSHIPS WITH COMMUNITY LEADERS AND BUSINESSES TO REBUILD TROUBLED NEIGHBORHOODS
	CONTINUE COMMUNITY POLICING EFFORTS WITHIN DESIGNATED WEED & SEED SITES

1. **Hawaii Fugitive Task Force**
   The Hawaii Fugitive Task Force conducts investigations focusing on the arrest of felony fugitives remaining free in communities and neighborhoods who are responsible for continuing criminal activity, especially those wanted for violent drug trafficking offenses. Disproportionate shares of individuals in the State of Hawaii have multiple felony arrests and/or are felony fugitives.

2. **Safe Neighborhoods Task Force (PSN)**
   According to the State of Hawaii Uniform Crime Reports, firearms were used in 147 robberies and 159 aggravated assaults during year 2002. There were also 1,210 robberies and 71,976 property crimes during this period[7]. The majority of these crimes were committed by individuals who used the proceeds to support narcotics abuse. In addition, there was approximately $163,891.00 worth of firearms stolen during the year, with only 5.8 percent recovered.

   Removing guns from the street has a significant impact on the amount of crime occurring in Hawaii. Special emphasis is placed on stopping those who supply illegal firearms and narcotics to violent criminals, organizations and juveniles.

3. **Prosecutor's Initiative**
   Because of the way Hawaii's drug laws are written, a significant number of drug traffickers are identified but not prosecuted. The Prosecutorial Initiative works within the legislative process to propose model legislation to bring Hawaii's laws into harmony with federal statutes.

4. **Weed & Seed Initiative (proposed - supplemental)**
   The Weed & Seed Initiative is designed to reclaim, restore, and rebuild neighborhoods through community policing activities.

SECTION X.

GOAL 3

Improve the Efficiency and Effectiveness of Law Enforcement Organizations

The guiding theme of the HIDTA Program is to attack drug trafficking from all angles by combining all available resources from federal, state and local law enforcement organizations. The principle elements of coordinating this effort and facilitating efficient and effective operations fall under the Support Subsystem and the Intelligence Subsystem.

The main goal of the support initiatives, including the Management and Coordination Initiative, is to facilitate the efficient operation of all investigative and case support activities by providing oversight, administrative, and budgetary support in accordance with ONDCP and Hawaii HIDTA Executive Board policy and directives. The support initiatives coordinate resources and promote and encourage information sharing. The Hawaii HIDTA also provides a strong training program to enhance the knowledge and skills of participating personnel and staff.

Among the directives of the Intelligence Initiatives is providing analytical support, intelligence, enhanced case support, and access to open-source and closed-source information for participating agencies. Another is providing subject and event deconfliction to ensure officer and citizen safety during law enforcement activities and providing a secure electronic link to neighbor islands via WSIN intranet. The following is the combined Hawaii HIDTA strategy for addressing Goal 3:

COMBINED HAWAII HIDTA GOALS	Goal 3: Improve the Efficiency & Effectiveness of Law Enforcement Organizations
	ACHIEVE AND MAINTAIN 100% PARTICIPATION BY LAW ENFORCEMENT AGENCIES IN THE WSIN DECONFLICTION SERVICES
	PROVIDE ANALYTICAL CASE SUPPORT & PRODUCTS
	PROVIDE ELECTRONIC LINK FROM ISC TO NEIGHBOR ISLANDS VIA WSIN SECURE INTRANET
	SHARE INTELLIGENCE DATA WITH OTHER HIDTAS/LEAS WITHIN & OUTSIDE OF HAWAII
	DEVELOP AN ACTIVE MEANS OF COMMUNICATING WITH PACIFIC BASIN/RIM LAW ENFORCEMENT
	DEVELOP AND/OR SPONSOR TRAINING PROGRAMS THROUGHOUT THE REGION
	ESTABLISH CORRDINATION WITH CLAN LAB RESPONSE COORDINATORS AT FEDERAL, STATE, AND LOCAL AGENCIES
	PROVIDE COLLOCATION FOR HIDTA INITIATIVES
	DEVELOP PARTNERSHIPS WITH EXISTING TRAINING COORDINATORS AT FEDERAL, STATE, AND LOCAL AGENCIES
	MEET IN EXECUTIVE SESSION TO COORDINATE HAWAII HIDTA ACTIVITIES
	CONDUCT MEETINGS WITH HIDTA INITIATIVES & PARTICIPATING AGENCY SUPERVISORS
	ATTAIN 100% OF DEVELOPMENTAL STANDARDS
	MONITOR, REVIEW, AND TRACK FISCAL EXPENDITURES BY HIDTA INITIATIVES TO ENSURE COMPLIANCE WITH POLICIES
	IMPLEMENT & CONDUCT HAWAII HIDTA'S INTERNAL REVIEW PROGRAM
	PREPARE THE ANNUAL REPORT, THREAT ASSESSMENT, STRATEGY, AND BUDGET

1. **Investigative Support Center**
The ISC has primary responsibility for accomplishing Goal 3. The ISC is the communication infrastructure for the Hawaii HIDTA. The ISC facilitates information sharing, intelligence collection, analysis and dissemination. It provides technical and strategic support to HIDTA initiatives and participating agencies. The Hawaii HIDTA fully supports Title III investigations and gives all initiatives easy access to intelligence and analytical support because of its proximity to the ISC. It also allows the ISC to develop and provide operational support to investigations being conducted by HIDTA initiative personnel or their agencies. This support includes time sensitive analysis of Dialed Number Recorder (DNR) information, subpoenaed TOLL information, pager and clone pager data, post seizure analysis of documents and financial analysis.

The ISC consists of two intelligence groups. The Investigative Support Group focuses on supporting ongoing drug trafficking investigations primarily in the areas of communications analysis, association/link analysis, pre-seizure analysis, and event/subject deconfliction. The Strategic Support Group focuses on money laundering investigations and strategic reporting. The group collects, assembles, and disseminates data for the Hawaii HIDTA Threat Assessment and Annual Report. It tracks trends and authors intelligence bulletins.

2. **Western States Information Network (WSIN)**
The Hawaii HIDTA is part of the Regional Information Sharing System (RISS) through WSIN. WSIN allows law enforcement agencies to share information and coordinate efforts against criminal networks that operate across jurisdictional boundaries. The WSIN region also includes the states of Alaska, California, Oregon, and Washington, and has member agencies in Canada, Australia, and Guam.

WSIN provides the Hawaii HIDTA with subject/event deconfliction services, access to an automated criminal intelligence sharing database, and a secure intranet for electronic networking among participating agencies. Each of the initiatives has developed protocol to ensure event and subject deconfliction submission to the WSIN Watch Center located in Sacramento, California. Submissions can be made 24/7 by contacting the Watch Center via phone or fax, or through remote access via the secure RISSNET intranet connection.

3. **Combined Intelligence Unit (proposed – base line)**
The Hawaii HIDTA Combined Intelligence Unit initiative is comprised of sworn law enforcement personnel. It unites existing Criminal Intelligence Units within the four counties to Hawaii HIDTA participating federal, state, and local law enforcement agencies. It greatly enhances criminal intelligence analysis through a coordinated, unified statewide collection process that is based on current, updated, pro-active, and evaluated intelligence. The Criminal Intelligence Unit provides a comprehensive intelligence picture of illicit drug trafficking and organized crime activities in the four major Hawaiian Islands. The intelligence gathered is used to initiate or enhance priority HIDTA investigations and to produce HIDTA intelligence summaries, bulletins, and reports. This initiative furthers the concept of intelligence led policing.

4. **Financial Intelligence Unit** **(proposed – base line)**
The mission of the Financial Intelligence Unit collects, analyzes, and disseminates financial intelligence in support of the ISC. It provides financial investigative and intelligence assistance to Hawaii HIDTA initiatives and Organized Crime Drug Enforcement Task Force (OCDETF) investigations.

A recent review by the ONDCP resulted in concerns for the processing of financial intelligence and the utilization of financial investigation in the Hawaii HIDTA. The recommendation was that the Hawaii HIDTA establish a financial analysis unit to serve as a central analysis and coordination mechanism for financial intelligence and provide analytical support to the Money Laundering/Asset Forfeiture Initiative and all other initiatives conducting significant investigations.

5. **Pacific Rim Intelligence Unit** **(proposed - supplemental)**
The Hawaii HIDTA is unique to all other HIDTA's in that the Hawaii ISC is sponsoring the development of an intelligence/enforcement outreach program that provides direct narcotics law enforcement links with countries in the Pacific Basin and Pacific Rim. The Be On the Lookout (BOLO) developmental component, will be able to provide first hand, timely, actionable information from Pacific Rim/Basin countries for methodical investigation, targeting, and establishment of joint intelligence pools. Partnered with Australia and New Zealand, this information is available to all law enforcement agencies operating within the Hawaii HIDTA and HIDTAs across the country that are destination points for Asia/Pacific manufactured drugs.

6. **Clandestine Lab Coordination**
The Clandestine Lab Coordination initiative is a support initiative that has primary responsibility to provide consolidated training and coordination for first responders and investigators to clandestine laboratories.

7. **Management and Coordination**
The Management and Coordination initiative is responsible for providing the day to day oversight and management of the Hawaii HIDTA. A Director is assisted by a staff which implements the policy established by the ONDCP/ NHPO and the Hawaii HIDTA Executive Board. The Director and staff oversee an annual internal review and evaluation process of all initiatives to assess efficiency and effectiveness. The Management and Coordination initiative monitors, reviews, and tracks fiscal expenditures by the HIDTA initiatives to ensure compliance with policy. It facilitates efficient operation of initiatives by providing oversight, administrative, and budgetary support. It has primary responsibility for preparing the Annual Report, Threat Assessment, Strategy, and Budget.

8. **Training**
The Training Initiative is directed by a coordinator who provides oversight to on-site and off-site training. It tracks initiative training and budgets. The main goal of the training initiative is to provide resources that improve the ability of investigative and analytical personnel to counter drug trafficking and related criminal activity.

SECTION XI.

TARGETED OUTPUTS & OUTCOMES

A. GOAL ONE: REDUCE DRUG AVAILABILITY BY ELIMINATING OR DISRUPTING DRUG TRAFFICKING ORGANIZATIONS

1. Targeted Investigative Outcomes

COMBINED INVESTIGATIVE OUTCOMES	TARGET 10 OF IDENTIFIED INTERNATIONAL DTOS & DISRUPT OR DISMANTLE 7 OF THOSE TARGETED
	TARGET 2 OF IDENTIFIED CPOT LINKED DTOs & DISRUPT OR DISMANTLE 1 OF THOSE TARGETED
	TARGET 4 OF IDENTIFIED RPOT LINKED DTOs & DISRUPT OR DISMANTLE 4 OF THOSE TARGETED
	TARGET 48 OF IDENTIFIED LOCAL DTOs & DISRUPT OR DISMANTLE 34 OF THOSE TARGETED
	APPREHEND AND/OR CLEAR WARRANTS FOR 100 FUGITIVES WITH A NARCOTIC NEXUS
	ARREST 90 ARMED VIOLENT DRUG OFFENDERS
	SEIZE 90 KILOGRAMS OF ILLICIT DRUGS
	TARGET 25% (16) OF TARGETED DTOs FOR MONEY LAUNDERING CHARGES
	SEIZE $1.5 IN ILLICIT DRUG RELATED ASSETS (IN CONJUNCTION WITH INTERDICTION INITIATIVES)
	SEIZE 100 FIREARMS

2. Targeted Interdiction Outcomes

COMBINED INTERDICTION OUTCOMES	DISRUPT OR DISMANTLE 25 DTOs IDENTIFIED THROUGH INTERDICTION EFFORTS
	ARREST 60 DRUG TRAFFICKERS AND/OR COURIERS WHO SMUGGLE ILLICIT DRUGS THROUGH HAWAII'S AIRPORTS
	INSPECT 1000 PARCELS AND SEIZE 100 PARCELS CONTAINING ILLICIT DRUGS
	SEIZE 60 KILOGRAMS OF ILLICIT DRUGS
	SEIZE $1.5 IN ILLICIT DRUG RELATED ASSETS (IN CONJUNCTION WITH INVESTIGATIVE INITIATIVES)

3. Targeted Support Outcomes

COMBINED SUPPORT OUTCOMES	SECURE 25 HIDTA ASSISTED FEDERAL INDICTMENTS AGAINST DRUG TRAFFICKERS
	FORFEIT $1 MILLION IN DRUG RELATED ASSETS
	ERADICATE 370,000 MARIJUANA PLANTS

4. **Targeted Intelligence Outcomes**

COMBINED INTELLIGENCE OUTCOMES	IDENTIFY 3 CPOT LINKED DTOS STATEWIDE
	IDENTIFY 5 RPOT LINKED DTOS STATEWIDE

B. GOAL TWO: REDUCE THE HARMFUL CONSEQUENCES OF DRUG TRAFFICKING

1. **Targeted Investigative Outcomes**

COMBINED INVESTIGATIVE GOALS	SEIZE 100 FIREARMS FROM VIOLENT DRUG TRAFFICKERS
	CLEAR 250 FELONY WARRANTS AND APPREHEND 100 DRUG FUGITIVES
	PROPOSE MODEL LEGISLATION TO INCREASE INVESTIGATIVE METHODS
	DEVELOP & MAINTAN RELATIONSHIPS WITH COMMUNITY LEADERS AND BUSINESSES TO REBUILD TROUBLED NEIGHBORHOODS
	CONTINUE COMMUNITY POLICING EFFORTS WITHIN DESIGNATED WEED & SEED SITES

C. GOAL THREE: IMPROVE THE EFFICIENCY AND EFFECTIVENESS OF LAW ENFORCEMENT ORGANIZATIONS

1. **Targeted Hawaii HIDTA Initiative Outcomes**

COMBINED INVESTIGATIVE GOALS	ACHIEVE AND MAINTAIN 100% PARTICIPATION BY LAW ENFORCEMENT AGENCIES IN THE WSIN DECONFLICTION SERVICES
	SUBMIT 9000 CASE/SUBJECT DECONFLICTIONS AMONG HIDTA INITIATIVES AND PARTICIPATING AGENCIES
	SUBMIT 1400 EVENT DECONFLICTIONS AMONG HIDTA INITIATIVES AND PARTICIPATING AGENCIES

2. **Targeted Intelligence Outcomes**

COMBINED INTELLIGENCE GOALS	ISC TO CONDUCT 4000 DATABASE QUERIES & PROVIDE 100 INTELLIGENCE REPORTS
	COMPLETE 30 REQUESTS FOR CASE ASSISTANCE
	PROVIDE 3000 ANALYTICAL PRODUCTS (TOLL ANALYSES, LINK ANALYSES, GRAPHS, CHARTS, PROFILES, ETC)
	PARTICIPATE, HOST, AND PROMOTE QUARTERLY INTELLIGENCE SHARING MEETINGS, EXCHANGES & FORUMS
	DEVELOP AN ACTIVE MEANS OF COMMUNICATING WITH PACIFIC BASIN/RIM LAW ENFORCEMENT
	PROVIDE ELECTRONIC LINK FROM ISC TO NEIGHBOR ISLANDS VIA WSIN SECURE INTRANET
	FORWARD 5 INTELLIGENCE LEADS TO HAWAII HIDTA INITIATIVES FOR CASE DEVELOPMENT & INVESTIGATION
	IDENTIFY THE THREAT POSED BY ASIAN, MEXICAN, AND COLOMBIAN DTOs
	DEVELOP IN-HOUSE "COMPUTER FORENSIC" CAPABILITY BY CERTIFYING 2 ISC PERSONNEL
	PROVIDE DATA ACCESS AND INPUT INTO REGIONAL ASSESSMENTS AND THE NATIONAL DRUG THREAT ASSESSMENT

3. Targeted Support Outcomes

COMBINED SUPPORT GOALS	FACILITATE 42 TRAINING PROGRAMS/PRESENTATIONS TO HIDTA INITIATIVES AND PARTICIPATING AGENCIES
	TRAIN 100 OFFICERS ON SAFE CLAN LAB INVESTIGATIONS
	TRAIN 30 OFFICERS ON "JETWAY" AND/OR REFRESHER INTERDICTION COURSE
	DEVELOP PARTNERSHIPS WITH EXISTING TRAINING COORDINATORS AT FEDERAL, STATE, AND LOCAL AGENCIES
	PROVIDE LEGAL TRAINING FOR 200 LAW ENFORCEMENT OFFICERS/AGENTS
	DISSEMINATE EXISTING TRAINING OPPORTUNITIES FROM OTHER AGENCIES TO HIDTA PERSONNEL
	DEVELOP ADVANCED TRAINING FACILITIES & MEDIA SUPPORT
	DEVELOP & MAINTAIN HIDTA TRAINING DATABASE
	HOLD QUARTERLY STRATEGIC PLANNING MEETINGS
	MEET QUARTERLY WITH RESPONSE TEAM STAFF
	PROVIDE TECHNICAL EXPERTISE AND ASSISTANCE TO DISRUPT 5 CLAN LAB OPERATIONS
	INCREASE COLLOCATION FOR HIDTA INITIATIVES BY EXPANDING CURRENT OFFICE SPACE
	EXPAND TITLE III CAPACITY FROM 8 LINES TO 18 LINES
	CONVENE QUARTERLY WITH FEDERAL, STATE AND COUNTY PROSECUTORS TO RESOLVE PROBLEMS
	MEET IN EXECUTIVE SESSION A MINIMUM OF 8 TIMES TO COORDINATE HAWAII HIDTA ACTIVITIES
	ATTAIN 100% COMPLIANCE WITH THE HIDTA PMP IN 2004
	IDENTIFY, COLLECT, DISSEMINATE AND ANALYZE TIMELY, RELIABLE DATA TO SUPPORT THE HIDTA PMP IN 2004
	COMPLETE AND TRACK A FULL INVENTORY OF ACCOUNTABLE EQUIPMENT PURCHASED WITH HIDTA FUNDS
	MONITOR, REVIEW, AND TRACK FISCAL EXPENDITURES BY HIDTA INITIATIVES TO ENSURE COMPLIANCE WITH POLICIES
	CONDUCT FISCAL AUDITS OF ALL INITIATIVES
	IMPLEMENT & CONDUCT HAWAII HIDTA'S INTERNAL REVIEW PROGRAM
	HOLD QUARTERLY OVERSIGHT COMMITTEE MEETINGS (BUDGET, ADMIN, INTEL, & INITIATIVE REVIEW)
	COLLECT & ANALYZE STATISTICAL DATA & SIGNIFICANT ACTIVITY REPORTS
	PREPARE THE ANNUAL REPORT, THREAT ASSESSMENT, STRATEGY AND BUDGET
	DEVELOP BUDGETS TO COVER EXISTING INITIATIVE SHORTFALLS
	DEVELOP PACIFIC BASIN/RIM INITIATIVE
	DEVELOP EDUCATION & PREVENTION INITIATIVE
	DEVELOP MARIJUANA ERADICATION INITIATIVE

SECTION XII.

APPENDICES

APPENDIX A; HAWAII HIDTA ORGANIZATIONAL CHART

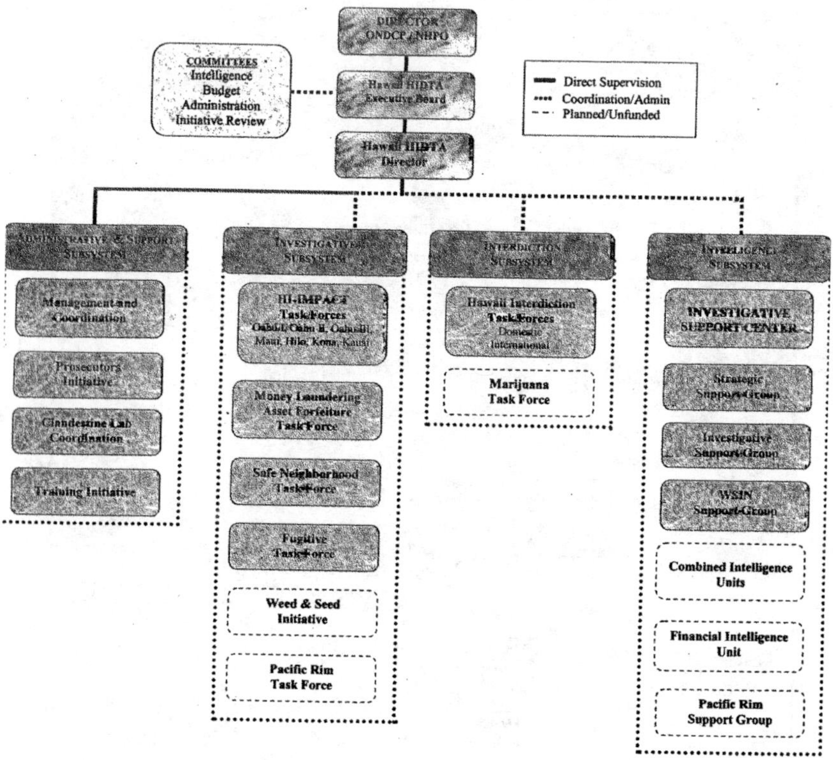

APPENDIX B: ENDNOTES

[1] "How Hawaii is really different," *Pacific Business News*, February 16, 2004; Asia-Pacific Distance Calculator, http://russia.shaps.hawaii.edu
[2] Source: United States Census Bureau, State and County Quick Facts 2000
[3] *The State of Hawaii Data Book 2002*, Table 13.04 and 7.03, respectively.
[4] *The State of Hawaii Data Book 2002*, Table 10.03
[5] Hawaii Agriculture Statistics Service, *Agriculture Contributions to Hawaii's Economy2000*
[6] Hawaii HIDTA Threat Analysis, "Transportation of Drugs into Hawaii."
[7] Hawaii State Department of the Attorney General, Crime Prevention & Justice Assistance Division, *Crime in Hawaii 2002*.

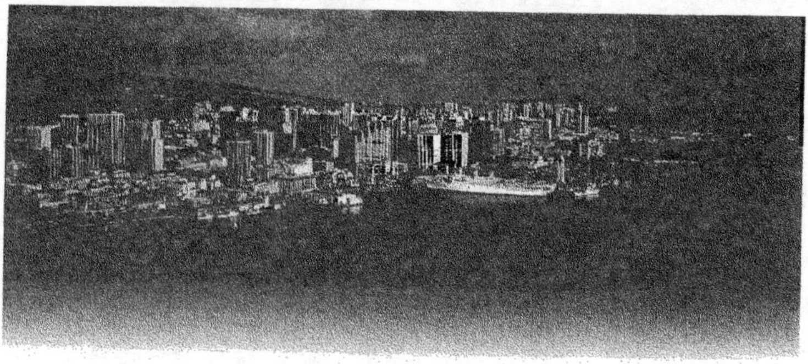

2005 THREAT ASSESSMENT

HAWAII HIDTA PMP MATRIX

GOAL 1 - REDUCE DRUG AVAILABILITY BY ELIMINATING OR DISRUPTING DRUG TRAFFICKING ORGANIZATIONS

GEOGRAPHIC AREA	THREATS	THREAT DESCRIPTION	SOURCE	DESIRED OUTPUTS
Honolulu City/County	PRIMARY THREAT	20 DRUG DISTRIBUTION ORGANIZATIONS IDENTIFIED AS OF 12/03	FIELD SURVEY	TARGET 3 DISTRIBUTION ORGANIZATIONS AND DISRUPT OR DISMANTLE 3 OF THOSE TARGETED
		5 DRUG MANUFACTURING OPERATIONS IDENTIFIED AS OF 12/03		TARGET 1 MANUFACTURING ORGANIZATIONS AND DISRUPT OR DISMANTLE 1 OF THOSE TARGETED
		3500 ACTIVE DRUG WARRANTS STATEWIDE		CLEAR 250 WARRANTS FOR DRUG CHARGES
		100 ARMED VIOLENT DRUG OFFENDERS OPERATE IN AND THROUGH THE REGION		ARREST 50 ARMED VIOLENT OFFENDERS WITH A DRUG NEXUS
		MULTI-POUND QUANTITIES OF ILLEGAL NARCOTICS ARE SMUGGLED THROUGH HONOLULU INTERNATIONAL AIRPORT	THREAT ASSESSMENT	ARREST 50 INDIVIDUALS WHO SMUGGLE NARCOTICS THROUGH THE AIRPORT
		SHIPMENT OF 1000 ILLICIT PARCELS ANNUALLY TO/THROUGH HONOLULU VIA MAIL AND EXPRESS SERVICES		INSPECT 750 PARCELS AND SEIZE 100 PARCELS
				SEIZE 90 KILOGRAMS OF ILLICIT DRUGS ENTERING THE AIRPORT
		A SIGNIFICANT AMOUNT OF ILLEGAL DRUG MONEY FLOW THROUGH THE REGION VIA BULK CASH SHIPMENTS, WIRE TRANSFER SERVICES, FINANCIAL INSTITUTIONS, AND COMMERCIAL BUSINESSES		TARGET ONE MONEY REMITTANCE ESTABLISHMENT FOR MONEY LAUNDERING CHARGES
				SEIZE $1,000,000 IN ILLICIT DRUG RELATED ASSETS
				FORFEIT $1,000,000 IN ILLICIT DRUG RELATED ASSETS
		USE OF PUBLIC LANDS FOR THE CULTIVATION AND PRODUCTION OF MARIJUANA		ERADICATE 50,000 MARIJUANA PLANTS
		WEAPONS ASSOCIATED WITH DRUG TRAFFICKING		SEIZE 50 FIREARMS
Maui County		10 DRUG DISTRIBUTION ORGANIZATIONS IDENTIFIED AS OF 12/03	FIELD SURVEY	TARGET 2 DISTRIBUTION ORGANIZATIONS AND DISRUPT OR DISMANTLE 2 OF THOSE TARGETED
		3 DRUG MANUFACTURING OPERATIONS IDENTIFIED AS OF 12/03		TARGET 1 MANUFACTURING ORGANIZATIONS AND DISRUPT OR DISMANTLE 1 OF THOSE TARGETED
		3500 ACTIVE DRUG WARRANTS STATEWIDE		CLEAR 250 WARRANTS FOR DRUG CHARGES
		100 ARMED VIOLENT DRUG OFFENDERS OPERATE IN AND THROUGH THE REGION		ARREST 50 ARMED VIOLENT OFFENDERS WITH A DRUG NEXUS
		A SIGNIFICANT AMOUNT OF ILLEGAL DRUG MONEY FLOW THROUGH THE REGION VIA BULK CASH SHIPMENTS, WIRE TRANSFER SERVICES, FINANCIAL INSTITUTIONS, AND COMMERCIAL BUSINESSES	THREAT ASSESSMENT	SEIZE $250,000 IN ILLICIT DRUG RELATED ASSETS
		USE OF PUBLIC LANDS FOR THE CULTIVATION AND PRODUCTION OF MARIJUANA		ERADICATE 75,000 MARIJUANA PLANTS
		WEAPONS ASSOCIATED WITH DRUG TRAFFICKING		SEIZE 15 FIREARMS
Hawaii County (Big Island)		10 DRUG DISTRIBUTION ORGANIZATIONS IDENTIFIED AS OF 12/03	FIELD SURVEY	TARGET 3 DISTRIBUTION ORGANIZATIONS AND DISRUPT OR DISMANTLE 3 OF THOSE TARGETED
		3 DRUG MANUFACTURING OPERATIONS IDENTIFIED AS OF 12/03		TARGET 3 MANUFACTURING ORGANIZATIONS AND DISRUPT OR DISMANTLE 3 OF THOSE TARGETED
		3500 ACTIVE DRUG WARRANTS STATEWIDE		CLEAR 250 WARRANTS FOR DRUG CHARGES
		100 ARMED VIOLENT DRUG OFFENDERS OPERATE IN AND THROUGH THE REGION		ARREST 50 ARMED VIOLENT OFFENDERS WITH A DRUG NEXUS
		A SIGNIFICANT AMOUNT OF ILLEGAL DRUG MONEY FLOW THROUGH THE REGION VIA BULK CASH SHIPMENTS, WIRE TRANSFER SERVICES, FINANCIAL INSTITUTIONS, AND COMMERCIAL BUSINESSES	THREAT ASSESSMENT	SEIZE $250,000 IN ILLICIT DRUG RELATED ASSETS
		USE OF PUBLIC LANDS FOR THE CULTIVATION AND PRODUCTION OF MARIJUANA		ERADICATE 300,000 MARIJUANA PLANTS
		WEAPONS ASSOCIATED WITH DRUG TRAFFICKING		SEIZE 35 FIREARMS
Kauai County		5 DRUG DISTRIBUTION ORGANIZATIONS IDENTIFIED AS OF 12/03	FIELD SURVEY	TARGET 2 DISTRIBUTION ORGANIZATIONS AND DISRUPT OR DISMANTLE 2 OF THOSE TARGETED
		1 DRUG MANUFACTURING OPERATIONS IDENTIFIED AS OF 12/03		TARGET 1 MANUFACTURING ORGANIZATIONS AND DISRUPT OR DISMANTLE 1 OF THOSE TARGETED
		3500 ACTIVE DRUG WARRANTS STATEWIDE		CLEAR 250 WARRANTS FOR DRUG CHARGES
		100 ARMED VIOLENT DRUG OFFENDERS OPERATE IN AND THROUGH THE REGION		ARREST 50 ARMED VIOLENT OFFENDERS WITH A DRUG NEXUS
		A SIGNIFICANT AMOUNT OF ILLEGAL DRUG MONEY FLOW THROUGH THE REGION VIA BULK CASH SHIPMENTS, WIRE TRANSFER SERVICES, FINANCIAL INSTITUTIONS, AND COMMERCIAL BUSINESSES	THREAT ASSESSMENT	SEIZE $100,000 IN ILLICIT DRUG RELATED ASSETS
		USE OF PUBLIC LANDS FOR THE CULTIVATION AND PRODUCTION OF MARIJUANA		ERADICATE 80,000 MARIJUANA PLANTS
		WEAPONS ASSOCIATED WITH DRUG TRAFFICKING		SEIZE 10 FIREARMS
	SECONDARY THREAT	INTER ISLAND TRANSPORTATION OF ILLEGAL NARCOTICS VIA AIR AND SEA		LAW ENFORCEMENT SENSITIVE ISSUE CURRENTLY UNDER CONSIDERATION
		PACIFIC RIM TRANSPORTATION OF ILLEGAL NARCOTICS		LAW ENFORCEMENT SENSITIVE ISSUE CURRENTLY UNDER CONSIDERATION
		IDENTIFYING ASIAN AND PACIFIC ISLANDER ORGANIZED CRIME GROUPS		LAW ENFORCEMENT SENSITIVE ISSUE CURRENTLY UNDER CONSIDERATION
		IDENTIFY CROSS POLLINATION AND DEVELOPERS OF SUPER HYBRID MARIJUANA PLANTS		LAW ENFORCEMENT SENSITIVE ISSUE CURRENTLY UNDER CONSIDERATION
		IDENTIFY INDOOR AND HYDROPONIC GROWS		LAW ENFORCEMENT SENSITIVE ISSUE CURRENTLY UNDER CONSIDERATION
		IDENTIFY TRANSPORTATION OF MARIJUANA SEEDS		LAW ENFORCEMENT SENSITIVE ISSUE CURRENTLY UNDER CONSIDERATION

* Includes 211,100 marijuana plants attributed to the Hawaii Department of Land and Natural Resources

	INVESTIGATIVE									INTERDICTION		ERADICATION	SUPPORT		INTELLIGENCE			ADMINISTRATIVE	
	HI-IMPACT																		
ACTUAL OUTPUTS	OAHU II	OAHU III	MAUI	HILO	KONA	KAUAI	SAFE NEIGHBORHOOD	FUGITIVE	MONEY LAUNDERING/ ASSET FORFEITURE	DOMESTIC	INTERNATIONAL	MARIJUANA	CLAN LAB	PROSECUTORS	INVESTIGATIVE	STRATEGIC	WSIN	MANAGEMENT AND COORDINATION	TRAINING
DISRUPTED/DISMANTLED 10 DTOS	X	X																	
DISRUPTED/DISMANTLED 1 DTO	X	X								X	X								
CLEARED 250 WARRANTS (STATEWIDE)								X											
ARRESTED 95 ARMED OFFENDERS (STATEWIDE)							X												
ARRESTED 47 INDIVIDUALS										X	X								
INSPECTED 16,000 & SEIZED 59 PARCELS										X	X								
SEIZED 59 KILOS OF DRUGS										X	X								
TARGETED 1 ESTABLISHMENT									X										
SEIZED $2,910,896 (STATEWIDE)	X	X							X	X	X								
FORFEITED $1,237,749 (STATEWIDE)														X					
ERADICATED 14,001 PLANTS												X							
SEIZED 162 (PSN) & 41 (OAHU HI-IMPACT) FIREARMS	X	X					X												
DISRUPTED/DISMANTLED 9 DTOS			X																
DISRUPTED/DISMANTLED 3 DTOS			X																
CLEARED 250 WARRANTS (STATEWIDE)								X											
ARRESTED 95 ARMED OFFENDERS (STATEWIDE)							X												
SEIZED $2,910,896 (STATEWIDE)			X						X										
ERADICATED 79,106 PLANTS												X							
SEIZED 162 (PSN) & 6 (MAUI HI-IMPACT) FIREARMS			X				X												
DISRUPTED/DISMANTLED 6 DTOS				X	X														
DISRUPTED/DISMANTLED 3 DTOS				X	X														
CLEARED 250 WARRANTS (STATEWIDE)								X											
ARRESTED 95 ARMED OFFENDERS (STATEWIDE)							X												
SEIZED $2,910,896 (STATEWIDE)				X	X				X										
ERADICATED 394,644 PLANTS*												X							
SEIZED 162 (PSN) & 47 (HAWAII HI-IMPACT) FIREARMS				X	X		X												
DISRUPTED/DISMANTLED 3 DTOS						X													
DISRUPTED/DISMANTLED 0 DTOS						X													
CLEARED 250 WARRANTS (STATEWIDE)								X											
ARRESTED 95 ARMED OFFENDERS (STATEWIDE)							X												
SEIZED $2,910,896 (STATEWIDE)						X			X										
ERADICATED 33,349 PLANTS												X							
SEIZED 162 (PSN) & 16 (KAUAI HI-IMPACT) FIREARMS						X	X												

OUTCOMES: SEE SECTIONS VIII, IX, AND X FOR THIS INFORMATION

GOAL 2 - REDUCE THE HARMFUL CONSEQUENCES OF DRUG TRAFFICKING

GEOGRAPHIC AREA	HARMFUL CONSEQUENCES	SOURCE	DESIRED OUTPUTS
HAWAII HIDTA AREA	VIOLENCE ASSOCIATED WITH DRUG TRAFFICKING	THREAT ASSESSMENT	SEIZE X FIREARMS FROM VIOLENT DRUG TRAFFICKERS
			CLEAR 200 WARRANTS FOR DRUG CHARGES
			PROPOSE MODEL LEGISLATION TO INCREASE INVESTIGATIVE METHODS

GOAL 3 - IMPROVE THE EFFICIENCY AND EFFECTIVENESS OF LAW ENFORCEMENT ORGANIZATIONS

GEOGRAPHIC AREA		REGIONAL NEEDS	DESIRED OUTPUTS
HAWAII HIDTA AREA	INFORMATION SHARING	PROVIDE FOR OFFICER AND GENERAL PUBLIC SAFETY DURING ONGOING ENFORCEMENT OPERATIONS	ACHIEVE AND MAINTAIN 100% PARTICIPATION BY LAW ENFORCEMENT AGENCIES IN THE WSIN DECONFLICTION SERVICES
		PROVIDE CASE/SUBJECT DECONFLICTION PARTICIPATION AMONG HIDTA INITIATIVES AND PARTICIPATING AGENCIES	SUBMIT 8000 CASE/SUBJECT DECONFLICTIONS AMONG HIDTA INITIATIVES AND PARTICIPATING AGENCIES
		PROVIDE EVENT DECONFLICTION UTILIZING WSIN	SUBMIT 1400 CRITICAL EVENT DECONFLICTIONS AMONG HIDTA INITIATIVES AND PARTICIPATING AGENCIES
		PROVIDE LAW ENFORCEMENT PERSONNEL ACCESS TO CRIMINAL, OPEN SOURCE INFORMATION & INTELLIGENCE	ISC TO CONDUCT 4000 DATABASE QUERIES & PROVIDE 100 INTELLIGENCE PROFILES
		INCREASE ANALYTICAL CASE SUPPORT TO HIDTA INITIATIVES	COMPLETE 20 REQUESTS FOR CASE ASSISTANCE
			PROVIDE 3000 ANALYTICAL PRODUCTS (TOLL ANALYSES, LINK ANALYSES, GRAPHS, CHARTS, PROFILES, ETC)
		ESTABLISH & MAINTAIN AN INTELLIGENCE OUTREACH PROGRAM	DEVELOP AN ACTIVE MEANS OF COMMUNICATING WITH PACIFIC BASIN/RIM LAW ENFORCEMENT
			PROVIDE ELECTRONIC LINK FROM ISC TO NEIGHBOR ISLANDS VIA WSIN SECURE INTRANET
		IMPROVE INFORMATION & INTELLIGENCE SHARING BETWEEN HAWAII HIDTA AND OTHER HIDTAS/LEAS	SHARE INTELLIGENCE DATA WITH HIDTAS/LEAS OUTSIDE OF HAWAII
	TRAINING	IMPROVE THE SKILLS OF PERSONNEL AT PARTICIPATING AGENCIES AND COOPERATING INSTITUTIONS WITHIN THE HAWAII HIDTA REGION	SPONSOR QUARTERLY TRAINING PROGRAMS FOR REGIONAL AND/OR SPECIALIZED TRAINING
			SPONSOR QUARTERLY CLANDESTINE LAB TRAINING PROGRAMS
		INFORM LAW ENFORCEMENT PERSONNEL OF TRAINING OPPORTUNITIES	DISSEMINATE EXISTING TRAINING OPPORTUNITIES FROM OTHER AGENCIES & BUT SOURCES TO HIDTA PERSONNEL
		TRACK & REPORT COURSES CONDUCTED, PERSONNEL TRAINED, & AGENCIES INVOLVED	DEVELOP & MAINTAIN HIDA TRAINING DATABASE
	COORDINATION	IMPROVE COORDINATION AMONG LAW ENFORCEMENT AGENCIES AND HIDTA INITIATIVES	COORDINATE WITH CLAN LAB RESPONSE COORDINATORS AT FEDERAL, STATE, AND LOCAL AGENCIES
			PROVIDE COLLOCATION FOR HIDTA INITIATIVES
			DEVELOP PARTNERSHIPS WITH EXISTING TRAINING COORDINATORS AT FEDERAL, STATE, AND LOCAL AGENCIES
			MEET IN EXECUTIVE SESSION A MINIMUM OF 4 TIMES TO COORDINATE HAWAII HIDTA ACTIVITIES
		ADDRESS DRUG ENFORCEMENT OR PROSECUTION ISSUES	CONDUCT MONTHLY MEETINGS WITH HIDTA INITIATIVES
	OVERSIGHT	IMPLEMENT HIDTA DEVELOPMENTAL STANDARDS	ATTAIN 100% OF DEVELOPMENTAL STANDARDS
		ACCOUNT FOR USE OF HIDTA FUNDS	COMPLETE AND TRACK A FULL INVENTORY OF ACCOUNTABLE EQUIPMENT PURCHASED WITH HIDTA FUNDS
			MONITOR, REVIEW, AND TRACK FISCAL EXPENDITURES BY HIDTA INITIATIVES TO ENSURE COMPLIANCE WITH POLICIES
			CONDUCT FISCAL AUDITS OF ALL INITIATIVES
		ENSURE INITIATIVES ARE ADDRESSING THE IDENTIFIED THREATS & THEIR INTENDED MISSION	IMPLEMENT & CONDUCT HAWAII HIDTA'S INTERNAL REVIEW PROGRAM
			HOLD QUARTERLY MEETINGS WITH INITIATIVE AND PARTICIPATING AGENCY SUPERVISORS
		ENSURE COMPLIANCE WITH ONDCP REPORTING REQUIREMENTS	PREPARE THE ANNUAL REPORT, THREAT ASSESSMENT, STRATEGY AND BUDGET

** ONDCP assumptions apply to 4 task forces because of Hawaii's island makeup and costly office rental market

INVESTIGATIVE									INTERDICTION		ERADICATION	SUPPORT		INTELLIGENCE			ADMINISTRATIVE			OUTCOMES: SEE SECTIONS VIII, IX, AND X FOR THIS INFORMATION
HI-IMPACT																				
OAHU II	OAHU III	MAUI	HILO	KONA	KAUAI	SAFE NEIGHBORHOOD	FUGITIVE	MONEY LAUNDERING/ASSET FORFEITURE	DOMESTIC	INTERNATIONAL	MARIJUANA	CLAN LAB	PROSECUTORS	INVESTIGATIVE	STRATEGIC	WSIN	MANAGEMENT AND COORDINATION	TRAINING	ACTUAL OUTPUTS	
						X													SEIZED 142 FIREARMS	
							X												CLEARED 259 WARRANTS	
													X						PROPOSED 2 PIECES OF LEGISLATION	

INVESTIGATIVE									INTERDICTION		ERADICATION	SERVICES		INTELLIGENCE			ADMINISTRATIVE			OUTCOMES: SEE SECTIONS VIII, IX, AND X FOR THIS INFORMATION
HI-IMPACT																				
OAHU II	OAHU III	MAUI	HILO	KONA	KAUAI	SAFE NEIGHBORHOOD	FUGITIVE	MONEY LAUNDERING/ASSET FORFEITURE	DOMESTIC	INTERNATIONAL	MARIJUANA	CLAN LAB	PROSECUTORS	INVESTIGATIVE	STRATEGIC	WSIN	MANAGEMENT AND COORDINATION	TRAINING	ACTUAL OUTPUTS	
X	X	X	X	X	X	X	X	X	X	X	X	X		X	X				ACHIEVED 100% PARTICIPATION	
X	X	X	X	X	X	X	X	X	X	X				X	X	X			SUBMITTED 6365 CASE/SUBJECT DECONFLICTIONS	
X	X	X	X	X	X	X	X	X	X	X						X			SUBMITTED 1533 EVENT DECONFLICTIONS	
														X	X				CONDUCTED 3302 DATABASE QUERIES & PROVIDED 369 PROFILES	
														X	X				COMPLETED 34 REQUESTS	
														X	X				PROVIDED 4,830 PRODUCTS	
														X	X	X	X		ACHIEVED BY 39%	
																X			ACHIEVED BY 100%	
														X	X				DAILY COMMUNICATION WITH OTHER HIDTAS/LEAS	
																		X	SPONSORED 16 PROGRAMS	
												X							SPONSORED 3 PROGRAMS	
																		X	100% DISSEMINATION OF TRAINING OPPORTUNITIES	
																		X	DATABASE DEVELOPED & MAINTAINED	
												X							100% COORDINATION WITH AGENCIES	
																	X		COLLOCATION PROVIDED*	
																		X	PARTNERSHIPS DEVELOPED	
																	X		MET 6 TIMES	
													X						MEETINGS NOT CONDUCTED	
																	X		ATTAINED 99% OF STANDARDS	
																	X		INVENTORY TRACKED & COMPLETED	
																	X		FISCAL EXPENDITURES REVIEWED & TRACKED	
																	X		FISCAL AUDITS COMPLETED	
																	X		REVIEW PROGRAM IMPLEMENTED & COMPLETED	
																	X		MET QUARTERLY	
																	X		REPORTS PREPARED & SUBMITTED	

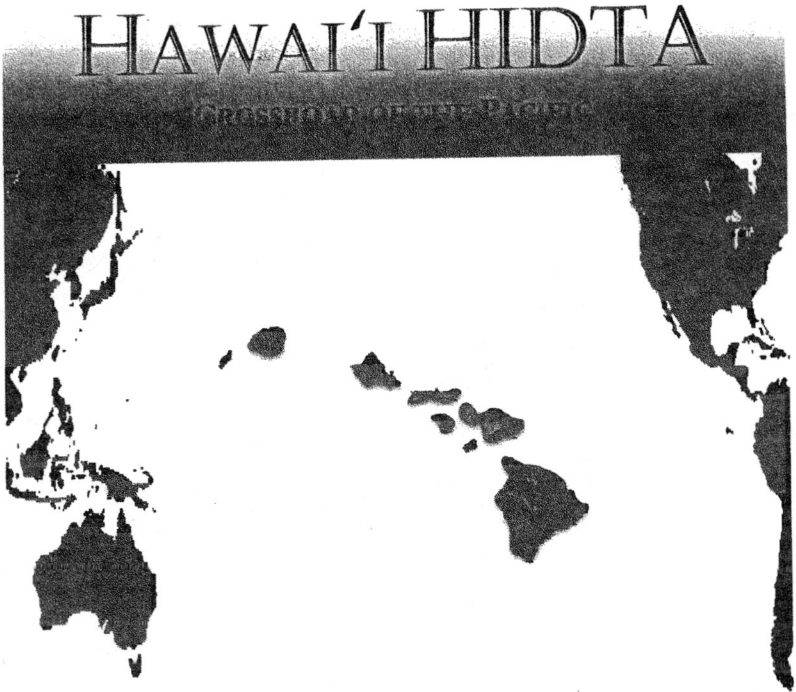

A LOOK AT THE THREAT POSED TO THE HAWAII HIDTA REGION BY ILLICIT DRUG TRAFFICKING

This document and the information contained herein are unclassified.
Produced in conjunction with the National Drug Intelligence Center.

Table of Contents

Introduction

The state of Hawaii and U.S. Territories of the Pacific are currently under attack from crystal methamphetamine, commonly called "ICE".[1] The rampant abuse of crystal methamphetamine, along with the violence and dangers associated with the drug, is the single most significant drug problem afflicting the state, a point that cannot be overemphasized. This problem, which threatens the well-being of Hawaii's citizens and challenges its law enforcement personnel, could not have reached such epidemic proportions if not for the constant pressure of the traffickers supplying crystal methamphetamine, as well as other illicit drugs, to the region. This constant pressure fuels a market that generates larceny, theft, burglary, homicides, abuse, and endangerment. Consequently, Drug Trafficking Organizations (DTOs) — international and local — are a focus of law enforcement and pose a significant drug threat to Hawaii. This 2005 Threat Assessment among other issues highlights the DTO problem within the region. A case in point was during Operation Shave Ice a Mexican national was placed in Hilo by a DTO and subsequently removed when pressure by law enforcement officials became too "hot", only to be arrested in Tennessee where the same DTO had moved him to transport drugs inland from the Gulf Coast.

Executive Summary

A multitude of illicit drugs are available to varying degrees in Hawaii, as in any populated area; however, these drugs can be categorized in three tiers based on the severity of the problems they pose to Hawaii's law enforcement and citizens. In the first tier are the two drugs causing the most serious problems—crystal methamphetamine and marijuana. Arrest and seizure data for both these drugs indicate that availability is high, while demand data suggest that use of both

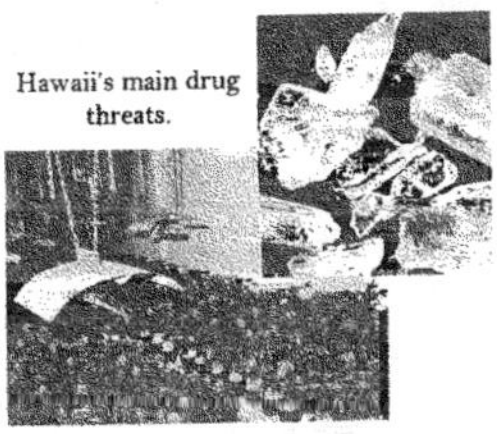

Hawaii's main drug threats.

drugs, along with the consequences of that use, is high and increasing. Nonetheless, the magnitude of the crystal methamphetamine problem in Hawaii—a far more socially disruptive problem—overshadows marijuana, which has seen an increase in associated violence, but not nearly to the same extent.

The second-tier drugs are cocaine (usually crack cocaine) and heroin which, although they remain problems in Hawaii, appear to rank well behind crystal methamphetamine and marijuana in contributing to the state's drug troubles. Cocaine-related arrests and seizures are on an upswing, but demand data suggest declining prevalence and consequences of use. At the same time, heroin distribution and abuse appear to be diminishing in light of indicators suggesting declines in arrests, seizures,

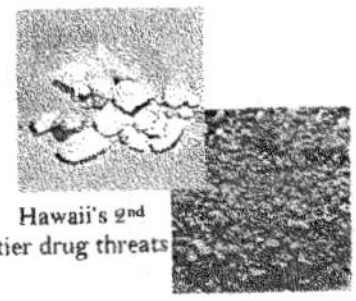

Hawaii's 2nd tier drug threats

reported use, and treatment.

In the third tier are drugs such as MDMA, GHB, steroids, and diverted pharmaceuticals, which are available and abused in Hawaii but to a much lesser extent. While it is imperative to continue combating these drugs and thus preventing them from becoming a larger problem in the future, it is the trafficking and abuse of primarily crystal methamphetamine as well as marijuana, cocaine, and heroin that currently pose

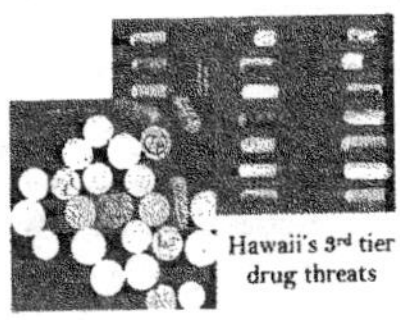

Hawaii's 3rd tier drug threats

the most viable drug threats to Hawaii.

International and local DTOs have ample opportunity to traffic those four drugs to, through, and from the area because of Hawaii's high volume of international and domestic air and sea traffic including passengers, cargo, and mail. Hawaii is the destination for crystal methamphetamine, cocaine, and heroin supplied from the West Coast and Mexico by Mexican Consolidated Priority Organization Targets (CPOTs) and DTOs; for crystal methamphetamine and heroin transported from Asia, Canada, and the West Coast by Asian DTOs; and for marijuana transported from Canada and the Pacific Northwest by local DTOs. Hawaii is a trans-shipment point for methamphetamine transported from the West Coast to locations in the Pacific Basin, such as Guam, by local DTOs supplied by Mexican DTOs.[2] It also is a trans-shipment point for methamphetamine transported from the West Coast or Asia to locations in the Pacific Basin by Asian DTOs. Finally, Hawaii is the source of high potency marijuana transported to the U.S. mainland, Canada and, to a lesser extent, Mexico by local DTOs.

The region covered by the Hawaii HIDTA comprises four counties. The description of the drug threats posed to these four geographic regions is nearly identical (see Matrix). In addition to the threat from the presence of international and local DTOs; drug fugitives, armed violent drug offenders; smuggling, money laundering, and the use of public lands for cannabis cultivation plague the counties. Because of the way Hawaii's drug laws are written, a significant number of drug traffickers are identified but not prosecuted. Among the differences from county to county is that law enforcement in the County of Honolulu, far more than in the other counties, faces the challenge of illicit drug shipments by parcels through Honolulu International Airport and the International Mail Branch. DTOs in Kauai County, unlike in the other three, currently are not linked to CPOTs.

Through its many initiatives the Hawaii HIDTA and its participating agencies are disrupting and dismantling the DTOs responsible for trafficking illicit drugs in Hawaii through the interdiction of crystal methamphetamine, marijuana, cocaine, heroin, and other illicit drugs as they are transported to, through, and from Hawaii. It is disrupting and dismantling these DTOs by seizing the money they use to operate and the assets they acquire with illicit drug proceeds.

The Hawaii HIDTA and its federal and state/local law enforcement partners are removing weapons from the street and bringing drug offenders and fugitives to justice to in its efforts to cripple the drug trade and reduce drug-related crime in Hawaii. The future impact of Hawaii HIDTA initiatives will be measured in the continuing and increasing seizures of illicit drugs and proceeds as well as the arrests and successful prosecutions of those responsible for transporting drugs and drug proceeds through Hawaii's airports, parcel facilities, and ports.

HIDTA Matrix

The Office of National Drug Control Policy (ONDCP) has established three goals for the HIDTA program:

Goal 1- Reduce Drug Availability by Eliminating or Disrupting Drug Trafficking Organizations
Goal 2- Reduce the Harmful Consequences of Drug Trafficking
Goal 3- Improve the Efficiency and Effectiveness of Law Enforcement Organizations

The National HIDTA Program Office (NHPO) is mandated by the Office of Management and Budget (OMB) to accurately account for the performance of the HIDTA program. In doing so, the NHPO has developed the Performance Management Process (PMP), which measures program efficiency and effectiveness. The cornerstone of this effort is the PMP Matrix, a tool designed to illustrate the performance process and keep it simple, direct and understandable. The Matrix is a grid system that:

1. Identifies primary threats by geographic area;
2. Develops desired goals to counter the threats;
3. Assigns responsibility to accomplish the desired goals;
4. Captures output measurements;
5. Illustrates the program's outcomes.

The left side of the Matrix contains a description of the primary threats and desired outputs (strategy) by geographic region. The right side of the Matrix lists the entities responsible for addressing the threats and outputs/outcomes.

The Hawaii HIDTA sits on the National HIDTA PMP Development Committee and is among a select few using the PMP Matrix in the submission of its CY2003 Annual Report and development of its CY2005 Drug Threat Assessment. We expect the PMP Matrix to be fully implemented by the end of CY2004. When fully implemented, each calendar year's Annual Report, Threat Assessment and Strategy will be illustrated by the data included in the matrix.

The Matrix reflects information from CY2004 Initiative Submissions and the CY2003 Annual Report. The desired outcomes and responsibility sections are based on the expected outputs as indicated by each of the initiatives in their initial submission package.

The matrix based system establishes a mechanism that measures each HIDTA's performance and holds them accountable for what they do. Standardized threat measurements have yet to be finalized by the NHPO. For this assessment, threats have been identified using monthly initiative statistics, field interviews, open source data, intelligence briefs, and agency surveys.

HAWAII HIDTA MATRIX

→

Overview of HIDTA Region

GEOGRAPHY

The State of Hawaii encompasses eight main islands and a 1,500-mile chain of islets covering more than 6,400 square miles in the north central Pacific Ocean. It is perhaps the most geographically isolated populated place in the world, situated approximately 2,500 miles from California, almost 4,000 miles from Guam and Japan, and more than 5,000 miles from Taiwan, Australia, the Philippines, and Hong Kong.[3] Yet it is Hawaii's remote location, situated as it is in the expanse of the Pacific Ocean, that makes Hawaii an ideal transshipment point for illicit drugs to and from Asia and North America or to Pacific Basin locations, where profits two-four times higher are realized.

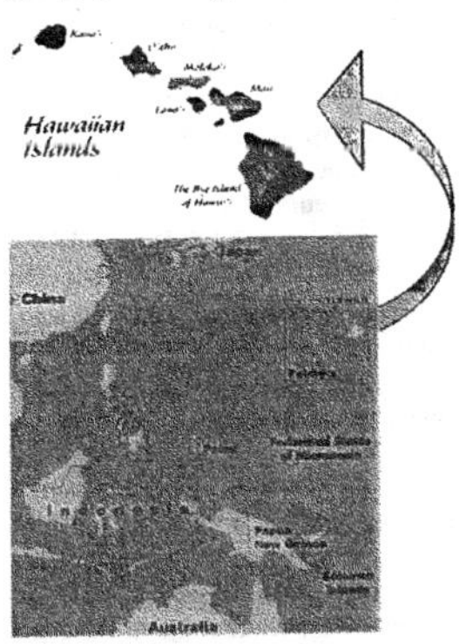

The State of Hawaii's population resides in four counties. Honolulu, Hawaii, Maui, and Kauai Counties are themselves separated by miles of ocean, and the drug situation in each is often controlled by DTOs that supply and distribute illicit drugs statewide. While Hawaii is a geographically expansive state, three-quarters of the population reside on Oahu, and, to a large extent, circumstances in the City and County of Honolulu drive the drug situation statewide.

HIDTA REGION

The region covered by the Hawaii HIDTA comprises all four counties. The demand for illicit drugs in all counties is high, particularly in regards to crystal methamphetamine and marijuana, and the description of the drug threats posed to these four geographic regions is nearly identical (see Matrix). The drug situation in all four counties includes the presence of international DTOs, drug fugitives, and armed violent drug offenders; the smuggling, transportation, and distribution of multi-pound quantities of illicit drugs; significant numbers of drug traffickers identified but not prosecuted; significant drug money laundering activity; the use of public lands for cannabis cultivation; and the presence of weapons associated with drug trafficking. The few differences from county to county are that law enforcement in the City and County of Honolulu, far more than in the other counties, faces the challenge of illicit drug shipments by parcels through Honolulu International Airport and that DTOs in Kauai County, unlike in the other three, currently are not linked to CPOTs.

The Hawaii HIDTA's mission is to measurably reduce drug trafficking, to which end it strives to dismantle, disrupt, arrest, and prosecute DTOs, drug gangs, and organized crime groups involved in the manufacturing, transportation, and distribution of illicit drugs as well as drug-related crimes, including money laundering. Because of Hawaii's remote location in the Pacific Ocean, much of the Hawaii HIDTA's efforts focus on the transportation to, through, and from Hawaii of illicit drugs (at least one of which—marijuana—is produced in significant quantities in the state) and drug proceeds. As an interdiction HIDTA, the Hawaii HIDTA is not engaged in prevention or treatment initiatives; however, selected data relevant to the prevalence and consequences of illicit drug use in Hawaii are provided in the Appendix as supplementary information.

ECONOMICS

Tourism, military, and agriculture are Hawaii's leading economic industries and play an important role in the State's drug threat. With over 6 million visitors arriving annually[4], the daily profusion of tourists can make it difficult for law enforcement to interdict drug couriers at Hawaii's airports.

Military personnel and their dependents contribute nearly 87,000 individuals to the State's population[5]. According to military law enforcement agencies, there has been an increase in the use of predatory drugs, such as MDMA and GHB among personnel. Because these drugs are not detectable in the body after a day or two, service members use the drugs over the weekend when they know they will not be tested.

Agriculture is Hawaii's third largest industry generating $1.07 billion to the State's economy each year[6]. Crops such as exotic fruits, coffee, macadamia nuts, flowers, and foliage not only provide products for Hawaii's markets but have become exports to destinations around the world. These products, especially flowers and foliage, may be used to conceal drug exports such as marijuana.

TRANSPORTATION

Hawaii's island makeup eliminates land-based border threats and allows law enforcement to concentrate on air and sea chokepoints. Airborne package delivery services and commercial aircraft are the most significant threats for transporting illicit drug to and from the State. Monitoring the flow of parcels and people is difficult for law enforcement due to lack of resources and the enormous amount of activity. In 2003, FedEx, UPS, and the U.S. Postal Service delivered over 28 million packages into the State. In addition, there were over one million takeoffs and landings at Hawaii's airports. Local law enforcement agencies estimate that more than 50 percent of the State's illicit drugs arrive by package delivery services with the majority of the remainder transported by couriers on commercial aircraft.

CLIMATE

Hawaii is an optimal location for marijuana cultivation because of its weather conditions and rich volcanic soil. Ample morning rain and afternoon sunlight provide growing favorable conditions. Marijuana cultivators often use public lands to produce large outdoor grows.

Goal 1: Reduce Drug Availability by Eliminating or Disrupting Drug Trafficking Organizations

DTOs are a significant drug threat to Hawaii. Hawaii HIDTA participating agencies identified their top 10 DTOs—groups defined by Continuing Criminal Enterprise Statute 21 USC 848 as consisting of five or more persons committing a continuing series of violations and obtaining substantial income or resources—operating throughout Hawaii in 2003. Hawaii HIDTA initiatives also reported disrupting or dismantling approximately 34 DTOs in 2003. Of the remaining operational DTOs, approximately 7 are considered priority targets for the Hawaii HIDTA and 6 have been linked to CPOTs.[7]

Most of Hawaii's DTOs are local DTOs, usually consisting of 5 to 50 individuals of mixed ethnicity including, but not limited to, those of native Hawaiian, Japanese, Chinese, Filipino, Korean, Hispanic, and Caucasian descent. Members of local DTOs typically are connected through family and/or social ties and often include family members, extended family members, neighbors, and childhood friends who work together to transport and distribute illicit drugs. The composition and fluidity of local DTOs help facilitate a loose cooperation among themselves and with international DTOs, and local DTOs are linked to CPOTs largely through their associations with Mexican DTOs based in Hawaii and the U.S. mainland. Because of the cooperation among organizations and the heavy reliance on sources of supply outside Hawaii, particularly for crystal methamphetamine, cocaine, and heroin, the majority of Hawaii's DTOs could be considered international or national in scope; however, for the purposes of this report, the discussion of international DTOs will be limited to those whose membership is primarily of foreign origin including Mexican, Asian, and Pacific Islander DTOs.

INTERNATIONAL

Mexican DTOs are transportation and distribution organizations. They supply wholesale quantities of illicit drugs to local DTOs or independent distributors who, because of their stronger family and social ties within Hawaii's communities, can facilitate quick retail sales. The Mexican DTOs based in the state typically are located in counties with larger Hispanic populations such as Hawaii and Maui. Mexican DTOs typically are organized around family ties and operations are highly compartmentalized; that is, individual cells within the organization manage production, transportation, distribution, money laundering, communications, and security separately to protect organization leaders. Of all the international DTOs in Hawaii, Mexican DTOs likely pose the most formidable

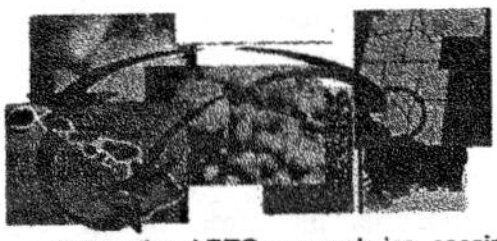

International DTOs smuggle ice, cocaine and heroin

drug threat because of their established and extensive transportation network. As in many other areas of the country, in Hawaii Mexican DTOs usually focus on the movement of illegal drugs in wholesale quantities, not on controlling lower level distribution.

Mexican DTOs transport crystal methamphetamine, cocaine, and heroin to Hawaii as well as supply these illicit drugs to local, other Mexican, and Pacific Islander DTOs who also transport them to Hawaii for distribution. These organizations transport crystal methamphetamine to Hawaii from the West Coast, primarily California, although Las Vegas has been the origin of some of the shipments seized. Transport typically involves mailed parcels and couriers on commercial flights arriving at Honolulu International Airport. Most of the crystal methamphetamine available in the state appears to be produced in Mexican DTO-controlled clandestine laboratories in Mexico and California: analysis of crystal methamphetamine samples from 47 federal cases in 2002 determined that 97 percent were of Californian, Mexican, or South American origin.[8]

Mexican DTOs supply cocaine to local, Mexican, and Pacific Islander DTOs that travel to the U.S. mainland to obtain the drug and then transport it to Hawaii, often flying out of Los Angeles, Oakland, and San Francisco. In addition, Mexican DTOs are the primary transporters of heroin to Hawaii, where black tar is the predominant type available. While Hawaii is a consumer market for Mexico-produced heroin transported from Los Angeles, San Diego, and Mexico, it is possible that some of the heroin is transshipped to the Pacific Basin given that local DTOs have already established distribution routes to locations such as Guam for the crystal methamphetamine supplied to them by Mexican DTOs.

Given their roles as principal suppliers, transporters, and wholesale distributors of illicit drugs in Hawaii, Mexican DTOs are significant money launderers. Mexican DTOs typically smuggle drug proceeds generated in the U.S. out of the country to be laundered through foreign financial systems, which generally are less regulated than the U.S. financial system. To that end, Mexican DTOs send bulk drug proceeds generated in Hawaii to Mexico via mailed parcels, couriers on commercial flights, and maritime freight. Funds are transported from points throughout Hawaii either directly to Mexico or through major collection points in the U.S. such as cities in California, Texas, and Arizona en route to Mexico. Mexican DTOs also launder illegal drug proceeds through money service businesses and front companies as well as by purchasing tangible assets such as real estate, vehicles, and jewelry.

Asian DTOs, which often consist of ethnic Japanese, Chinese, Korean, Filipino, and members of other Asian groups from Thailand, Laos, Cambodia, and Vietnam, are transportation and distribution organizations. Intelligence reporting indicates that several Asian DTOs operate in Hawaii, including Chinese and Korean DTOs in the City and County of Honolulu, Filipino DTOs in Hawaii County, and Chinese DTOs in Kauai County. Asian DTOs are highly cohesive and traditionally have been difficult for law enforcement to penetrate because of strong family, social, and/or tribal ties.

Law enforcement authorities in Hawaii report that some Asian DTOs transport Asia-produced crystal methamphetamine to Hawaii indirectly (such as through California or Canada), while others smuggle crystal methamphetamine into Hawaii directly from source countries in Asia. In fact, Asian DTOs are known to transship methamphetamine from the West Coast through Hawaii to locations in the Pacific Basin.[9]

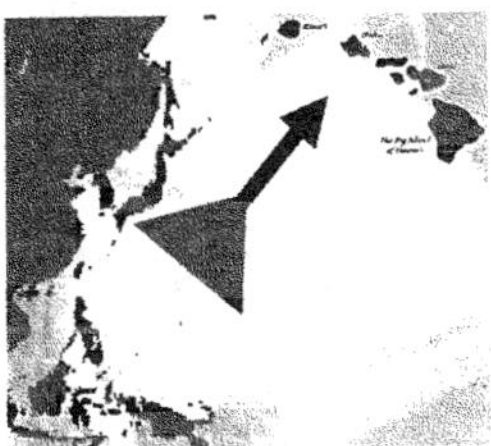

Some ice comes directly to Hawaii from Asian countries

Asian DTOs also transport cocaine to Hawaii from the West Coast, although to a lesser extent than Mexican DTOs, and the small quantities of Asian heroin (China White) available in Hawaii are supplied by Asian DTOs as well. In addition, shipments of opium, typically from Laos and Cambodia, are seized at the International Mail Facility at Honolulu International Airport when they transit Hawaii en route to the U.S. mainland, primarily California.

Asian DTOs generate considerable profits from drug distribution in Hawaii, and these funds must be laundered in order to minimize the risk of detection and seizure. Asian DTOs typically send bulk drug proceeds generated in Hawaii to their country of origin, where the money is used to purchase businesses or real property. Law enforcement is aware, however, of individual drug traffickers who are associated with DTOs based in Asia and the U.S. mainland laundering drug proceeds through the purchase of high-priced residential real estate throughout the state of Hawaii.

Pacific Islander DTOs, mainly consisting of Samoan and Tongan members, are primarily transportation and distribution organizations. Pacific Islander DTOs maintain ties to California, primarily in the Los Angeles and San Francisco areas, and use these ties to obtain cocaine and crystal methamphetamine in California for transportation to Hawaii; the source of some of these drugs obtained in California has been traced to Mexico. Past law enforcement investigations also have linked Pacific Islander DTOs in Hawaii with Pacific Islander DTOs in Utah, where there is a large Tongan population.

Pacific Islander DTOs are, to a lesser degree, production organizations as well. They are involved in cannabis cultivation in Hawaii, and they convert most of the powder cocaine they transport to Hawaii into crack.

Pacific Islander DTOs generally use simple methods to launder their drug proceeds. They often either transport bulk cash out of Hawaii via mailed parcels or couriers on commercial flights to their source of supply or launder drug proceeds through the purchase of postal money orders or tangible assets.

Consolidated Priority Organization Targets

Consolidated Priority Organization Targets (CPOTs) are Department of Justice-identified national priority targets. CPOTs are linked to Hawaii's local and Pacific Islander DTOs through high-level Mexican polydrug traffickers. Currently there are 6 identified CPOT-linked DTOs out of the DTOs identified in Hawaii in 2003. The link between CPOTs and Hawaii's DTOs exists largely because of the heavy reliance on sources of supply outside Hawaii and the trafficking patterns that emerge as a consequence. Some of the principal source areas supplying Hawaii are California and Mexico for crystal methamphetamine, South America for cocaine, and Mexico for heroin; therefore, the trafficking patterns that result from these outside source areas necessitate associations between DTOs in Hawaii and CPOTs that control the production of methamphetamine and heroin in, as well as the transportation of South American cocaine through, Mexico.

Regional Priority Organization Targets

Regional Priority Organization Targets (RPOTs) are HIDTA-identified priority targets that conduct operations over an expanded area in the region, minimally defined as two or more of Hawaii's ocean-separated counties. Currently there are 5 identified RPOTs out of the DTOs identified in Hawaii in 2003. Identified RPOTs include Asian, Pacific Islander, and local DTOs. Hawaii's RPOTs are prosecuted in conjunction with the Organized Crime Drug Enforcement Task Force (OCDETF).

Because drugs in Hawaii are typically double the price found on the mainland the state is a highly profitable market for drug trafficking organizations. Moreover, drugs prices in Guam and Saipan are twice as much as Hawaii creating an even more lucrative market for Tongan and Samoan organizations who operate in the region.

Local Drug Trafficking Organizations

Local DTOs are transportation, distribution, and production organizations, although as the principal midlevel and retail distributors of crystal methamphetamine, cocaine, heroin, and marijuana throughout Hawaii, they are perhaps involved primarily in distribution. Local DTOs typically obtain their supplies through loose connections to international DTOs, including CPOTs and RPOTs. The distinction between distributor and transporter often is blurred, however, and local DTOs also transport crystal methamphetamine, cocaine and, at times, marijuana (typically BC Bud from Canada or similar high potency domestic marijuana, often from Oregon or Washington) from the U.S. mainland to Hawaii via mailed parcels and commercial air. While neither method permits the transportation of large amounts of illicit drugs at any one time, the frequency with which local DTOs travel to and from the U.S. mainland helps maintain adequate supplies for their distribution networks. Local DTOs transship some methamphetamine supplied by Mexican DTOs from the West Coast to the Pacific Basin, primarily Guam. It is possible they use the same distribution routes for heroin supplied by Mexican DTOs, although currently there are no quantifiable data to support this possibility.

Local DTOs also cultivate cannabis in Hawaii and thus are production organizations as well. Their role as marijuana producers has enabled some local DTOs to become not only statewide wholesale, midlevel, and retail distributors but also national, regional, or even international transporters of marijuana. Local DTOs transport marijuana produced in Hawaii to the U.S. mainland, Mexico and, to a lesser extent, Canada. Transport typically occurs via mailed parcels; however, the Hawaii County Police Department has reported that large quantities of marijuana are transported from the island of Hawaii to the U.S. mainland via maritime methods. Some intelligence indicates that local DTOs may exchange Hawaii-produced marijuana for methamphetamine or other illicit drugs on the U.S. mainland.[10]

Like international DTOs, local DTOs also frequently transport their drug proceeds out of Hawaii. The funds usually are destined for the U.S. mainland (often Las Vegas, which is a popular vacation destination for Hawaii residents) or to their source of supply, and larger local DTOs transport drug proceeds in bulk to the U.S. mainland usually via mailed parcels or couriers on commercial flights. Some local DTOs, however, launder drug proceeds through the purchase of postal money orders or tangible assets such as vehicles and personal watercraft.

Independent Distributors

Hawaii also has many local independent drug distributors involved in primarily retail-level sales. Independent distributors are not affiliated with any DTOs and therefore usually sell illicit drugs outside any structured distribution network. Independent distributors are mostly associated with drugs such as marijuana, ecstasy (or MDMA), GHB, steroids, and diverted pharmaceuticals.

Drugs of Choice in Hawaii

The two drugs causing the most serious problems for Hawaii's law enforcement and citizens are crystal methamphetamine and marijuana. Crystal methamphetamine is the most widely abused illicit drug in Hawaii, and it is also the drug believed to contribute to the most serious consequences.[11] The magnitude of the crystal methamphetamine problem in Hawaii overshadows the difficulties posed to law enforcement and society by the production and use of marijuana. However, Hawaii is a principal domestic source area for marijuana, and the drug's widespread availability and use contribute to its ranking as the second biggest drug problem in the state.

Crack cocaine and heroin remain problems in Hawaii, but they appear to rank well behind crystal methamphetamine and marijuana in contributing to Hawaii' drug troubles. Other drugs such as MDMA, GHB, steroids, and diverted pharmaceuticals are available in Hawaii but are abused to a lesser extent.

Most of the crystal methamphetamine available throughout Hawaii appears to be produced in Mexico and California. Asia-produced crystal methamphetamine is available to a lesser extent, as is a limited amount of locally produced crystal methamphetamine. Clandestine methamphetamine laboratory seizures have been relatively low in recent years; in fact, Hawaii HIDTA initiatives reported seizing only one laboratory in 2003. Laboratory seizures likely have been underreported, however, and should increase as more of Hawaii's law enforcement personnel and citizens are educated in laboratory identification (see Outlook and Predictions on page 29).

Mexican DTOs typically transport crystal methamphetamine directly to the City and County of Honolulu, as well as to Hawaii and Maui Counties, from the West Coast, primarily California, although Las Vegas also has been the origin of some crystal methamphetamine seized in Hawaii. Local and Pacific Islander DTOs transport crystal methamphetamine, usually supplied by Mexican DTOs, to Hawaii also primarily from California. Law enforcement in Hawaii reports that some Asian RPOTS and DTOs (primarily Filipino, Vietnamese, and Korean) transport Asia-produced crystal methamphetamine to Hawaii via California or Canada, attempting to avoid the strict U.S. Customs inspections given to international mail or flights at Hawaii ports of entry, particularly mail or flights originating in known source countries. Others, however, smuggle crystal methamphetamine into Hawaii directly from source countries such as the Philippines, Korea, and Thailand.

Hawaii law enforcement estimates that approximately 80–90 percent of the crystal methamphetamine seized in the state is smuggled through Honolulu International Airport via mailed parcels and couriers on commercial flights. The Hawaii HIDTA Airport Task Force reported seizing nearly 20 kilograms of crystal methamphetamine transported via parcels or couriers on domestic flights in 2003;[12] several of the parcels seized were routed to Hawaii out of California (Los Angeles and Oakland areas) and Tennessee (Memphis). The Airport Task Force reported seizing approximately 21 kilograms of crystal methamphetamine at Honolulu International Airport in 2002.[13]

The Hawaii HIDTA Foreign Interdiction Task Force, which focuses on interdicting illicit drugs smuggled from international sources by air, sea, and mail, reported seizing nearly 7 kilograms of crystal methamphetamine that had been smuggled largely via international mail and couriers on international flights in 2003. The vast majority of this ice—approximately 6 kilograms—originated in Canada (Vancouver and Ottawa connections), at least 4 kilograms of which were smuggled by Asian traffickers.[14]

Marijuana also is widely available and used, but because of the rampant abuse of crystal methamphetamine in the state, Hawaii is one of the few places in the U.S. where marijuana might not be considered the most widely abused illicit drug.[15] Hawaii is, however, a principal domestic source for marijuana, particularly high potency marijuana,[16] and most of what is available in the state is produced locally, throughout the islands but largely in Hawaii County. The vast majority of cultivation occurs

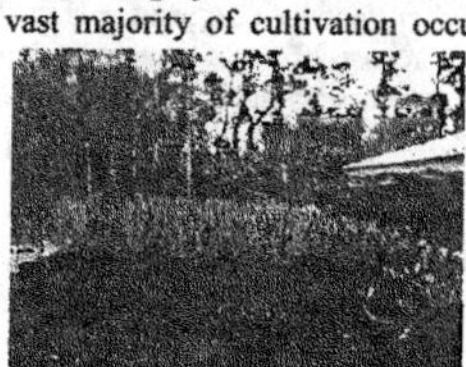

Outdoor Marijuana Grow

outdoors and, frequently, on public lands.

More than half (54%) of the 392,276 cannabis plants eradicated from outdoor plots under DEA's Domestic Cannabis Eradication and Suppression Program (DCE/SP) in 2003 were eradicated by the Department of Land and Natural Resources (DLNR), which is responsible for eradication on Hawaii's public lands.[17] While a breakdown of DLNR seizures by county is unavailable, nearly 70 percent of the forest reserve lands and natural areas administered by the DLNR are in Hawaii County and another 12 percent (second most) are in Maui County.[18] In addition, Hawaii and Maui Counties accounted for most of the eradicated plants removed from lands other than those administered by DLNR.[19]

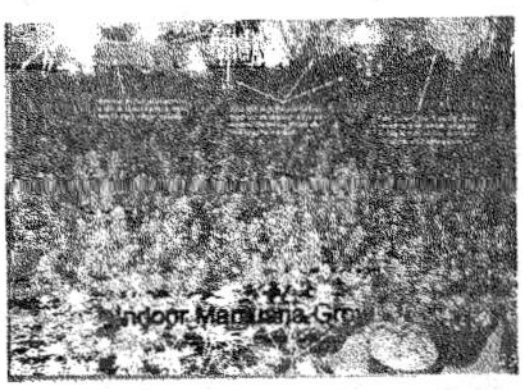

Although the agricultural and weather conditions are optimal for outdoor cannabis cultivation, indoor marijuana grows do exist in Hawaii. These operations generally are small and located in private residences, and the marijuana produced is usually for personal use or limited distribution in a small area. Yet while indoor eradication figures in Hawaii are still very low compared with other states—DCE/SP reported eradicating 3,519 cannabis plants from 9 indoor grow operations in 2003—these figures represent a considerable increase for the state from just 314 plants eradicated and 3 grow operations seized in 2002.[20] Interestingly, the increase in indoor plant eradication parallels a decline in outdoor plant eradication from 2002 to 2003 (see Table 1). Moreover, there are some indications that suggest indoor cultivation operations in Hawaii could continue to increase either in number or in productivity (see Other Issues: Marijuana Production on page 28).

Table 1: Hawaii DCE/SP Totals, 2002–2003

Year	Outdoor Plants	Outdoor Plots	Indoor Plants	Indoor Grows
2003	392,276	9,662	3,519	9
2002	435,789	9,865	314	3

While local production accounts for most of the marijuana available in Hawaii by far, some marijuana is transported to the state, and amounts seized have increased. Available statistics for the Hawaii HIDTA Airport Task Force indicate that approximately 25 kilograms of marijuana were intercepted in 2003, transported primarily via parcels but also in luggage transported on commercial flights from the U.S. mainland.[21] Almost 20 kilograms of the marijuana seized from parcels and luggage in 2003 originated in Seattle and Portland. The Airport Task Force reported seizing nearly 10 kilograms of cannabis in 2002.[22]

The Hawaii HIDTA Foreign Interdiction Task Force intercepted approximately 10 more kilograms of marijuana, an estimated 85 percent of which originated in Canada. The remaining 15 percent originated in the Netherlands and consisted mostly of seeds. Virtually all the marijuana seized by the Foreign Interdiction Task Force is smuggled via international mail.[23] The task force reported seizing approximately 5½ kilograms of marijuana in 2002.[24]

The primary producers of marijuana in Hawaii, local and Pacific Islander DTOs, also are the primary wholesale and retail distributors. They usually transport marijuana produced on neighbor islands to Oahu in multi-ounce to multi-pound quantities typically via inter-island commercial flights. The distribution of marijuana as compared with that of other illicit drugs is the least structured, however, and nearly anyone with access to seeds and a cultivation site can become a marijuana producer, and potentially, a marijuana distributor.

The trafficking and abuse of cocaine and crack cocaine remain a threat to Hawaii, although the cocaine problem does not rise to the level of either crystal methamphetamine or marijuana. Mexican DTOs supply local and Pacific Islander DTOs with most of the cocaine transported to Hawaii; Asian DTOs transport cocaine to a lesser extent. According to the Honolulu Police Department, local and Pacific Islander DTOs with ties to sources in California, particularly Los Angeles and San Francisco, transport cocaine from California to Hawaii; they also transport cocaine from Utah, which has a large Tongan population.

Most cocaine is transported to Hawaii in powder form via mailed parcels or couriers on commercial flights; couriers typically use checked luggage for cocaine transportation. The Hawaii HIDTA Airport Task Force reported seizing nearly 8 kilograms of powder cocaine and 30 grams of crack cocaine in 2003. The Airport Task Force reported seizing less than 2 kilograms of cocaine in 2002.[25]

The Hawaii HIDTA Foreign Interdiction Task Force reported seizing another 1.22 kilograms of powder cocaine smuggled via international mail in 2003. One seizure involved a 1-kilogram parcel that originated in Antigua.[26] In 2002, the Foreign Interdiction Task Force reported seizing approximately 4 kilograms of cocaine.[27]

While the cocaine transported to Hawaii is mostly powder, most cocaine available at street level is in the form of crack, which accounted for 80 percent of all cocaine-related cases (crack and powder combined) and 76 percent of all cocaine-related arrests in 2003, according to Honolulu Police Department statistics (see Table 2). Pacific Islander and local DTOs that control retail distribution convert the powder cocaine into crack before distributing the drug in Hawaii's communities at locations such as at night clubs, bars, open-air drug markets, as well as private residences.

Table 2: Crack Cocaine to All Cocaine* Cases & Arrests, Honolulu Police Department, 2002–2003

Year	All Cocaine Cases	Crack Cocaine Cases	All Cocaine Arrests	Crack Cocaine Arrests
2003	202	163	185	141
2002	122	98	100	74

* "All cocaine" refers to crack and powder combined.

Heroin is available and abused in Hawaii; however, decreasing arrests and treatment admissions suggest that heroin distribution, as well as the consequences associated with heroin abuse, is a diminishing problem in the state. It is possible that local DTOs are transshipping heroin supplied by Mexican DTOs from the West Coast, primarily Los Angeles, through Hawaii to other Pacific Basin locations as they do for crystal methamphetamine, although currently there are no quantifiable data to support this possibility. Asian DTOs supply Hawaii with small quantities of Asian heroin (China White) as well.

As it is for other illicit drugs, Honolulu International Airport appears to be the primary entry point for heroin transported to Hawaii. Nearly all the heroin seized by the Hawaii HIDTA Airport Task Force in 2003—more than 2½ kilograms of black tar and brown heroin and another 190 grams of heroin powder—was transported via mailed parcels. While most of the heroin transported to and available in Hawaii is black tar, at least 0.23 kilogram was brown powder heroin seized from a parcel destined for Hawaii County.[28] The Airport Task Force reported seizing less than 2 kilograms of heroin in 2002.[29] The Hawaii HIDTA Foreign Interdiction Task Force reported seizing approximately 19 kilograms of opium from international mail in 2003; however, Hawaii usually is not the destination for opium.[30] Shipments of opium, usually from Laos and Cambodia, typically are seized at the International Mail Facility at Honolulu International Airport en route to the U.S. mainland, primarily California.

Despite the best efforts of Hawaii HIDTA initiatives and law enforcement to stop the flow of drugs at the state's airports and parcel facilities, shipments do make it through the front-line defenses. The Hawaii Interagency Mobile Police Apprehension Crime Task Force (HI-IMPACT), staffed by all the Hawaii HIDTA participating agencies, has been extremely effective in removing illicit drugs from Hawaii's streets since its inception (see Table 3).

Table 3: HI-IMPACT Seizures of Hawaii's Drugs of Choice, in kilograms, 2002–2003

Year	Methamphetamine (ice & powder)	Marijuana (processed)	Cocaine (crack & powder)	Heroin (black tar, brown, & powder)
2003	52.9	23.4	6.1	0.7
2002	16.5	20.5	4.4	0.9

Goal 2: Reduce the Harmful Consequences of Drug Trafficking

As an interdiction HIDTA, the Hawaii HIDTA targets the violence associated with drug trafficking and drug offenders largely by seizing firearms from violent drug offenders and apprehending drug fugitives. Regrettably, there remain, at this time, legal and legislative barriers to the effective prosecution of drug offenders in Hawaii.

An estimated 90 percent of property crime in the state is believed to be drug-related,[31] a cause for considerable concern given that Hawaii ranked second highest in the U.S. for the property index crime rate (5,135.5) in 2001, the latest year for which national figures are available.[32] What is more, the state's ranking could rise since this rate increased 12.7 percent in 2002, driven largely by a motor vehicle theft rate that rose dramatically in that year as well as a perennially high larceny-theft rate.

While violent crime is comparatively low in Hawaii—the state ranked forty-second highest in the U.S. for the violent index crime rate (254.6) in 2001—it is problematic and likely attributable, to a large extent, to Hawaii's prevailing drug of choice.[33] While drug-related crime statistics are not captured by the State of Hawaii, many homicides and high-profile cases of violence, including hostage situations, have been associated with crystal methamphetamine, and in 2002 the U.S. Attorney stated that crystal methamphetamine had been associated with 90 percent of confirmed child abuse cases.[34] More recently, media articles in 2004 have reported that assaults on Maui police officers have increased fivefold over the past 5 years and that the violence associated with crystal methamphetamine abuse is a contributing factor in that increase.[35]

According to data from the Arrestee Drug Abuse Monitoring (ADAM) program, almost half of adult male arrestees in Hawaii tested positive for crystal methamphetamine in 2002, ranking the state first among all ADAM sites reporting in that year as in the previous two years. As illustrated in Table 4, while the percentages of male arrestees testing positive for Hawaii's two most problematic illicit drugs have increased, those for the "second-tier" drugs in Hawaii—cocaine and heroin (opiates)—have declined sharply.

Table 4: Percentage of Adult Male Arrestees in Hawaii Testing Positive, Arrestee Drug Abuse Monitoring Program, 2000 & 2002

Year	Methamphetamine	Marijuana	Cocaine	Opiates (usually heroin)
2002	46.1	31.7	8.9	3.4
2000	35.9	30.4	15.8	6.8

SEIZING WEAPONS FROM VIOLENT DRUG OFFENDERS

According to statistics from the Bureau of Alcohol, Tobacco, Firearms and Explosives (ATF), 90% (86 of 95) of all cases investigated by the ATF in Hawaii in 2003 were drug-related. Of those drug-related cases, 79 involved firearms and 7 involved ammunition. Crystal methamphetamine was involved in 66 drug-related cases, followed by marijuana (23), and cocaine (11).[36]

Project Safe Neighborhoods
The HIDTA Executive Board approved the addition of the Safe Neighborhoods Initiative for FY2003. It is a joint effort with the Department of Justice's Project Safe Neighborhoods initiative that targets gun crime and violent offenders to remove guns from the street and keep communities safe. HIDTA supplements the Project Safe Neighborhoods endeavor with resources needed to reduce the harmful consequences of drug trafficking by taking a hard line against armed criminals.

Hawaii HIDTA initiatives reported seizing 162 weapons in 2003; most on the islands of Oahu and Hawaii.[37] Another 25 weapons were seized during DCE/SP eradication operations on the islands of Hawaii (23) and Kauai (2). Of note is that 6 of the 25 weapons seized during DCE/SP operations in 2003 were removed from the limited number (9) of indoor grow operations seized that year, while seizures of the remaining 19 weapons were spread over more than 3,500 outdoor operations.[38]

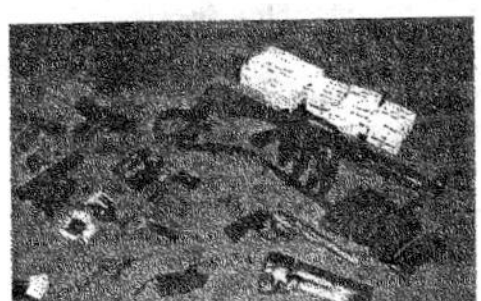
Firearms seizure

APPREHENDING DRUG FUGITIVES

According to the State Attorney General's *Crime in Hawaii 2002* report,[39] 503 adults were arrested in Hawaii in 2002 for drug sale/manufacturing, compared with 578 in 2001. "Opium or cocaine" has accounted for most drug sale/manufacturing arrests among adults since 1993; however, the number of opium- or cocaine-related arrests has declined steadily overall and, in 2002, was just slightly ahead of the number of nonnarcotic-related arrests, which has risen steadily overall from 1993 to 2002.[40] Because of the groupings used in Uniform Crime Reports (such as combining opium and cocaine) it is impossible to analyze drug-specific trends from these arrest data. Arrests reported by the Honolulu Police Department in Table 5 are perhaps more illustrative of drug-specific trends in the state. Hawaii HIDTA initiatives reported over 1,600 arrests resulting from more than 2,100 initiated cases.[41]

Table 5: Number of Arrests by Hawaii Drug of Choice, Honolulu Police Department, 2001–2003

Year	Crystal methamphetamine	Detrimental (includes Marijuana)	Crack Cocaine	Black Tar Heroin
2003	641	78	141	27
2002	477	82	74	23
2001	507	75	74	30

Barriers to Effective Prosecution

In addition to the harmful consequences of drug-related violence that challenge law enforcement and diminish the quality of life in Hawaii, state law sometimes impedes the ability of law enforcement to effectively combat drug offenders. For example, evidence obtained from federal wiretap and consensual encounters remain, at this time, inadmissible in Hawaii state courts. While evidence found during a federal investigation can be used in federal court, federal thresholds for drug possession are higher than at the state level, and arrested offenders not meeting federal thresholds are released without prosecution. Two of the larger barriers to effective prosecution of drug offenders in the state involve the "challenger provision" to Hawaii's electronic surveillance law and the state law governing consensual encounters.

The challenger provision, which is not in federal statutes, requires that an in-camera adversarial hearing be held before a judge before an order authorizing or approving a wiretap is issued. A defense attorney is appointed to the hearing and is provided with the application for the wiretap as well as all supporting documents. Moreover, at the hearing, the defense attorney has the right to cross-examine all witnesses.

The argument for the challenger provision is that the adversarial hearing protects against rubber stamping by judges, or having decisions based on a distorted view of evidence and arguments supporting an application. This argument is flawed, however, since judges grant search warrants, which are more invasive than electronic surveillance. Also, the challenger provision's requirements for dissemination of information regarding potential targets, witnesses, and evidence create many problems for local law enforcement. This additional dissemination not only increases the risk that the target of an investigation will find out about the investigation but also increases the potential danger to any informants and witnesses. Furthermore, evidence obtained from federal wiretaps is inadmissible in Hawaii courts since federal statutes lack the challenger provision. As a result, many lower level drug distributors who do not meet federal thresholds go unprosecuted in state courts. It is not uncommon to find individuals with 30-plus arrests still free on city streets in Hawaii (see Outlook and Predictions on page 30).

Consensual encounters commonly referred to as "walk and talks," are not permited under the Hawaii State Constitution. In 1996 the Hawaii Supreme Court ruled that simply approaching someone in the airport violated the state constitution. Even if an investigator informs the person being approached that a drug investigation is being conducted, that he or she is talking to a police officer, and that he or she is free to leave at any time, that person cannot be prosecuted in Hawaii courts for any drugs discovered.

Despite the state law governing consensual encounters, they are conducted at Hawaii airports because local law enforcement officers are cross-designated with federal authority to conduct such encounters. Unfortunately, any evidence of an offense discovered through this technique can be used only in a federal court—evidence obtained from federal consensual encounters is inadmissible in Hawaii courts. Again, many lower level distributors that do not meet federal thresholds go unprosecuted in state courts.

Weed and Seed

Weed and Seed is a United States Department of Justice initiative that takes a multi-faceted proactive to fight crime by "weeding" out the criminal element and "seeding" the community with services that support neighborhood revitalization. The program relies on the collaboration of community residents, law enforcement, social service providers, educators, area businesses and a variety of other resources. Since its official recognition in 1997, Honolulu Weed and Seed reports a 66% reduction in Part I Crimes and a 75% reduction in Part II Crimes. Because of the program's success and impact on Hawaii's neighborhoods the Hawaii HIDTA is joining forces with Honolulu Weed and Seed. Through cooperative involvement the Hawaii HIDTA can measurable reduce the harmful consequences associated with drug trafficking.

Goal 3: Improve the Efficiency and Effectiveness of Law Enforcement Organizations

Information Sharing

The Hawaii HIDTA Investigative Support Center (ISC) gathers, analyzes, and disseminates intelligence relating to drug trafficking and money laundering activities and is thus able to continually provide information and intelligence, analytical support, and enhanced case support to participating agencies to advance ongoing law enforcement initiatives. The ISC also continues to provide subject and event deconfliction, ensuring officer and citizen safety during law enforcement activities, and to maintain connectivity among task forces in the City and County of Honolulu, Hawaii, Maui, and Kauai Counties; Hawaii HIDTA participating agencies; other regional law enforcement agencies; and other HIDTAs nationwide. As illustrated in Table 6, the ISC's development is continuing strongly.

Table 6: Hawaii HIDTA Investigative Support Center Activity, 2001–2003

Year	Analytical Products*	Deconfliction (subject & event)	DEA Support ("6's" & subpoenas)	Wire Support Cases
2003	8,474	420	152	3
2002	7,521	450	0	0
2001	318	0	0	0

* "Analytical products" include charts/graphs, telephone tolls, document/link/statistical analysis, intelligence profiles, database searches, geo-mapping, photographs, and presentations.

The ISC also provides, via email, information items of interest relating to drug abuse within the state and across the nation to HIDTA initiatives and participating agencies. Such items range from specific case-related information to background information relating to health, legalization, legislation, and enforcement activities. The ISC anticipates making this information available through a website in the near future.

Information sharing works both ways, and the Hawaii HIDTA has benefited greatly from intelligence supplied by other agencies. Many of the Hawaii Airport Task Force cases are derived from intelligence supplied by both international and U.S.-based agencies. In turn, the task force shares intelligence regarding outgoing parcel interdiction cases either with the proper jurisdictional HIDTAs or with non-HIDTA jurisdictions.

Training

The Hawaii HIDTA continually identifies training needs to improve the ability of its initiatives and participating agencies to counter drug trafficking and related criminal activity. The Hawaii HIDTA provides on-site training, coordinates other agency and out-source training, and disseminates information about training opportunities to increase the knowledge, skills, and abilities of investigative and analytical personnel directly involved in the drug suppression effort. HIDTA management and support operations maintain and improve their efficiency through appropriate in-service training.

Some of the most important training the Hawaii HIDTA is involved in is in the area of clandestine laboratory safety. Clan Lab Safety Recertification was completed by 76 personnel with the Honolulu, Hawaii, Maui, and Kauai Police Departments in 2003 and by 79 in 2004. Another 23 personnel with the Hawaii, Maui, and Kauai Police Departments completed Clan Lab Confined Space Training in 2003. HIDTA and law enforcement officials believe the number of clandestine laboratories operating in Hawaii has been significantly underreported because of a lack of training on laboratory identification in the past.

Coordination

Through a central manager the Hawaii HIDTA's Clandestine Laboratory Response Team coordinates and supports all "first responders" to clandestine laboratory calls. The HIDTA ensures that all county teams are completely certified and fully outfitted with operational equipment; provides certified personnel for clandestine laboratory operations; and supports personnel in sampling and recovering laboratory evidence.

The Hawaii HIDTA Prosecutorial Initiative is supporting current model legislation to amend the state's electronic surveillance and consensual encounter laws to more conform to federal laws. The success of this legislation will do much to provide law enforcement with the tools necessary to convict those individuals responsible for countless drug offenses who have previously gone unprosecuted.

Oversight

To achieve and exceed developmental standards, the Hawaii HIDTA has established a self-review policy and conducts an annual internal audit. The reviews address the effectiveness of the Hawaii HIDTA in the following areas: its support of the National Drug Control Strategy, its accomplishment of its mission; its use of and accountability for resources; and its compliance with HIDTA, ONDCP, and NHPO policies and directives.

The Hawaii HIDTA fiscal officer monitors, reviews, and tracks expenditures to ensure compliance with ONDCP and NHPO policies. Each Hawaii HIDTA initiative provides detailed quarterly reports identifying its budget and documenting expenses. The information is used to track the overall Hawaii HIDTA budget.

Funding

The Hawaii HIDTA ISC is sponsoring the development of an intelligence/enforcement outreach program that provides direct narcotics law enforcement links with countries in the Pacific Basin and Pacific Rim. Through its BOLO (Be On the Lookout) developmental component, the ISC will be able to provide first-hand, timely, actionable information from Pacific Basin/Rim countries for investigation, targeting, and the establishment of joint intelligence pools. This information will be available to all law enforcement agencies operating within the Hawaii HIDTA's area and to those under other HIDTAs whose jurisdictions are destinations for drug shipments originating in Asia or the Pacific.

Other Issues

Several other issues challenge the Hawaii HIDTA in its mission to measurably reduce drug trafficking, reduce the impact of illicit drugs to society, and increase citizen safety. Such issues include the transshipment of illicit drugs through Hawaii (including inter-island transshipment) to Pacific Basin locations, the prevalence of drug smuggling via international parcels; money laundering; and marijuana production methods that suggest that cannabis cultivators on the islands may be shifting toward more indoor operations or attempting to refine their techniques to produce even better quality marijuana that will fill user demand and yield higher profits.

Transshipment

Large quantities of illicit drugs shipped to the state of Hawaii—usually methamphetamine, cocaine, and heroin—typically arrive on Oahu at Honolulu International Airport. An unknown percentage of these drugs are in turn transported via inter-island flights from Oahu to neighbor islands. Law enforcement officials suspect that neighbor island airports such as Keahole-Kona International (Hawaii) and Kahului (Maui),[42] which now service flights to and from the West Coast, are being used to transport illicit drugs directly. At this time, however, quantifying the use of these alternate entry points is impracticable. Conversely, local and Pacific Islander DTOs who produce marijuana on neighbor islands usually transport their product to Oahu via inter-island commercial flights.

Hawaii also serves as an international transshipment point for illicit drugs transported to and from locations in North America, Asia, and the Pacific Basin. Intelligence indicates that an unknown percentage of crystal methamphetamine transported to Hawaii is destined for locations in the Pacific Basin, primarily Guam, while shipments of opium are transported to Hawaii en route to the U.S. mainland, primarily California.

Seizure data do indicate that the principal means of transporting illicit drugs and drug proceeds to and from Hawaii are mailed parcels and couriers on commercial flights. In fact, law enforcement estimates that approximately 90 percent of the illicit drugs seized in Hawaii are transported in parcels or in baggage and personal effects of couriers. The key limitation to seizure data, however, is that such data only provide insight into what was seized—the amount of illicit drugs transported to Hawaii but not seized is unknown.

A considerable amount of illicit drugs transported to and from Hawaii are potentially not seized from maritime vessels and freight. Nearly 80 percent of the legitimate goods consumed in Hawaii are commercial maritime imports yet maritime seizures of illicit drugs have been extremely limited. But even infrequent seizures of both drugs and bulk cash suggest that maritime smuggling may be more common than seizure data imply (see Outlook and Predictions on page 29).

International Parcels

Since September 11, 2001, most drug seizures in Hawaii have come from mailed parcels. Airborne mail and package delivery services delivered more than 28 million parcels to Hawaii in 2003 alone. While it is difficult to determine the actual volume of illicit drugs transported to Hawaii—again, what is not seized is unknown—it has been estimated by some local law enforcement that more than 50 percent of illicit drugs transported to Hawaii come via mailed parcels. Seizure data suggest that this method also appears to be used equally to transport, in bulk, the proceeds generated through drug distribution.

Money Laundering

Money laundering is the act of hiding the source and/or destination of illegally obtained funds, usually so that the profits of criminal activity—whether from theft, drug sales, or some other crime—will appear to have originated from a legitimate transaction. The sale of illicit drugs in Hawaii generates considerable sums of money that, instead of being used to build schools or roads, exit the local economy with no benefit to the state. Indeed, the international DTOs operating in Hawaii most often smuggle their illicit drug proceeds from the state to their country of origin. Most local DTOs, too, transport their proceeds from Hawaii to the U.S. mainland, likely to their source of supply.

Reporting from Hawaii HIDTA initiatives suggests that many seizures of illegal drug proceeds transported out of Hawaii via package delivery services in 2003 often involved amounts ranging from $20,000 to $50,000 destined for California and Las Vegas. Many incidents also involved circumstances whereby the individual wishing to mail the parcel often was willing to pay a fee that would seem unjustifiable given the weight of the parcel or the value of the item that was claimed to be inside the parcel. Seizures involving bulk cash carried by couriers on commercial flights were reported less often but also involved U.S. currency destined for California and Las Vegas; however, amounts seized from couriers were more disparate, ranging from $20,000 to as much as $200,000.[43]

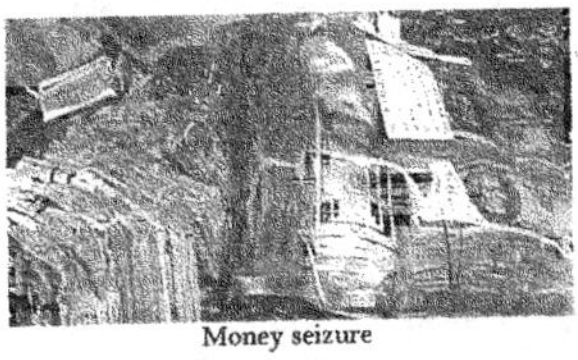

Money seizure

The Hawaii HIDTA Money Laundering Task Force initiated 56 cases and made 11 arrests in 2003, up significantly from 2002 when just 18 significant criminal cases were initiated and 5 arrests were made. Also in 2003 the Money Laundering Task Force seized seven automobiles, $175,000 in U.S. currency, and $966,000 in assets, again showing dramatic improvement over 2002 seizures of one automobile and $205,000 in U.S. currency.[44] Reporting from all other Hawaii HIDTA initiatives combined shows additional seizures of more than 50 automobiles, over $2½ million more in U.S. currency, and assets including a boat, two motorcycles, a plasma television, a DVD player, surveillance equipment, and more than $350,000 worth of jewelry.[45]

MARIJUANA PRODUCTION

Hawaii has long been one of the foremost production areas for marijuana and for high potency marijuana in particular. With the growing demand for better quality marijuana nationwide, cannabis cultivators in Hawaii can only gain in the lucrative marijuana market by continually refining ongoing methods of cultivation. Cultivators, especially those involved with indoor operations, appear to be ready to maximize the productivity of growing environments and to experiment with different strains of cannabis plants to increase potency and yield higher profits.

Despite agricultural and weather conditions that make Hawaii an optimal location to cultivate cannabis outdoors, small indoor marijuana grow operations do exist in Hawaii. These operations typically have yielded only enough marijuana for personal use or very limited distribution; however, intelligence indicates that some cannabis cultivators in Hawaii are using hydroponic equipment, importing marijuana seeds, and cross-pollinating plants, likely attempting to increase the quality, quantity, and value of their product. The Hawaii HIDTA is working to identify these indoor and hydroponic operations, the cultivators involved, and the sources of the marijuana seeds supplied.

According to the State Attorney General's *Crime in Hawaii 2002* report, marijuana has accounted for most drug sale/manufacturing arrests among juveniles since 1993. What is notable, however, is that after fluctuating relatively narrowly during most of that period with a low of 27 (2001) and a high of 56 arrests (2000), juvenile marijuana-related arrests escalated to 144 in 2002.[46] The escalation in drug sale/manufacturing arrests for marijuana accounts for the large increase in juvenile arrests for all drug sale/manufacturing in 2002 when 165 juveniles were arrested in Hawaii compared with just 54 in 2001.

Marijuana as Medicine

In 2000 the Governor of Hawaii signed into law a measure to approve the possession and use of marijuana for medical purposes. The use and enforcement of this law has caused problems for law enforcement, particularly in differentiating illegal and legitimate marijuana grow operations and in ascertaining whether medical users are legitimately prescribed. Moreover, law enforcement in many states that allow patients to use marijuana for medical purposes believes the promotion of marijuana as medicine is an important contributing factor in increased marijuana use.[47] Interestingly, a study by the Hawaii Department of Health, Alcohol and Drug Abuse Division, shows that between 2000 and 2002 the prevalence of daily marijuana use among Hawaii's students did rise for eighth (1.5% to 1.6%), tenth (3.4% to 4.4%), and twelfth graders (4.6% to 4.8%).[48]

Outlook and Predictions

Seizures of methamphetamine laboratories will increase in Hawaii as training of law enforcement results in the identification of laboratories previously unrecognized as such. The Hawaii HIDTA and participating agencies have worked diligently to train law enforcement in methamphetamine laboratory identification and clandestine laboratory safety, and reaction from newly trained personnel indicates that methamphetamine laboratories had been encountered often but not recognized for what they were.[49] In addition, the training has alerted law enforcement to concealment methods that, because they were previously unknown to law enforcement, likely resulted in hidden methamphetamine laboratories being overlooked.

The HIDTA's Clandestine Laboratory Response Team continues to work to ensure that all county teams are completely certified and fully outfitted with operational equipment; however, as the number of methamphetamine laboratories seized rises, law enforcement resources—personnel and financial—will be spread thin. Another consequence to the state of Hawaii will be concurrent increases in health costs as previously "ignored" victims also are identified and treated.

Maritime seizures of illicit drugs will increase. Many in law enforcement consider that a large volume of drugs are potentially transported to Hawaii by sea. After all, Hawaii's economy is dependent on commercial maritime imports for nearly 80 percent of the goods consumed in the state,[50] and even conservative estimates suggest that 20–30 percent of illicit drugs are transported to the state via maritime means, including commerical vessels, containerized cargo, crew member or passenger couriers, private yachts, fishing vessels, and inter-island vessels. While the Hawaii HIDTA has received increased intelligence regarding maritime transportation of illicit drugs in general, actual drug seizures have proven difficult to achieve without specific intelligence because of the volume of maritime traffic through Hawaii and the low rate of ship container inspections.

This should change following the July 1, 2004, deadline given to U.S. and global ports to create counterterrorism systems and to implement all measures required by the Maritime Transportation Security Act (MTSA).[51] The MTSA requires numerous measures designed to improve port security, and if a port does not meet security standards, ships leaving that port will not be allowed to enter U.S. ports. Also, if a ship does not meet security standards, or has visited a port that does not meet standards in its last 10 stops, it will not be allowed to enter U.S. ports.[52]

Although the MTSA is designed to counter terrorism, a collateral effect will be an increase in drug seizures in the near term as the implementation of MTSA measures will necessitate a rise in the rate of ship and container inspections. Also, while physically searching every container that arrives at the Port of Honolulu or one of Hawaii's nine other commercial ports[53] is impractical, both from a manpower and economic standpoint, the increased frequency of inspections likely will result in the development of indicators to help identify high-risk containers, thus facilitating seizures without the need for specific intelligence.

Successful prosecutions of drug distributors will increase provided that a proposed bill that would make it easier for law enforcement to use wiretaps against suspected criminals becomes law. The Hawaii State Senate and House have been deliberating the bill, putting it in position to move out of the legislature and become law. Although the latest draft of the bill no longer contains a section that would allow law enforcement to conduct "emergency" wiretapping and has dropped other model legislation provisions, the main thrust of the bill, eliminating the requirement for an adversarial hearing before authorizing a wiretap, is intact. Successful passing of the wiretap bill into law would also allow the use of evidence gathered in a federal investigation to be used in state cases, which will result in the prosecution of many drug distributors who do not meet federal thresholds.[54]

Recognition of the dangers crystal methamphetamine poses to public health and safety has caused many in Hawaii to open up to the idea that reducing the problems associated with crystal methamphetamine and other illicit drugs requires not only treatment and prevention for drug users but meaningful consequences for those supplying the drugs. The future impact of Hawaii HIDTA initiatives will be measured in the continuing and increasing seizures of illicit drugs and proceeds as well as the arrests and successful prosecutions of those responsible for transporting drugs and drug proceeds through Hawaii's airports, parcel facilities, and ports.

Appendix

Selected Substance Abuse Indicators for Hawaii

Table A1: Estimated Numbers (in thousands) Reporting Past Month Use of Marijuana and Past Year Use of Cocaine in Hawaii National Household Survey on Drug Abuse, 2000 & 2001*

Drug	12–17	18–25	26 or older	12 or older
Marijuana (past month)	9	18	29	55
Cocaine (past year)	2	4	6	12

* Data are compiled from 24 months of reporting. Figures in this table for marijuana and cocaine cannot be compared against one another because of the different prevalence rates reported.

Table A2: Percentages Reporting Past Month Use of Marijuana and Past Year Use of Cocaine in Hawaii National Household Survey on Drug Abuse, 2001*

Drug/Year	12–17	18–25	26 or older	12 or older
Marijuana (past month)				
00–01	9.32	15.11	3.95	5.82
99–00	8.72	14.35	4.48	6.07
Cocaine (past year)				
00–01	1.69	3.79	0.078	1.23
99–00	1.61	3.72	1.54	1.81

* Figures in this table for marijuana and cocaine cannot be compared against one another because of the different prevalence rates reported.

Table A3: Percentage of High School Students Reporting Lifetime*/Current Use Hawaii Youth Risk Behavior Survey, 2001**

Drug	Lifetime Use		Drug	Current Use
Methamphetamine	6.5		Marijuana	20.5
Heroin	2.5		Cocaine	2.4

* Current use data are not provided for methamphetamine or heroin. Figures for methamphetamine and heroin cannot be compared those for marijuana and cocaine because of the different prevalence rates reported.

** YRBS data for 1999, the last year in which the biennial survey was conducted, are not included in this table because Hawaii results in that year were weighted, while data for 2001 are unweighted, thus precluding any trend analysis.

Table A4: Hawaii Treatment Admissions by Primary Substance of Abuse, 2001–2002

Year	Amphetamines*	Marijuana	Cocaine (smoked)	Cocaine (other route)	Heroin
2002	2,238	1,432	268	70	217
2001	2,089	1,429	297	63	196
2000	1,833	1,344	338	78	371

* Category comprises methamphetamine, including ice, and other amphetamines (e.g., Ritalin). Nationally, methamphetamine accounted for more than 80 percent of amphetamine-related treatment admissions.

Table A5: Hawaii Drug Prices, 2003[55]

	Gram	1/8th oz	Oz	Pound	Kilo
Crystal methamphetamine	$200-$300	$300-$600	$1,700-$,3000	$20,000-$30,000	$40,000-$70,000
Marijuana	$25	$100-$200	$400-$800	$6,000-$9,000	N/A
Powder cocaine	$100-$120	$250-$350	$1,000-$1,500	$13,500-$25,000	$24,000-$52,000
Crack cocaine	$100-$250	N/A	$1,000-$1,500	$24,000	N/A
Heroin	$200-$300	N/A	$2,500-$5,000	$50,000	$100,000

The Hawaii HIDTA would like to thank the following agencies that were instrumental in the development of the 2005 Threat Assessment. A special thank you to the National Drug Intelligence Center for their assistance in preparing this report.

Bureau of Alcohol, Tobacco and Firearms
Bureau of Immigration and Customs Enforcement
Community Epidemiology Work Group
Department of Defense
Department of Public Safety, Narcotics Enforcement Division
Drug Enforcement Administration
Federal Bureau of Investigation
Hawaii County Police Department
Hawaii State Department of the Attorney General
Hawaii State Department of Health
Hawaii State Department of Public Safety
Hawaii National Guard
Honolulu City & County Prosecutor's Office
Honolulu Police Department
Honolulu Weed and Seed Program
Internal Revenue Service
Kauai County Police Department
Maui Police Department
National Drug Intelligence Center
Naval Criminal Investigative Service
Office of National Drug Control Policy
United States Attorney's Office
United States Coast Guard
United States Marshall Service
United States Postal Inspection Service
Western States Information Network

Endnotes

[1] Ice methamphetamine, also known as glass, shabu, or batu, is a pure, highly addictive form of methamphetamine resembling shards of ice. It is the product of the process of recrystallizing powdered methamphetamine in a solvent such as water, methanol, ethanol, isopropanol, or acetone to remove impurities. Ice typically is smoked using either a glass pipe, an empty aluminum can, a piece of aluminum foil, or a light bulb. NDIC, *National Drug Threat Assessment 2004*, April 2004. Definition supplied by the Drug Enforcement Administration.
[2] Hawaii HIDTA Threat Analysis, "Transportation of Drugs into Hawaii."
[3] "How Hawaii is really different," *Pacific Business News*, February 16, 2004; Asia-Pacific Distance Calculator, http://russia.shaps.hawaii.edu
[4] *The State of Hawaii Data Book 2002*, Table 13.04 and 7.03, respectively.
[5] *The State of Hawaii Data Book 2002*, Table 10.03
[6] Hawaii Agriculture Statistics Service, *Agriculture Contributions to Hawaii's Economy2000*
[7] Given the fluidity of Hawaii's DTOs, particularly local DTOs, among which membership changes continually, new organizations are established, or an existing organization merges with another, these numbers are by no means concrete, but they do represent a reasonable attempt at quantification.
[8] Hawaii HIDTA 2002 Annual Report, April 2003. South America is not considered a source area for methamphetamine. It may be included in these results as part of a category. The methamphetamine samples tested likely were for either California or Mexico only.
[9] Hawaii HIDTA Threat Analysis, "Transportation of Drugs into Hawaii."
[10] Hawaii HIDTA Annual Threat Assessment 2004.
[11] Office of National Drug Control Policy, Pulse Check, November 2002.
[12] Hawaii HIDTA CY 2003 Initiative Stats, Drug Seizures spreadsheet, "HATF" Year End Totals; HATF submission of accomplishments, emailed March 25, 2004.
[13] Hawaii HIDTA 2002 Annual Report, April 2003.
[14] Hawaii HIDTA CY 2003 Initiative Stats, Drug Seizures spreadsheet, "International" Year End Totals; FITF/AG submission of accomplishments.
[15] Office of National Drug Control Policy, Pulse Check, November 2002.
[16] NDIC, *National Drug Threat Assessment 2003*, January 2003.
[17] Data for 2003 from Hawaii DCE/SP Coordinator, Hawaii; data for 2002 from the *Sourcebook of Criminal Justice Statistics 2002*, Table 4.38.
[18] *The State of Hawaii Data Book 2002*, Table 20.01.
[19] Data for 2003 from Hawaii DCE/SP Coordinator, Hawaii; data for 2002 from the *Sourcebook of Criminal Justice Statistics 2002*, Table 4.38.
[20] Data for 2003 from Hawaii DCE/SP Coordinator, Hawaii; data for 2002 from the *Sourcebook of Criminal Justice Statistics 2002*, Table 4.38.
[21] Hawaii HIDTA CY 2003 Initiative Stats, Drug Seizures spreadsheet, "HATF" Year End Totals; HATF submission of accomplishments, emailed March 25, 2004.
[22] Hawaii HIDTA 2002 Annual Report, April 2003.
[23] Hawaii HIDTA CY 2003 Initiative Stats, Drug Seizures spreadsheet, "International" Year End Totals; FITF/AG submission of accomplishments; Telephone conversation with BICE SSA.
[24] Hawaii HIDTA 2002 Annual Report, April 2003.
[25] Hawaii HIDTA CY 2003 Initiative Stats, Drug Seizures spreadsheet, "HATF" Year End Totals; HATF submission of accomplishments, emailed March 25, 2004; Hawaii HIDTA 2002 Annual Report, April 2003.
[26] Hawaii HIDTA CY 2003 Initiative Stats, Drug Seizures spreadsheet, "International" Year End Totals; FITF/AG submission of accomplishments.
[27] Hawaii HIDTA 2002 Annual Report, April 2003.
[28] Hawaii HIDTA CY 2003 Initiative Stats, Drug Seizures spreadsheet, "HATF" Year End Totals; HATF submission of accomplishments, emailed March 25, 2004.
[29] Hawaii HIDTA 2002 Annual Report, April 2003.

[30] Hawaii HIDTA CY 2003 Initiative Stats, Drug Seizures spreadsheet, "International" Year End Totals; FITF/AG submission of accomplishments; Telephone conversation with BICE SSA.
[31] Hawaii HIDTA 2002 Annual Report, April 2003. Drug-related crime statistics are not captured by the State of Hawaii.
[32] Hawaii State Department of the Attorney General, Crime Prevention Justice Prevention Assistance Division, *Crime in Hawaii 2002*, October 2003, Executive Summary. Crime rates are based on the number of crimes per 100,000 residents. The Uniform Crime Reporting program uses resident population to calculate crime rates for all states; however, because of Hawaii's relatively small resident population and large de facto population (includes residents, tourists, and non-resident military personnel), crime rates based on resident population are much higher than rates based on the actual number of people in the state.
[33] Hawaii State Department of the Attorney General, Crime Prevention Justice Prevention Assistance Division, *Crime in Hawaii 2002*, October 2003, Executive Summary. The violent index crime rate in Hawaii rose 2.7 percent in 2002.
[34] "Aiona is gathering forces to form isle "ice" battle plan," *Honolulu Star-Bulletin*, June 6, 2003.
[35] "Maui officer shoots and kills man at Kihei beach," *Honolulu Advertiser*, March 2, 2004.
[36] Drug-related cases can involve more than one drug; hence, the sum of cases broken out by specific drug total more than the number of all drug-related cases.
[37] Hawaii HIDTA CY 2003 Initiative Stats, Drug Seizures spreadsheet, Year End Totals.
[38] Data for 2003 from Hawaii DCE/SP Coordinator, Hawaii.
[39] Hawaii State Department of the Attorney General, Crime Prevention Justice Prevention Assistance Division, *Crime in Hawaii 2002*, October 2003, Part II Arrests by Offense, State of Hawaii, 1993-2002 Adults & Juveniles. The data compiled in this report is based on Uniform Crime Reporting.
[40] Four different drug categories are reported in Uniform Crime Reporting: opium or cocaine (or their derivatives, including morphine, heroin, and codeine), marijuana, synthetic narcotics (including Demerol and methadone), and nonnarcotic drugs (such as barbiturates and Benzedrines). Because of the groupings (such as combining opium and cocaine) as well as the variation in reporting (LSD, for example, might be included in either "synthetic narcotics" or "nonnarcotics"), it is impossible to analyze trends except for marijuana as a proportion of all drug arrests. Nonetheless, the decline in opium or cocaine-related arrests in Hawaii and the concurrent rise in the nonnarcotic-related arrests may be suggestive of a demand shift away from more traditional drugs of abuse (e.g., heroin and cocaine) and toward drugs perceived as safer or "softer" (e.g., designer and prescription drugs).
[41] Hawaii HIDTA CY 2003 Initiative Stats, Case Info spreadsheet. Arrest and initiated case totals reflect the sum of those reported only by the Hawaii Airport Task Force and the HI-IMPACT groups on the islands of Oahu, Hawaii, Maui, and Kauai.
[42] Kahului Airport provides domestic overseas and inter-island commercial service.
[43] Hawaii HIDTA CY 2003 Initiative Stats, Drug Seizures spreadsheet, "HATF" Year End Totals; HATF submission of accomplishments, emailed March 25, 2004.
[44] Hawaii HIDTA CY 2003 Initiative Stats, Drug Seizures/Case Info spreadsheets, "Money Laundering" Year End Totals.
[45] Hawaii HIDTA CY 2003 Initiative Stats, Drug Seizures spreadsheet, Year End Totals.
[46] Hawaii State Department of the Attorney General, Crime Prevention Justice Prevention Assistance Division, *Crime in Hawaii 2002*, October 2003, Part II Arrests by Offense, Juveniles, State of Hawaii, 1993-2002. The data compiled in this report is based on Uniform Crime Reporting.
[47] Office of National Drug Control Policy, Pulse Check, January 2004.
[48] State of Hawaii Department of Health, Alcohol and Drug Abuse Division, *The 2002 Hawaii Student Alcohol, Tobacco, and Other Drug Study (1987-2002): Hawaii Adolescent Prevention and Treatment Needs Assessment*, 2003, Tables 3 & 4. The 2002 rates for daily prevalence among eighth and tenth graders in Hawaii (1.6% & 4.4%, respectively) are higher than the nationwide rates for those grades (1.2% & 3.9%). Daily rates for Hawaii's twelfth graders are lower (4.8% vs. 6.0%).
[49] Presentation by Investigator Dean Yamamoto, Narcotics and Enforcement Division, State of Hawaii, March 2004.
[50] Hawaii HIDTA Threat Analysis, "Transportation of Drugs into Hawaii." Over 95 percent of the volume of legitimate imports arrives from Pacific Rim nations as a natural consequence of Hawaii's location in the Pacific Ocean.

[51] President Bush signed the MTSA into law on November 25, 2002, as part of the U.S. response to the September 11, 2001, terrorist attacks The United Nations International Maritime Organization adopted a global code shortly after the law was signed.

[52] "Protecting America's Ports: Maritime Transportation Security Act of 2002," U.S. Department of Homeland Security, Office of the Press Secretary, press release and fact sheets, July 1, 2003.

[53] *The State of Hawaii Data Book 2002*, Table 18.45.

[54] "Bill to ease wiretaps advances," *Honolulu Advertiser*, April 2, 2004; "House, Senate panels OK bills to ease wiretap use," *Honolulu Star-Bulletin*, March 5, 2004. On March 4, 2004, the Senate Judiciary Committee killed a proposed bill to allow consensual encounters.

[55] Prices as indicated in *Narcotics Digest Weekly*, "Illicit Drug Prices, July 2003-December 2003," Volume 2, Number 50, NDIC

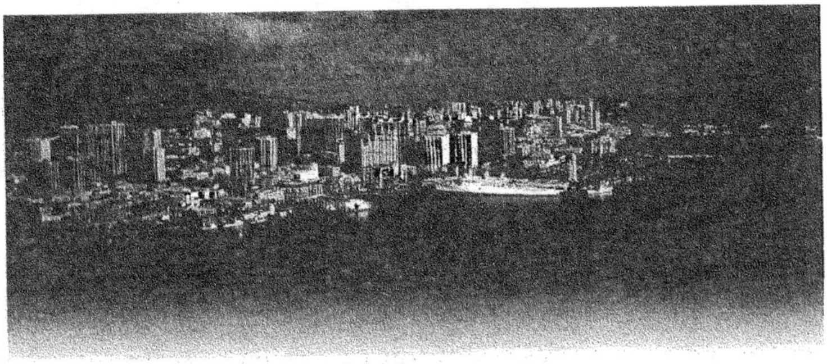

2003 ANNUAL REPORT

Dedication

ANO`AI! MAI KA `AINA NUI AKU A KA MOKUPUNI NEI ME NA AHUPUA`A MAI UKA A KE KAI I NA KANAKA WIWO`OLE APAU. E HEA MAI NEI I IA MAHALO NUI NO KO `OUKOU HANA KUPONO ME KA `IKE PONO I `OLE PAU `AI KA HANA `INO, KE KAUMANA, A ME KA NA`AU PO I HO`OKUKULI `IA E NA KANAKA E LAWE HEWA `ANA I NA LA`AU INO I HAWAI`I NEI

"`O ka hana `ole `ana o na kanaka kupono ka mea i pono `ai no ka lanakila`ana i ka mea `ino."........*Edmund Burke*

ENGLISH TRANSLATION:

TO THE MANY STATE, LOCAL, & FEDERAL PARTNERS WHO TOGETHER SHAPED THE HAWAII HIDTA; AND THE GOOD MEN AND WOMEN ACTIVELY ENGAGED IN RIDDING OUR ISLAND HOME FROM THE SCOURGE, VIOLENCE AND HUMAN MISERY TIED TO ILLICIT DRUG TRAFFICKING.

"The only thing necessary for the triumph of evil is for good men to do nothing."........*Edmund Burke*

HAWAI'I HIDTA

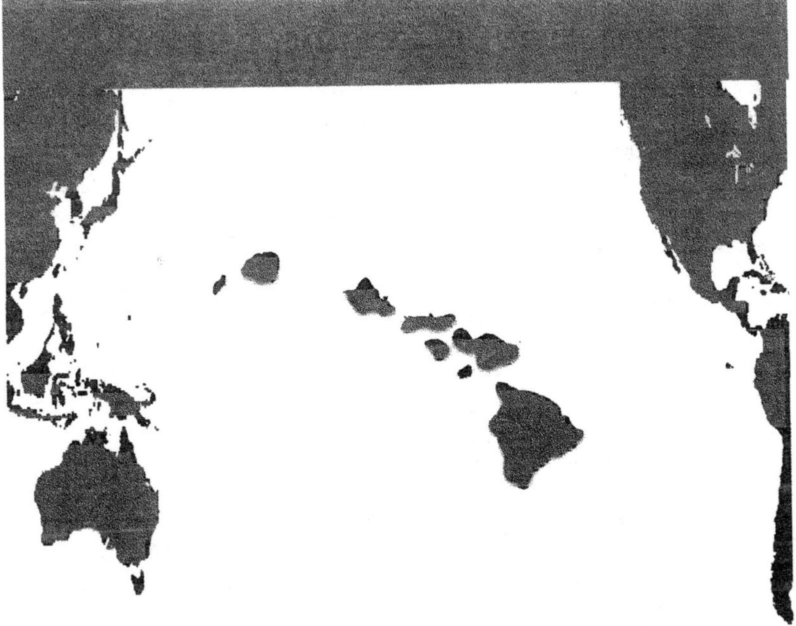

A LOOK AT THE MISSION, PROGRAMS, & ACHIEVEMENTS OF THE HAWAII HIDTA FOR CALENDAR YEAR 2003

This document and the information contained herein are unclassified.

Table of Contents

Introduction

Section I.

A. By design, significant effort is made to collocate and commingle Hawaii HIDTA resources. In fostering interagency cooperation and sharing of strategic and tactical information, the Hawaii HIDTA provides a comprehensive response to illicit drug activity by bringing together all available law enforcement resources in a united front. Success of the Hawaii HIDTA is measured in part by its ability to facilitate greater efficiency, effectiveness and cooperation among external participating agencies at the local, state and federal level, thereby yielding tangible, measurable results.

B. Data covers the period of *January 1 to December 31, 2003 (CY 2003)*

C. FY *2003* (*last full fiscal year*) Budget: *$ 2.5 million*
Supplemental for Title III and ISC enhancement: $ 1 million

D. Designated in *June 1999*

E. Geographic Area of Responsibility: *State of Hawaii- Hawaii, Honolulu, Kauai & Maui counties*

F. Mission Statement:

At the crossroad of the Pacific and gateway into the continental United States, the Hawaii HIDTA's participating agencies work together through enhanced coordination and integrated initiatives to disrupt and dismantle illicit drug distribution, production, money laundering, transportation, & trafficking within the region.

Executive Summary

Section II.

The year in review has seen Hawaii and the U.S. Territories of the Pacific beset with a myriad of illicit drug challenges. Illegal use and trafficking of crystal methamphetamine, commonly referred to as ICE, has reached epidemic proportions straining resources to the breaking point. State Legislators held hearings to explore the problem. The Governor and Lieutenant Governor crisscrossed the state in a series of town hall meetings. Communities fed up with the problems, violence, and crime associated with crystal methamphetamine addiction waved signs and demonstrated. In September a statewide Drug Control Strategy Summit was convened involving law enforcement, educators, treatment providers, and community leaders. The summit was followed by an unprecedented hour long simulcast of a documentary that ran, commercial free, on 11 television stations statewide. The award winning documentary addressed the "ICE epidemic" and its associated violence/crime, domestic abuse, child endangerment, and the drain on public resources. In CY2003 the 21 voting and advisory law enforcement agencies that make up the Hawaii HIDTA were highlighted as one of the few bright spots; for encouraging greater efficiency, interagency cooperation, sharing of information, and providing a unified front in combating drug trafficking.

TO GENERATE MOMENTUM, HIDTA HAS IDENTIFIED THREE GOALS TO ACCOMPLISH ITS MISSION OF REDUCING DRUG AVAILABILITY. THESE GOALS ARE SUPPORTED BY INTELLIGENCE DRIVEN DRUG TASK FORCES AIMED AT ELIMINATING OR REDUCING DOMESTIC DRUG TRAFFICKING AND ITS HARMFUL CONSEQUENCES, THROUGH ENHANCEMENT AND COORDINATION OF DRUG TRAFFICKING CONTROL EFFORTS AMONG FEDERAL, STATE AND LOCAL LAW ENFORCEMENT AGENCIES.

GOAL ONE. REDUCE DRUG AVAILABILITY BY ELIMINATING OR DISRUPTING DRUG TRAFFICKING ORGANIZATIONS.

The illegal drug market in the United States is one of the most profitable in the world. The prices in Hawaii and the Pacific Region are twice to four times as high as the continental U.S., which creates an attractive market for drug traffickers and organizations from both the continental U.S. and Asian countries.

GOAL TWO. REDUCE THE HARMFUL CONSEQUENCES OF DRUG TRAFFICKING

Drug trafficking causes various problems in the community and negatively impacts the quality and safety of life for citizens exposed to the dangers of the drug culture.

GOAL THREE. IMPROVE THE EFFICIENCY AND EFFECTIVENESS OF LAW ENFORCEMENT ORGANIZATIONS.

The guiding theme of the HIDTA Program is to attack drug trafficking from all angles, combining available resources from federal, state and local law enforcement organizations.

MATRIX

The Office of National Drug Control Policy (ONDCP) and the National HIDTA Program Office are mandated by the Office of Management and Budget (OMB) to accurately account for the performance of the HIDTA program. The performance measurement process can be very complex and, at times, overwhelming. The HIDTA Matrix is designed to keep the process simple, direct and understandable. The Matrix is a grid system based on the three goals. The grid system:

1. Identifies primary threats by geographic area;
2. Develops desired goals to counter the threats;
3. Assigns responsibility to accomplish the desired goals;
4. Captures output measurements;
5. Illustrates the program's outcomes.

The matrix based system is designed to hold HIDTAs accountable for what they do and establish a mechanism to measure their performance. The Hawaii HIDTA Matrix is located in section III. Parts of the matrix, as appropriate, are consolidated and/or broken out for the various sections of this annual report.

INVESTIGATIVE SUBSYSTEM

The investigative subsystem consists of eight investigative groups, two interdiction groups, one fugitive task force, and one safe neighborhoods strike force. Accomplishing goal one is one of the primary responsibilities of the Investigative Subsystem. The investigative task forces are most closely aligned with law enforcement goals of impacting the crime rate through arrests and seizures, and thereby reducing drug availability.

COMBINED HAWAII HIDTA GOALS	matrix – goal 1 (consolidated)	Goal	Actual	%
	TARGET DRUG DISTRIBUTION ORGANIZATIONS AND DISMANTLE OR DISRUPT THOSE TARGETED	10	34	340%
	TARGET DRUG MANUFACTURING ORGANIZATIONS AND DISMANTLE OR DISRUPT THOSE TARGETED	4	4	100%
	CLEAR WARRANTS FOR DRUG CHARGES	100	290	290%
	ARREST ARMED VIOLENT OFFENDERS WITH A NARCOTICS NEXUS	45	95	211%
	ARREST INDIVIDUALS WHO SMUGGLE NARCOTICS THROUGH AIRPORTS	50	47	94%
	INSPECT PARCELS	1000	10,000	1000%
	SEIZE PARCELS	100	60	60%
	TARGET DTOs FOR MONEY LAUNDERING CHARGES	1	1	100%
	SEIZE ILLICIT DRUG RELATED ASSETS	$1,000,000	2,510,906	251%
	ERADICATE MARIJUANA PLANTS	50,000	392,276	784.5%
	SEIZE FIREARMS	110	162	147.2%

Section 3 HIDTA Matrix – consolidated goals and outcomes for all Investigative Initiatives

COMBINED HAWAII HIDTA GOALS	matrix – goal 2 (consolidated)	Goal	Actual	%
	SEIZE FIREARMS FROM VIOLENT DRUG TRAFFICKERS	110	162	147.2%
	CLEAR WARRANTS FOR DRUG CHARGES	100	290	290%

Section 3 HIDTA Matrix – consolidated goals and outcomes for community consequences

COMBINED HAWAII HIDTA GOALS	matrix – goal 3 (consolidated)	Goal	Actual	%
	ACHIEVE AND MAINTAIN 100% PARTICIPATION BY LAW ENFORCEMENT AGENCIES IN THE WSIN DECONFLICTION SERVICES	100%	100%	100%
	SUBMIT CASE/SUBJECT DECONFLICTIONS AMONG HIDTA INITIATIVES AND PARTICIPATING AGENCIES	9000	9393	104.3%
	SUBMIT EVENT DECONFLICTIONS AMONG HIDTA INITIATIVES AND PARTICIPATING AGENCIES	1400	1333	95.2%

Section 3 HIDTA Matrix- consolidated goals and outcomes for oversight and support

HI-IMPACT

The HI-IMPACT initiative is the central investigative element of the Hawaii HIDTA whose focus is to disrupt and dismantle drug trafficking organizations (DTOs). HI-IMPACT utilizes state-of-the-art techniques to conduct complex multi-jurisdictional investigations.

INTERDICTION

The two Hawaii Interdiction Task Forces are charged with stopping the transport of illicit drugs as they enter through Hawaii's airports and harbors. The Interdiction initiative focuses on chokepoints and is the region's first line of defense.

MONEY LAUNDERING/ASSET FORFEITURE

The Money Laundering initiative disrupts and dismantles DTOs by making an impact on their ability to function, by seizing the money they use to operate and the assets they acquire with illicit drug proceeds.

SAFE NEIGHBORHOODS

By removing guns from the street, the Safe Neighborhoods Initiative targets chronic violent drug offenders who have a significant impact on the amount of crime occurring in Hawaii.

FUGITIVE INITIATIVE

The Fugitive Task Force assists other HIDTA initiatives in crippling the drug trade and related crime in Hawaii and throughout the Pacific region by bringing fugitives to justice.

SUPPORT INITIATIVES

The Hawaii HIDTA's support initiatives, one that oversees clandestine lab readiness and one that concentrates on successfully prosecuting drug traffickers, provide support for specific aspects of all three goals. The support initiatives are broad based and provide services and support to other initiatives and HIDTA functions.

COMBINED HAWAII HIDTA GOALS	matrix – goal 1 (consolidated)	Goal	Actual	%
	ASSIST IN THE INDICTMENT AND PROSECUTION OF DRUG TRAFFICKING AND/OR MONEY LAUNDERING ORGANIZATIONS	2	0	0
	FORFEIT $1,000,000 IN ILLICIT DRUG RELATED ASSETS	$1,000,000	$1,237,740	123.7%

Section 3 HIDTA Matrix – consolidated goals and outcomes for all Investigative Initiatives

COMBINED HAWAII HIDTA GOALS	matrix – goal 2 (consolidated)	Goal	Actual	%
	PROPOSE MODEL LEGISLATION	2	2	100%

Section 3 HIDTA Matrix – consolidated goals and outcomes for community consequences

COMBINED HAWAII HIDTA GOALS	matrix – goal 3 (consolidated)	Goal	Actual	%
	ACHIEVE AND MAINTAIN 100% PARTICIPATION BY LAW ENFORCEMENT AGENCIES IN THE WSIN DECONFLICTION SERVICES	100%	100%	100%
	COORDINATE WITH CLAN LAB RESPONSE COORDINATORS AT FEDERAL, STATE, AND LOCAL AGENCIES	100%	100%	100%
	SPONSOR QUARTERLY CLANDESTINE LAB TRAINING PROGRAMS	4	3	75%
	CONDUCT MONTHLY MEETINGS WITH HIDTA INITIATIVES	12	0	0

Section 3 HIDTA Matrix – consolidated goals and outcomes for oversight and support

CLANDESTINE LAB COORDINATION

The Clan Lab support initiative works with law enforcement personnel throughout the State of Hawaii to provide oversight, consolidated training and coordination for a first response to clandestine laboratories involved in manufacturing and/or converting crystal methamphetamine and other illicit drugs.

PROSECUTORIAL INITIATIVE

A number of Hawaii state laws impede the ability of local law enforcement agencies to effectively counter drug trafficking. During CY2003, the county prosecutor assigned to the Prosecutorial Initiative prepared testimony for the state legislature and various committees in support of legislation to conform the state's electronic surveillance and consensual encounter laws to federal statute.

INTELLIGENCE SUBSYSTEM

The intelligence subsystem is the main focus of the Hawaii HIDTA. It provides a communication infrastructure that promotes information sharing between participating law enforcement agencies. The analysis and deconfliction of strategic and operational intelligence is critical for effectively attacking drug traffickers and reducing drug availability. The Investigative Support Center (ISC) is the main body of the intelligence subsystem and consists of the Investigative Support Group and the Strategic Intelligence Support Group. In addition, the Regional Western States Information Network (WSIN) Coordinator and staff are housed under the intelligence subsystem umbrella.

COMBINED HAWAII HIDTA GOALS	matrix – goal 3 (consolidated)	Goal	Actual	%
	ACHIEVE AND MAINTAIN 100% PARTICIPATION BY LAW ENFORCEMENT AGENCIES IN THE WSIN DECONFLICTION SERVICES	100%	100%	100%
	SUBMIT CASE/SUBJECT DECONFLICTIONS AMONG HIDTA INITIATIVES AND PARTICIPATING AGENCIES	9000	9393	104.3%
	ISC TO CONDUCT DATABASE QUERIES	4000	3202	80%
	ISC TO PROVIDE INTELLIGENCE PROFILES	100	390	390%
	COMPLETE REQUESTS FOR CASE ASSISTANCE	20	24	120%
	PROVIDE ANALYTICAL PRODUCTS (TOLL ANALYSES, LINK ANALYSES, GRAPHS, CHARTS, PROFILES, ETC)	3,000	4030	134.3%
	DEVELOP AN ACTIVE MEANS OF COMMUNICATING WITH PACIFIC BASIN/RIM LAW ENFORCEMENT	100%	25%	25%
	PROVIDE ELECTRONIC LINK FROM ISC TO NEIGHBOR ISLANDS VIA WSIN SECURE INTRANET	100%	100%	100%
	SHARE INTELLIGENCE WITH HIDTAS/LEAS OUTSIDE OF HAWAII	*	*	*

Section 3 HIDTA Matrix – consolidated goals and outcomes for oversight and support

*All three HIDTA subsystems shared intelligence with HIDTAs/LEAs on the continental U.S. relating to controlled deliveries and joint investigations. Contacts with counterparts on the continental U.S. occur on a daily basis. This 2003 goal does not lend itself to measurement under the Matrix system.

INVESTIGATIVE SUPPORT CENTER (ISC)

The ISC facilitates information sharing, intelligence collection, analysis and dissemination among Hawaii HIDTA's participating agencies and initiatives. The ISC provides technical and strategic support to HIDTA participants and other stakeholders (law enforcement & non-law enforcement) engaged in the counterdrug effort. Intelligence led policing is the cornerstone of the ONDCP/HIDTA program.

WSIN

The Western States Information Network (WSIN) maintains a criminal intelligence database and provides subject and critical event deconfliction for the Hawaii HIDTA. WSIN serves as the intelligence communications platform and computer server/hub between islands. WSIN functions as the 24/7 HIDTA Watch Center via phone access through Sacramento and the San Diego HIDTA Narcotics Information Network.

ADMINISTRATIVE SUPPORT SUBSYSTEM

The administrative support subsystem has two components- the Management and Coordination Initiative and the Training Initiative. Efficiency of the Hawaii HIDTA largely results from the Management and Coordination Initiative while effectiveness is addressed in part by the Training Initiative. Both initiatives support all other Hawaii HIDTA initiatives in their efforts to combat drug trafficking and reduce its harmful consequences.

	matrix – goal 3 (consolidated)	Goal	Actual	%
COMBINED HAWAII HIDTA GOALS	ACHIEVE AND MAINTAIN 100% PARTICIPATION BY LAW ENFORCEMENT AGENCIES IN THE WSIN DECONFLICTION SERVICES	100%	100%	100%
	SPONSOR QUARTERLY TRAINING PROGRAMS FOR REGIONAL AND/OR SPECIALIZED TRAINING	4	10	250%
	DEVELOP PARTNERSHIPS WITH EXISTING TRAINING COORDINATORS AT FEDERAL, STATE AND LOCAL AGENCIES	100%	100%	100%
	DEVELOP & MAINTAIN HIDTA TRAINING DATABASE	100%	100%	100%
	DISSEMINATE EXISTING TRAINING OPPORTUNITIES FROM OTHER AGENCIES & OUT-SOURCES TO HIDTA PERSONNEL	100%	100%	100%
	PROVIDE COLLOCATION FOR HIDTA INITIATIVES	100%*	100%*	100%*
	MEET IN EXECUTIVE SESSION TO COORDINATE HAWAII HIDTA ACTIVITIES	6	6	100%
	ATTAIN ONDCP/NHPO DEVELOPMENTAL STANDARDS	100%	95%	95%
	TRACK FISCAL EXPENDITURES OF INITIATIVES TO ENSURE COMPLIANCE WITH POLICIES	100%	100%	100%
	CONDUCT FISCAL AUDITS OF ALL INITIATIVES	100%	100%	100%
	IMPLEMENT & CONDUCT HAWAII HIDTA INTERNAL REVIEW PROGRAM	100%	100%	100%
	MEET QUARTERLY WITH INITIATIVE AND PARTICIPATING AGENCY SUPERVISORS	4	4	100%
	PREPARE THE ANNUAL REPORT, THREAT ASSESSMENT, STRATEGY AND BUDGET	100%	100%	100%

Section 3 HIDTA Matrix – consolidated goals and outcomes for oversight and support

*ONDCP exemptions apply to 4 task forces, because of Hawaii's island makeup and costly office rental market.

MANAGEMENT AND COORDINATION INITIATIVE

The Management and Coordination initiative facilitates the efficient operation of all Hawaii HIDTA initiatives, providing oversight, administrative, and budgetary support in accordance with ONDCP and NHPO, and Hawaii HIDTA Executive Board policies and directives.

TRAINING

The Hawaii HIDTA Training Initiative provides on-site and coordinates off-site training, including training on the continental U.S. The main goal of the training initiative is to provide resources and improve the ability of investigative and analytical personnel to counter drug trafficking and related criminal activity.

Weed and Seed

Hawaii HIDTA Initiatives are sensitive to Operation Weed and Seed, a U.S. Department of Justice initiative designed to reclaim, restore, and rebuild neighborhoods, by "weeding" out the criminal element, then "seeding" the community with services that support neighborhood revitalization. The "weed" component of the strategy requires the active involvement and partnership between residents, businesses and law enforcement.

Organized Crime Drug Enforcement Task Force (OCDETF)

Routinely OCDETF designation is sought for all complex Hawaii HIDTA investigations.

OVERALL ACHIEVEMENT

Based on expected and actual outputs indicated by each Hawaii HIDTA initiative, this graph depicts the percentage of outputs achieved by each HIDTA Program goal. Goal Three has been broken down into two sub-sections: outputs quantified by numerical values and outputs quantified by percentages.

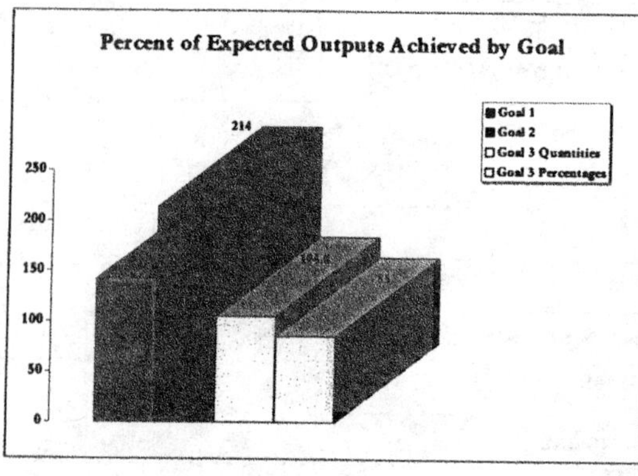

All three HIDTA Program goals have exceeded expectation with the exception of the percentages of Goal Three.

Hawaii HIDTA initiatives have more than doubled their Goal Two expected outputs for CY2003.

The Project Safe Neighborhood initiative and Hawaii Fugitive Task Force are already making their mark, by helping law enforcement and communities get criminals and firearms off the streets. Additionally, the Prosecutorial initiative continued to support legislation aimed at changing the State's wiretap and consensual encounter laws. Progress shown by these initiatives indicates that they are accomplishing their intended goals of reducing harmful consequences associated with drug trafficking.

Goal Three expected outputs measured with numerical values included WSIN deconfliction, information sharing, analytical products, and intelligence support. Actual outputs exceeded expectations and clearly show consistency among all Hawaii HIDTA participating agencies and the ISC in promoting efficient law enforcement efforts. Examined separately, WSIN activity by participating agencies throughout the State of Hawaii has significantly increased over the past two years, and intelligence products from the ISC have increased nearly 2800% since 2001. Realizing the value added by using WSIN and the ISC, each initiative and task force group will raise and surpass their expectations in the coming year.

CY 2004 OUTLOOK

Addition of new initiatives such as the Hawaii Fugitive Task Force and the Safe Neighborhoods Initiative will have a positive impact on the community as they helped to remove drug offenders and firearms from the streets. The "revolving door" of the criminal justice system will no longer apply to these individuals due to the stiff imposition of federal charges and sentences. As career criminals and drug traffickers are imprisoned violent crimes are expected to decline.

HI-IMPACT task force groups saw another successful year with the disruption and/or dismantling of 28 drug distribution and manufacturing organizations, an increase of 164.7% over 2002. By implementing the Performance Management Process and clearly defining goals, it is expected that HI-IMPACT as well as other Hawaii HIDTA initiatives will continue to exceed their expected outcomes. Cooperation among participating agencies will continue to be strong, increasing efficiency and effectiveness.

It is expected that package delivery and mail services will continue to be the primary methods of transporting crystal methamphetamine, heroin, and cocaine to Hawaii from the West Coast and sending drug proceeds back to the Continental U.S. The use of mail drops and private mail box rentals will continue with DTOs using associates or nominees to rent the mail boxes at locations that accept delivery from private parcel delivery services. Crystal methamphetamine will also continue to be smuggled into Hawaii from Asia. The Hawaii HIDTA Aiport Task Force and Foreign Interdiction Initiative will maintain control over their respective chokepoints for illicit drugs entering Hawaii. Continued coordination with law enforcement agencies on the continental U.S. and abroad is expected to lead to increased interdiction efforts and further disruption of drug trafficking organizations worldwide.

Educators, treatment providers, law enforcement, legislators, and communities throughout the State of Hawaii have begun coordinating their efforts to battle crystal methamphetamine trafficking and abuse. However, the methamphetamine-related deaths, number drug arrests, and arrestees testing positive for crystal methamphetamine continue to rise. This information, combined with consistently high purity levels and stable prices, indicates that Hawaii is still battling the "ICE epidemic."

Mandating the use of WSIN among all HIDTA initiatives has created a broad avenue for coordination and information sharing. Understanding the importance of this resource for officer safety and identifying duplications of effort promotes efficiency and effectivness. Developing and coordinating information through the ISC that was once inaccessible has positive implications for law enforcement personnel who may have otherwise lacked pertinent, prosecutable, information regarding drug trafficking organizations.

HIDTA Matrix

Section III.

In accordance with OMB accountability standards and policies, NHPO has developed the Performance Management Process (PMP), which measures program efficiency and effectiveness. The cornerstone of the process is the PMP Matrix, a tool designed to illustrate the Performance Management Process and keep it simple, direct and understandable. The Matrix is a grid system that measures the three main goals and:

1. Identifies primary threats by geographic area;
2. Develops desired goals to counter the threats;
3. Assigns responsibility to accomplish the desired goals;
4. Captures output measurements;
5. Illustrates the program's outcomes.

The matrix-based system establishes a mechanism that measures each HIDTA's performance and holds them accountable for what they do.

The Hawaii HIDTA sits on the National HIDTA PMP Development Committee and is using the PMP Matrix in its CY2003 Annual Report to jumpstart this new process. We expect the PMP Matrix to be fully implemented by the end of CY2004. When fully implemented, each calendar year's Annual Report, Threat Assessment and Strategy will be illustrated by the data included in the matrix.

Although section XIII of the revised HIDTA Program Policy and Procedure Manual identifies particular data sets to be used and measured in the PMP Matrix, the Hawaii HIDTA CY2003 Matrix is a hybrid using the designated PMP Matrix format and data generated prior to the policy revision. During the ONDCP review in early CY2004 a recommendation was made to separate the Safe Neighborhood and Fugitive initiatives from HI-IMPACT. This change is reflected in the Matrix and throughout this report.

The Executive Summary and subsequent sections of this report show relevant Matrix categories consolidated and/or individually highlighted in tables for ease of use and clarity.

The CY2003 Matrix reflects information from CY2003 Initiative Submissions and the CY2004 and CY2005 Hawaii HIDTA Threat Assessments. Desired Outcomes and responsibility sections are based on the expected outputs as indicated by each of the initiatives in their initial submission package.

Standardized outcome measurements have yet to be finalized by the NHPO. For this report outputs have been measured using monthly initiative statistics and field interviews, comparing expected outputs to actual outputs, and indicating how much of each output was achieved. Finally, the outcome section gives anecdotal information that supports the initiative's outputs.

HAWAII HIDTA PMP MATRIX

GOAL 1 - REDUCE DRUG AVAILABILITY BY ELIMINATING OR DISRUPTING DRUG TRAFFICKING ORGANIZATIONS

GEOGRAPHIC AREA	THREATS	THREAT DESCRIPTION	SOURCE	DESIRED OUTPUTS
Honolulu City/County	PRIMARY THREAT	20 DRUG DISTRIBUTION ORGANIZATIONS IDENTIFIED AS OF 12/03	FIELD SURVEY	TARGET 3 DISTRIBUTION ORGANIZATIONS AND DISRUPT OR DISMANTLE 3 OF THOSE TARGETED
		5 DRUG MANUFACTURING OPERATIONS IDENTIFIED AS OF 12/03		TARGET 1 MANUFACTURING ORGANIZATIONS AND DISRUPT OR DISMANTLE 1 OF THOSE TARGETED
		3000 ACTIVE DRUG WARRANTS STATEWIDE		CLEAR 200 WARRANTS FOR DRUG CHARGES
		100 ARMED VIOLENT DRUG OFFENDERS OPERATE IN AND THROUGH THE REGION		ARREST 60 ARMED VIOLENT OFFENDERS WITH A DRUG NEXUS
		MULTI-POUND QUANTITIES OF ILLEGAL NARCOTICS ARE SMUGGLED THROUGH HONOLULU INTERNATIONAL AIRPORT	THREAT ASSESSMENT	ARREST 60 INDIVIDUALS WHO SMUGGLE NARCOTICS THROUGH THE AIRPORT
		SHIPMENT OF 1000 ILLICIT PARCELS ANNUALLY TO/THROUGH HONOLULU VIA MAIL AND EXPRESS SERVICES		INSPECT 750 PARCELS AND SEIZE 100 PARCELS
				SEIZE 60 KILOGRAMS OF ILLICIT DRUGS ENTERING THE AIRPORT
		A SIGNIFICANT AMOUNT OF ILLEGAL DRUG MONEY FLOW THROUGH THE REGION VIA BULK CASH SHIPMENTS, WIRE TRANSFER SERVICES, FINANCIAL INSTITUTIONS, AND COMMERCIAL BUSSINESSES		TARGET ONE MONEY REMITTANCE ESTABLISHMENT FOR MONEY LAUNDERING CHARGES
				SEIZE $1,300,000 IN ILLICIT DRUG RELATED ASSETS
				FORFEIT $1,000,000 IN ILLICIT DRUG RELATED ASSETS
		USE OF PUBLIC LANDS FOR THE CULTIVATION AND PRODUCTION OF MARIJUANA		ERADICATE 60,000 MARIJUANA PLANTS
		WEAPONS ASSOCIATED WITH DRUG TRAFFICKING		SEIZE 30 FIREARMS
Maui County		10 DRUG DISTRIBUTION ORGANIZATIONS IDENTIFIED AS OF 12/03	FIELD SURVEY	TARGET 2 DISTRIBUTION ORGANIZATIONS AND DISRUPT OR DISMANTLE 2 OF THOSE TARGETED
		3 DRUG MANUFACTURING OPERATIONS IDENTIFIED AS OF 12/03		TARGET 1 MANUFACTURING ORGANIZATIONS AND DISRUPT OR DISMANTLE 1 OF THOSE TARGETED
		3000 ACTIVE DRUG WARRANTS STATEWIDE		CLEAR 250 WARRANTS FOR DRUG CHARGES
		100 ARMED VIOLENT DRUG OFFENDERS OPERATE IN AND THROUGH THE REGION		ARREST 60 ARMED VIOLENT OFFENDERS WITH A DRUG NEXUS
		A SIGNIFICANT AMOUNT OF ILLEGAL DRUG MONEY FLOW THROUGH THE REGION VIA BULK CASH SHIPMENTS, WIRE TRANSFER SERVICES, FINANCIAL INSTITUTIONS, AND COMMERCIAL BUSSINESSES	THREAT ASSESSMENT	SEIZE $250,000 IN ILLICIT DRUG RELATED ASSETS
		USE OF PUBLIC LANDS FOR THE CULTIVATION AND PRODUCTION OF MARIJUANA		ERADICATE 75,000 MARIJUANA PLANTS
		WEAPONS ASSOCIATED WITH DRUG TRAFFICKING		SEIZE 15 FIREARMS
Hawaii County (Big Island)		10 DRUG DISTRIBUTION ORGANIZATIONS IDENTIFIED AS OF 12/03	FIELD SURVEY	TARGET 3 DISTRIBUTION ORGANIZATIONS AND DISRUPT OR DISMANTLE 2 OF THOSE TARGETED
		3 DRUG MANUFACTURING OPERATIONS IDENTIFIED AS OF 12/03		TARGET 3 MANUFACTURING ORGANIZATIONS AND DISRUPT OR DISMANTLE 3 OF THOSE TARGETED
		3000 ACTIVE DRUG WARRANTS STATEWIDE		CLEAR 250 WARRANTS FOR DRUG CHARGES
		100 ARMED VIOLENT DRUG OFFENDERS OPERATE IN AND THROUGH THE REGION		ARREST 50 ARMED VIOLENT OFFENDERS WITH A DRUG NEXUS
		A SIGNIFICANT AMOUNT OF ILLEGAL DRUG MONEY FLOW THROUGH THE REGION VIA BULK CASH SHIPMENTS, WIRE TRANSFER SERVICES, FINANCIAL INSTITUTIONS, AND COMMERCIAL BUSSINESSES	THREAT ASSESSMENT	SEIZE $250,000 IN ILLICIT DRUG RELATED ASSETS
		USE OF PUBLIC LANDS FOR THE CULTIVATION AND PRODUCTION OF MARIJUANA		ERADICATE 300,000 MARIJUANA PLANTS *
		WEAPONS ASSOCIATED WITH DRUG TRAFFICKING		SEIZE 35 FIREARMS
Kauai County		5 DRUG DISTRIBUTION ORGANIZATIONS IDENTIFIED AS OF 12/03	FIELD SURVEY	TARGET 2 DISTRIBUTION ORGANIZATIONS AND DISRUPT OR DISMANTLE 2 OF THOSE TARGETED
		1 DRUG MANUFACTURING OPERATIONS IDENTIFIED AS OF 12/03		TARGET 1 MANUFACTURING ORGANIZATIONS AND DISRUPT OR DISMANTLE 1 OF THOSE TARGETED
		3000 ACTIVE DRUG WARRANTS STATEWIDE		CLEAR 250 WARRANTS FOR DRUG CHARGES
		100 ARMED VIOLENT DRUG OFFENDERS OPERATE IN AND THROUGH THE REGION		ARREST 50 ARMED VIOLENT OFFENDERS WITH A DRUG NEXUS
		A SIGNIFICANT AMOUNT OF ILLEGAL DRUG MONEY FLOW THROUGH THE REGION VIA BULK CASH SHIPMENTS, WIRE TRANSFER SERVICES, FINANCIAL INSTITUTIONS, AND COMMERCIAL BUSSINESSES	THREAT ASSESSMENT	SEIZE $100,000 IN ILLICIT DRUG RELATED ASSETS
		USE OF PUBLIC LANDS FOR THE CULTIVATION AND PRODUCTION OF MARIJUANA		ERADICATE 80,000 MARIJUANA PLANTS
		WEAPONS ASSOCIATED WITH DRUG TRAFFICKING		SEIZE 10 FIREARMS
	SECONDARY THREAT	INTER ISLAND TRANSPORTATION OF ILLEGAL NARCOTICS VIA AIR AND SEA		LAW ENFORCEMENT SENSITIVE ISSUE CURRENTLY UNDER CONSIDERATION
		PACIFIC RIM TRANSPORTATION OF ILLEGAL NARCOTICS		LAW ENFORCEMENT SENSITIVE ISSUE CURRENTLY UNDER CONSIDERATION
		IDENTIFYING ASIAN AND PACIFIC ISLANDER ORGANIZED CRIME GROUPS		LAW ENFORCEMENT SENSITIVE ISSUE CURRENTLY UNDER CONSIDERATION
		IDENTIFY CROSS POLLINATION AND DEVELOPERS OF SUPER HYBRID MARIJUANA PLANTS		LAW ENFORCEMENT SENSITIVE ISSUE CURRENTLY UNDER CONSIDERATION
		IDENTIFY INDOOR AND HYDROPONIC GROWS		LAW ENFORCEMENT SENSITIVE ISSUE CURRENTLY UNDER CONSIDERATION
		IDENTIFY TRANSPORTATION OF MARIJUANA SEEDS		LAW ENFORCEMENT SENSITIVE ISSUE CURRENTLY UNDER CONSIDERATION

* Includes 211,900 marijuana plants attributed to the Hawaii Department of Land and Natural Resources

INVESTIGATIVE									INTERDICTION		ERADICATION	SUPPORT		INTELLIGENCE			ADMINISTRATIVE		
HI-IMPACT																			
OAHU II	OAHU III	MAUI	HILO	KONA	KAUAI	SAFE NEIGHBORHOOD	FUGITIVE	MONEY LAUNDERING/ ASSET FORFEITURE	DOMESTIC	INTERNATIONAL	MARIJUANA	CLAN LAB	PROSECUTORS	INVESTIGATIVE	STRATEGIC	WSIN	MANAGEMENT AND COORDINATION	TRAINING	ACTUAL OUTPUTS
X	X																		DISRUPTED/DISMANTLED 16 DTOS
X	X								X	X									DISRUPTED/DISMANTLED 1 DTO
							X												CLEARED 300 WARRANTS (STATEWIDE)
						X													ARRESTED 94 ARMED OFFENDERS (STATEWIDE)
									X	X									ARRESTED 47 INDIVIDUALS
									X	X									INSPECTED 15,000 & SEIZED 65 PARCELS
									X	X									SEIZED 86 KILOS OF DRUGS
								X											TARGETED 1 ESTABLISHMENT
X	X							X	X	X									SEIZED $2,370,000 (STATEWIDE)
													X						FORFEITED $1,337,749 (STATEWIDE)
											X								ERADICATED 14,501 PLANTS
X	X					X													SEIZED 162 (PSN) & 41 (OAHU HI-IMPACT) FIREARMS
		X																	DISRUPTED/DISMANTLED 9 DTOS
		X																	DISRUPTED/DISMANTLED 2 DTOS
							X												CLEARED 300 WARRANTS (STATEWIDE)
						X													ARRESTED 94 ARMED OFFENDERS (STATEWIDE)
		X						X											SEIZED $2,990,000 (STATEWIDE)
											X								ERADICATED 78,100 PLANTS
		X				X													SEIZED 162 (PSN) & 6 (MAUI HI-IMPACT) FIREARMS
			X	X															DISRUPTED/DISMANTLED 9 DTOS
			X	X															DISRUPTED/DISMANTLED 3 DTOS
							X												CLEARED 300 WARRANTS (STATEWIDE)
						X													ARRESTED 94 ARMED OFFENDERS (STATEWIDE)
			X	X				X											SEIZED $2,990,000 (STATEWIDE)
											X								ERADICATED 204,944 PLANTS*
			X	X		X													SEIZED 162 (PSN) & 47 (HAWAII HI-IMPACT) FIREARMS
					X														DISRUPTED/DISMANTLED 2 DTOS
					X														DISRUPTED/DISMANTLED 8 DTOS
							X												CLEARED 299 WARRANTS (STATEWIDE)
						X													ARRESTED 92 ARMED OFFENDERS (STATEWIDE)
					X			X											SEIZED $2,990,000 (STATEWIDE)
											X								ERADICATED 33,243 PLANTS
					X	X													SEIZED 162 (PSN) & 16 (KAUAI HI-IMPACT) FIREARMS

OUTCOMES: SEE SECTIONS VIII, IX, AND X FOR THIS INFORMATION

GOAL 2 - REDUCE THE HARMFUL CONSEQUENCES OF DRUG TRAFFICKING

GEOGRAPHIC AREA	HARMFUL CONSEQUENCES	SOURCE	DESIRED OUTPUTS
HAWAII HIDTA AREA	VIOLENCE ASSOCIATED WITH DRUG TRAFFICKING	THREAT ASSESSMENT	SEIZE X FIREARMS FROM VIOLENT DRUG TRAFFICKERS
			CLEAR 250 WARRANTS FOR DRUG CHARGES
			PROPOSE MODEL LEGISLATION TO INCREASE INVESTIGATIVE METHODS

GOAL 3 - IMPROVE THE EFFICIENCY AND EFFECTIVENESS OF LAW ENFORCEMENT ORGANIZATIONS

GEOGRAPHIC AREA		REGIONAL NEEDS	DESIRED OUTPUTS
HAWAII HIDTA AREA	INFORMATION SHARING	PROVIDE FOR OFFICER AND GENERAL PUBLIC SAFETY DURING ONGOING ENFORCEMENT OPERATIONS	ACHIEVE AND MAINTAIN 100% PARTICIPATION BY LAW ENFORCEMENT AGENCIES IN THE WSIN DECONFLICTION SERVICES
		PROVIDE CASE/SUBJECT DECONFLICTION PARTICIPATION AMONG HIDTA INITIATIVES AND PARTICIPATING AGENCIES	SUBMIT 9000 CASE/SUBJECT DECONFLICTIONS AMONG HIDTA INITIATIVES AND PARTICIPATING AGENCIES
		PROVIDE EVENT DECONFLICTION UTILIZING WSIN	SUBMIT 1400 CRITICAL EVENT DECONFLICTIONS AMONG HIDTA INITIATIVES AND PARTICIPATING AGENCIES
		PROVIDE LAW ENFORCEMENT PERSONNEL ACCESS TO CRIMINAL, OPEN SOURCE INFORMATION & INTELLIGENCE	ISC TO CONDUCT 4000 DATABASE QUERIES & PROVIDE 100 INTELLIGENCE PROFILES
		INCREASE ANALYTICAL CASE SUPPORT TO HIDTA INITIATIVES	COMPLETE 30 REQUESTS FOR CASE ASSISTANCE
			PROVIDE 3000 ANALYTICAL PRODUCTS (TOLL ANALYSES, LINK ANALYSES, GRAPHS, CHARTS, PROFILES, ETC)
		ESTABLISH & MAINTAIN AN INTELLIGENCE OUTREACH PROGRAM	DEVELOP AN ACTIVE MEANS OF COMMUNICATION WITH PACIFIC [illegible] LAW ENFORCEMENT
			PROVIDE ELECTRONIC LINK FROM ISC TO NEIGHBOR ISLANDS VIA WSIN SECURE INTRANET
		IMPROVE INFORMATION & INTELLIGENCE SHARING BETWEEN HAWAII HIDTA AND OTHER HIDTAS/LEAS	SHARE INTELLIGENCE DATA WITH HIDTAS/LEAS OUTSIDE OF HAWAII
	TRAINING	IMPROVE THE SKILLS OF PERSONNEL AT PARTICIPATING AGENCIES AND COOPERATING INSTITUTIONS WITHIN THE HAWAII HIDTA REGION	SPONSOR QUARTERLY TRAINING PROGRAMS FOR REGIONAL AND/OR SPECIALIZED TRAINING
			SPONSOR QUARTERLY CLANDESTINE LAB TRAINING PROGRAMS
		INFORM LAW ENFORCEMENT PERSONNEL OF TRAINING OPPORTUNITIES	DISSEMINATE EXISTING TRAINING OPPORTUNITIES FROM OTHER AGENCIES & OUT-SOURCES TO HIDTA PERSONNEL
		TRACK & REPORT COURSES CONDUCTED, PERSONNEL TRAINED, & AGENCIES INVOLVED	DEVELOP & MAINTAIN HIDA TRAINING DATABASE
	COORDINATION	IMPROVE COORDINATION AMONG LAW ENFORCEMENT AGENCIES AND HIDTA INITIATIVES	COORDINATE WITH CLAN LAB RESPONSE COORDINATORS AT FEDERAL, STATE, AND LOCAL AGENCIES
			PROVIDE COLLOCATION FOR HIDTA INITIATIVES
			DEVELOP PARTNERSHIPS WITH EXISTING TRAINING COORDINATORS AT FEDERAL, STATE, AND LOCAL AGENCIES
			MEET IN EXECUTIVE SESSION A MINIMUM OF 4 TIMES TO COORDINATE HAWAII HIDTA ACTIVITIES
		ADDRESS DRUG ENFORCEMENT OR PROSECUTION ISSUES	CONDUCT MONTHLY MEETINGS WITH HIDTA INITIATIVES
	OVERSIGHT	IMPLEMENT HIDTA DEVELOPMENTAL STANDARDS	ATTAIN 100% OF DEVELOPMENTAL STANDARDS
		ACCOUNT FOR USE OF HIDTA FUNDS	COMPLETE AND TRACK A FULL INVENTORY OF ACCOUNTABLE EQUIPMENT PURCHASED WITH HIDTA FUNDS
			MONITOR, REVIEW, AND TRACK FISCAL EXPENDITURES BY HIDTA INITIATIVES TO ENSURE COMPLIANCE WITH POLICIES
			CONDUCT FISCAL AUDITS OF ALL INITIATIVES
		ENSURE INITIATIVES ARE ADDRESSING THE IDENTIFIED THREATS & THEIR INTENDED MISSION	IMPLEMENT & CONDUCT HAWAII HIDTA'S INTERNAL REVIEW PROGRAM
			HOLD QUARTERLY MEETINGS WITH INITIATIVE AND PARTICIPATING AGENCY SUPERVISORS
		ENSURE COMPLIANCE WITH ONDCP REPORTING REQUIREMENTS	PREPARE THE ANNUAL REPORT, THREAT ASSESSMENT, STRATEGY AND BUDGET

** ONDCP assumptions apply to 4 task forces because of Hawaii's island makeup and county office [illegible]

INVESTIGATIVE									INTERDICTION		ERADICATION	SUPPORT		INTELLIGENCE			ADMINISTRATIVE		
HI-IMPACT																			
OAHU II	OAHU III	MAUI	HILO	KONA	KAUAI	SAFE NEIGHBORHOOD	FUGITIVE	MONEY LAUNDERING/ASSET FORFEITURE	DOMESTIC	INTERNATIONAL	MARIJUANA	CLAN LAB	PROSECUTORS	INVESTIGATIVE	STRATEGIC	WSIN	MANAGEMENT AND COORDINATION	TRAINING	ACTUAL OUTPUTS
						X													SEIZED 562 FIREARMS
							X												CLEARED 389 WARRANTS
													X						PROPOSED 2 PIECES OF LEGISLATION

OUTCOMES: SEE SECTIONS VIII, IX, AND X FOR THIS INFORMATION

INVESTIGATIVE									INTERDICTION		ERADICATION	SERVICES		INTELLIGENCE			ADMINISTRATIVE		
HI-IMPACT																			
OAHU II	OAHU III	MAUI	HILO	KONA	KAUAI	SAFE NEIGHBORHOOD	FUGITIVE	MONEY LAUNDERING/ASSET FORFEITURE	DOMESTIC	INTERNATIONAL	MARIJUANA	CLAN LAB	PROSECUTORS	INVESTIGATIVE	STRATEGIC	WSIN	MANAGEMENT AND COORDINATION	TRAINING	ACTUAL OUTPUTS
X	X	X	X	X	X	X	X	X	X	X	X	X		X	X				ACHIEVED 100% PARTICIPATION
X	X	X	X	X	X	X	X	X	X	X				X	X	X			SUBMITTED 5333 CASE/SUBJECT DECONFLICTIONS
X	X	X	X	X	X	X	X	X	X	X						X			SUBMITTED 1333 EVENT DECONFLICTIONS
														X	X				CONDUCTED 2852 DATABASE QUERIES & PROVIDED 366 PROFILES
														X	X				COMPLETED 24 REQUESTS
														X	X				PROVIDED 4,836 PRODUCTS
														X	X	X	X		ACHIEVED BY 25%
																X			ACHIEVED BY 100%
														X	X				DAILY COMMUNICATION WITH OTHER HIDTAS/LEAS
																		X	SPONSORED 16 PROGRAMS
												X							SPONSORED 2 PROGRAMS
																		X	100% DISSEMINATION OF TRAINING OPPORTUNITIES
																		X	DATABASE DEVELOPED & MAINTAINED
												X							100% COORDINATION WITH AGENCIES
																	X		COLLOCATION PROVIDED**
																		X	PARTNERSHIPS DEVELOPED
																	X		MET 4 TIMES
													X						MEETINGS NOT CONDUCTED
																	X		ATTAINED 99% OF STANDARDS
																	X		INVENTORY TRACKED & COMPLETED
																	X		FISCAL EXPENDITURES REVIEWED & TRACKED
																	X		FISCAL AUDITS COMPLETED
																	X		REVIEW PROGRAM IMPLEMENTED & COMPLETED
																	X		MET QUARTERLY
																	X		REPORTS PREPARED & SUBMITTED

OUTCOMES: SEE SECTIONS VIII, IX, AND X FOR THIS INFORMATION

Overview of HIDTA Region

Section IV.

GEOGRAPHY

Given the fact that Hawaii is an island state, there are significant environmental risks associated with drug trafficking. The State of Hawaii encompasses eight main islands and a 1,500-mile chain of islets, covering 6,422.6 square miles in the North Central Pacific Ocean.

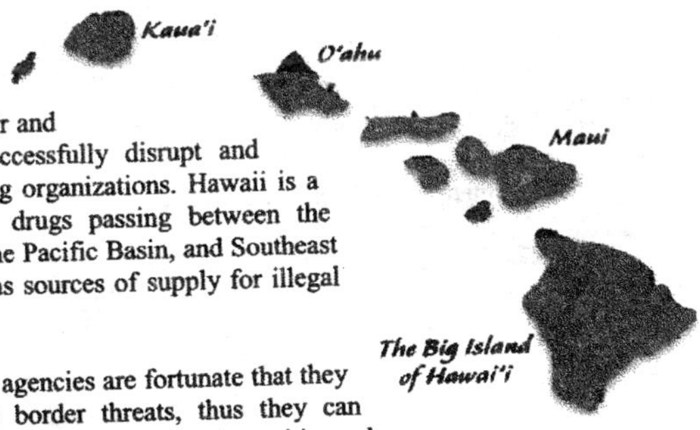

Hawaii's drug threat is unique in that concentrated efforts on air and sea chokepoints can successfully disrupt and dismantle drug trafficking organizations. Hawaii is a transshipment point for drugs passing between the Western United States, the Pacific Basin, and Southeast Asia, which are known as sources of supply for illegal narcotics.

Hawaii law enforcement agencies are fortunate that they do not face land-based border threats, thus they can concentrate efforts on disrupting air and maritime drug transportation. Unfortunately, being an island state and a popular tourist destination, it is difficult to identify drug couriers among the millions of passengers arriving at Hawaii's airports. It is also difficult to identify packages and cargo used to transport illicit drugs among the tons of mail/cargo received daily.

DEMOGRAPHICS

Hawaii has the most racially diverse population of any state in the nation with more than 1.2 million residents exposed to the influences of the illicit drug trade and the social costs associated with distribution and abuse. Asians account for 41.6 percent of the population, which includes Asian Indian (0.1), Chinese (4.7), Filipino (14.1), Japanese (16.7), Korean (1.9), Vietnamese (0.6), and other Asians (3.5). Caucasians represent 24.3 percent of the population, the lowest percentage of any state. Native Hawaiians account for 9.4 percent of the population, and African Americans account for 1.8 percent. Various mixed-racial groups account for most of the remaining 15.7 percent of the population[1]. A recent and

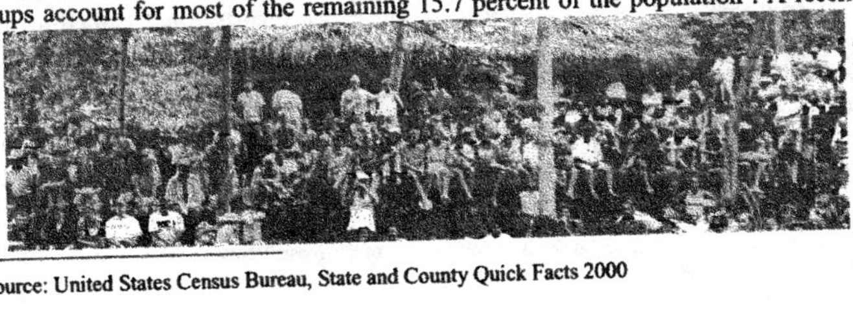
Photo: Unknown

[1] Source: United States Census Bureau, State and County Quick Facts 2000

significant change in Hawaii's population has been the increasing Mexican/Hispanic population, which now accounts for 7.2 percent of Hawaii's overall population. These Mexican/Hispanic communities are primarily located on the islands of Maui and Hawaii and have strong links to Mexico and South America.

Honolulu, located on Oahu, is the major population center of the State and home to approximately 80 percent of the State's permanent residents. Hawaii also has a large, possibility the largest, transient population in the United States, per capita. When military personnel and visitors are factored in, *the daily population of the state grows by as much as 20 percent.*

Military service members and their families contribute to Hawaii's diversity by adding nearly 87,000 individuals to its overall population[2]. The majority of military bases are concentrated on Oahu with several key installations housing large numbers of service members. These include Pearl Harbor Naval Base and Navy Yard; United States Pacific Command at Camp H.M. Smith; Hickam Air Force Base; Schofield Barracks; Kaneohe Marine Corps Base; and Fort Shafter. Bases on the neighbor islands include the Pacific Missile Range at Barking Sands on Kauai; and the Pohakuloa Army Training Area on the Big Island.

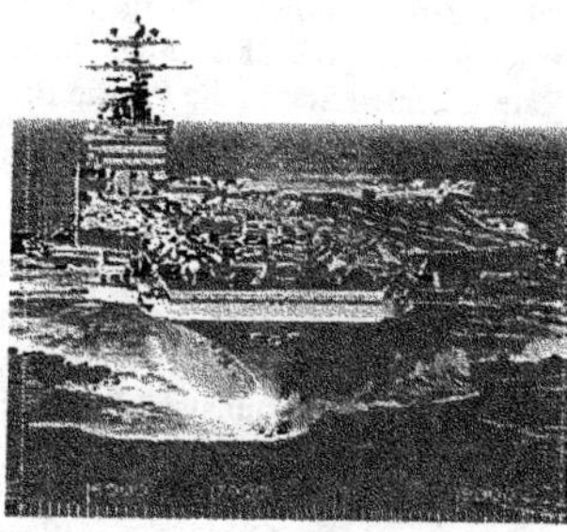
Photo: US Navy

According to military law enforcement agencies, there has been a significant increase in the use of predatory drugs, such as MDMA and GHB. The reason for the abuse of these drugs is that the drugs are not detectable in a person's system after a day or two. Therefore, service personnel can abuse the drug over the weekend when they know that they will not be drug tested. When military personnel test positive for illegal narcotics, they are discharged from military service. However, before doing so, interviews have been conducted that reveal these drugs are being sold to the military personal by civilian dealers, typically at off-base night clubs.

ECONOMICS

Economic trends in Hawaii are important to understand because Hawaii's leading economic industries—tourism, military, and agriculture—play an important role in Hawaii's drug threat. Tourism is Hawaii's number one industry. In FY2003, tourism grossed over $10.3 billion with over 6.4 million visitors arriving in the islands[3]. The flood of daily tourists can make it difficult for law enforcement to detect drug couriers and conduct drug interdiction at Hawaii's airports.

---

[2] Source: 2002 State of Hawaii Data Book, State Department of Business, Economic Development & Tourism, Table 10.03

[3] Source: 2002 State of Hawaii Data Book, State Department of Business, Economic Development & Tourism, Tables 13.04 and 7.03, respectively

Hawaii also relies on the U.S. Defense Department expenditures, which contributed $3.5 billion in CY2001 to Hawaii's economy[4]. The United States Pacific Command (USPACOM) is geographically the largest of the U.S. unified service commands. It covers 50 percent of the earth's surface from the U.S. West Coast to Africa's East Coast and from the Arctic to the Antarctic. Thus, with nearly 87,000 military personnel and dependents, Hawaii's economy benefits tremendously by the military presence.

This transient population can be linked to new drug trends and threats here in Hawaii. For example, MDMA and GHB are the predominate drug threats on military bases. This may indicate that Hawaii may start to see more MDMA and GHB cases throughout the State.

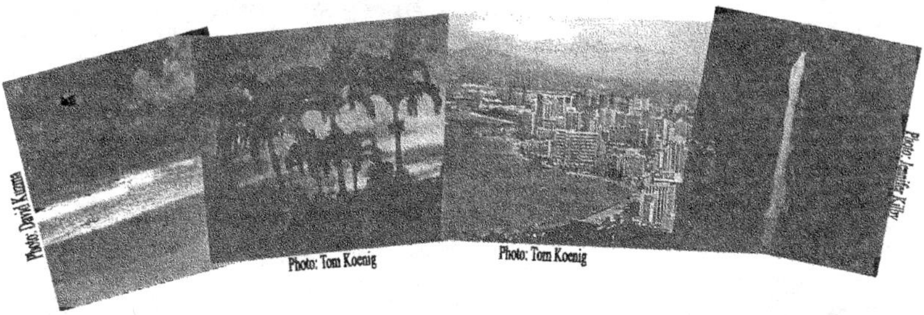

Hawaii's third largest industry is agriculture. It has always had a special place in Hawaii's history and continues to be an important industry, generating $1.07 billion to the State's annual economy[5] and directly and indirectly providing 42,000 jobs. With the decline of the sugar industry, these agricultural lands are returning to a new era of small farms growing diversified agricultural products. Crops such as exotic fruits, coffee, macadamia nuts, flowers, and foliage not only provide fresh produce and flowers to Hawaii's markets, but have also become major exports to destinations around the world. These agriculture products, especially fresh flowers and greenery, may be used as a way to conceal drug exports such as marijuana.

As with the rest of the United States, the effects of 9-11 on Hawaii's economy have been devastating. Only now is Hawaii experiencing some recovery. The unemployment rate is 4.2 percent, translating to over 28,000 residents unemployed, with over 126,000 residents living at or below the national poverty level[6]. According to some drug abuse counselors, many of the people they treat are unemployed and/or at the national poverty level. They also indicated that many have admitted to selling small quantities of illicit drugs to support their drug habit and raise income for their families.

---

[4] Source: 2002 State of Hawaii Data Book, State Department of Business, Economic Development & Tourism, Table 13.01

[5] Source: National Agriculture Statistics Service, Hawaii Agriculture Statistics Service, Agriculture Contributions to Hawaii's Economy, 2000

[6] Source: US Census Bureau, Poverty:1999, Table 3 State and Regional Poverty Rates, issued May 2003

TRANSPORTATION

Commercial Aircraft

The transportation of drugs into Hawaii by commercial aircraft represents a significant threat. Most of the seizures identified by law enforcement officers and agents involve drugs transported into Hawaii via aircraft. Seizures of drugs at the Honolulu International Airport in CY2003 include methamphetamine, marijuana, cocaine, heroin, and other illicit drugs.

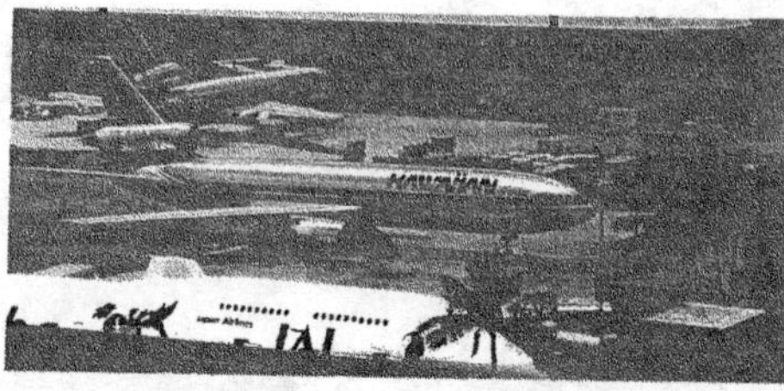

Photo: Hawaiian Airlines, Honolulu International Airport

Although other airports in Hawaii now receive flights from the Continental U.S., Canada, and Japan, the Honolulu International Airport remains the primary hub of Hawaii's travel industry and of illicit drugs transported into the State. However, according to Hawaii and Maui County law enforcement agencies, intelligence reveals that drugs are arriving via aircraft in these counties and then being transported to Oahu via package delivery service. This method has been used in an effort to avoid detection at the more secured airport in Honolulu.

Package Delivery Services

The threat posed by U.S. mail and parcel delivery services is the most significant transportation threat. Since 9/11/2001 airborne package delivery services such as FedEx, UPS, and the U.S. Postal Service have been the primary drug transportation method. The U.S. Postal Service delivered 18 million packages into Hawaii in 2003. FedEx and UPS added an additional 10 million packages. It is difficult to determine the actual volume of illegal drugs transported into Hawaii by these services. It has been estimated by some local law enforcement agencies that more than 50 percent of illegal narcotics transported into Hawaii come via package delivery services.

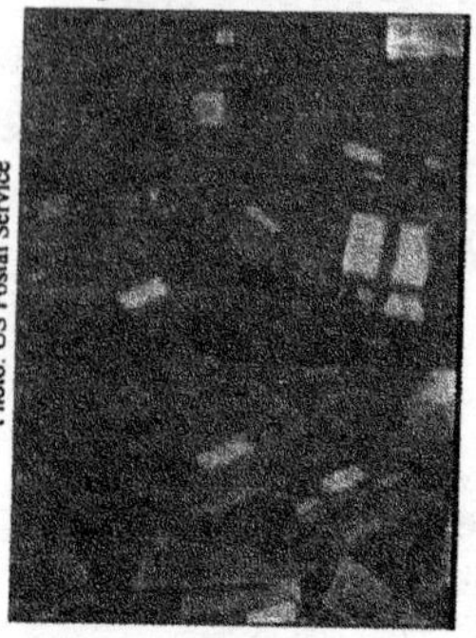

Photo: US Postal Service

There are many reasons why package delivery services are a popular method of drug transportation. In Hawaii, there are numerous private package delivery services as well as the U.S. Postal Service which maintains large domestic and international mail facilities at the Honolulu International Airport to process the heavy volume of incoming and outgoing parcels. Monitoring the flow of this commerce is difficult for law enforcement agencies due to a lack of law enforcement resources, high volume, and the existence of multiple processing facilities. Furthermore, the advantages of this method for DTOs are that it is fast, reliable, inexpensive, and fairly secure because customers can track their own packages. While there is always the possibility that law enforcement officers will intercept a shipment or an employee of the package delivery service would steal a shipment, these risks are relatively low, especially since DTOs often have contacts within the shipping agencies.

Air Freight

Air freight transported through Hawaii's airports is voluminous, with hundreds of thousands of tons transiting Hawaii every year. Concealment of small amounts of drugs in larger shipments, or even the forwarding of larger bulkier amounts presents minimal problems for DTOs. This is especially true for those DTOs that have established business or commercial covers to receive airfreight shipments on a regular basis. Investigations have detected incoming drugs in shipments of auto parts, paper materials, flowers, cooking supplies, and other products. Other investigations focused on outgoing drug shipments have revealed that marijuana is being transported out of Hawaii to the Continental U.S in exotic flower air packages such as orchids, Hawaiian fern, torch ginger, and bird of paradise. This intelligence comes mainly from the County of Hawaii, which produces the majority of the marijuana in the State in addition to many of Hawaii's exotic flowers for export. Air freight provides many of the same advantages as the smaller express or package delivery services such as relatively good security and low cost. Given the volume of air freight shipments each year and overall tonnage involved, the risk of drug detection in air freight is low to moderate.

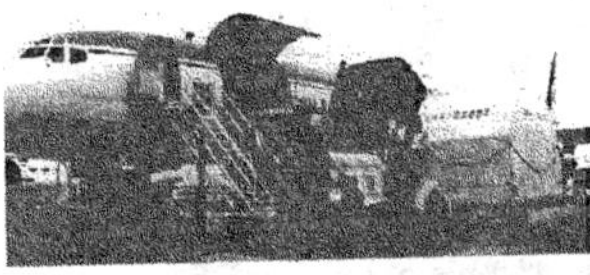

Photo: Air Freight Services

Maritime Shipping

There are many commercial vessels servicing Hawaii such as Matson, Horizon, Sause Brothers, and Young Brothers-Hawaii Tug and Barge. The statewide system of commercial harbors consists of ten harbors on six islands. This system plays a vital role in the State's economy as Hawaii imports about 80 percent of its consumed good, with 97 percent of large durable goods entering the state via the commercial harbor system. In FY2003 the commercial harbor facilities handled a total of 16.9 million tons of cargo. The threat of maritime smuggling of drugs is considered by many law enforcement agencies to be significant due to the large volume that can potentially be transported by sea vessels. In fact, the Honolulu Police Department has recently added a Marine Detail. However, due to the large volume of ships and containerized cargo entering Hawaii's harbors each day and the low rate of ship container inspections, actual drug seizures are very rare unless there is specific intelligence on a particular vessel or shipment.

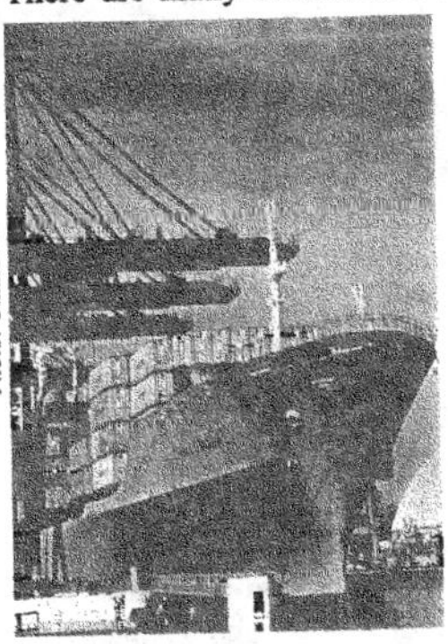

Adding to the maritime threat is the fact that Hawaii services a sizable international and domestic fishing fleet with over 3,400 commercial fishermen and over 750 miles of coast line. Domestic fishing fleets from California and international fishing fleets from Mexico and Asia are an irregular, but noteworthy drug threat to the State.

Cruise Ships

The current terrorism threat has been a significant boost for Hawaii's cruise industry.

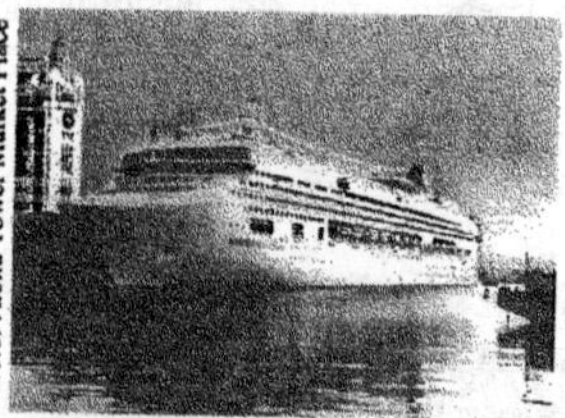

Photo: Aloha Tower Market Place

U.S. and non-U.S. flagged vessels have been forced to seek safe, yet exotic ports of call. Hawaii's tourism industry has stepped forward to promote cruising the state's tropical waters between islands as a safe passage. During CY2002 1,087,405 cruise ship passengers sailed these waters and came ashore through the State's system of harbors and ports of entry[7]. Intelligence indicates that employees of some of these cruise lines transport illegal narcotics into Hawaii or between the islands without the knowledge of their employer. Regularly scheduled dockings can make cruise ships almost as reliable as the post office or FedEx. An example of this is a DEA case, in which a cook and a steward on two separate vessels were indicted and arrested for transporting multi-pound quantities of cocaine on a regular basis to Hawaii.

CLIMATE CONDITIONS

Agricultural and weather conditions make Hawaii an optimal location to cultivate marijuana. Marijuana grown outdoors in Hawaii contains some of the highest THC levels in the nation because of growing conditions and the nutrient-mineral rich volcanic soil. The windward side of each of the islands provides an optimal location for marijuana growth due to ample morning rain showers and afternoon sunlight. Marijuana cultivators often use public lands such as national forests and state parks. The majority of marijuana is cultivated at remote jungle locations in Hawaii County.

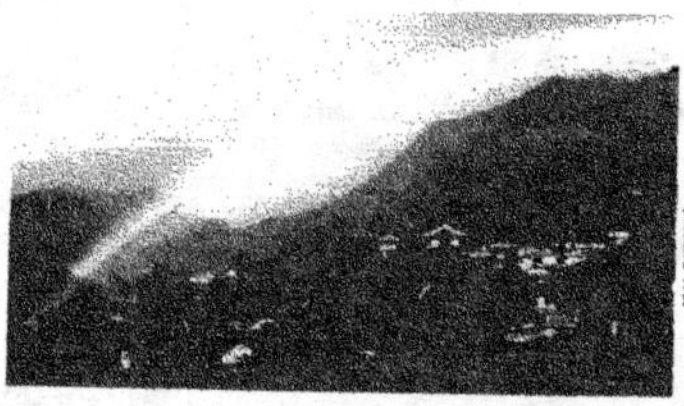

Photo: Unknown

DRUG TRAFFICKING ORGANIZATIONS

International drug trafficking organizations (DTOs), primarily linked to the Filipino, Vietnamese, Chinese, and Korean communities, transport illicit drugs into Hawaii. Law enforcement authorities in Hawaii report that International DTOs transport drugs to Hawaii from Asia and other source countries including Korea, Thailand, and the Philippines. Chinese DTOs have been known to transport drugs through Canada to Hawaii via California to avoid Hawaii's strict U.S. Customs inspections.

Mexican DTOs operating in Hawaii have been linked to Department of Justice Consolidated Priority Organization Targets (CPOT). These organizations transport Mexican-produced methamphetamine and methamphetamine produced in California directly to Hawaii and Maui Counties, as well as, the City and County of Honolulu.

---

[7] Source: State of Hawaii, Department of Transportation, Report to the Governor 2002

These DTOs transport crystal methamphetamine into Hawaii from the West Coast, primarily Southern California and Las Vegas, Nevada.

Local and Pacific Islander DTOs and street gangs distribute drugs at the retail level in the State. Retail distributors use pagers and cellular telephones when distributing. Crystal methamphetamine sold at the retail level is frequently packaged in plastic bags. Retail distribution occurs throughout Hawaii, primarily in nightclubs, bars, street corners, or from houses in residential communities using established tight-knit drug networks.

VIOLENCE

Violence related to illicit drug trafficking is a large concern for law enforcement officials and public health professionals. Crystal methamphetamine abusers can be violent and may endanger themselves and those around them. As the euphoric effects of crystal methamphetamine begin to diminish, abusers enter a stage called "tweaking" in which they are prone to violence, delusions, and paranoia. Many abusers try to buffer the effects of the "crash" with other drugs such as cocaine or Oxycontin. The effect of these drugs, combined with severe sleep deprivation, often results in unpredictable and uncontrollable behavior.

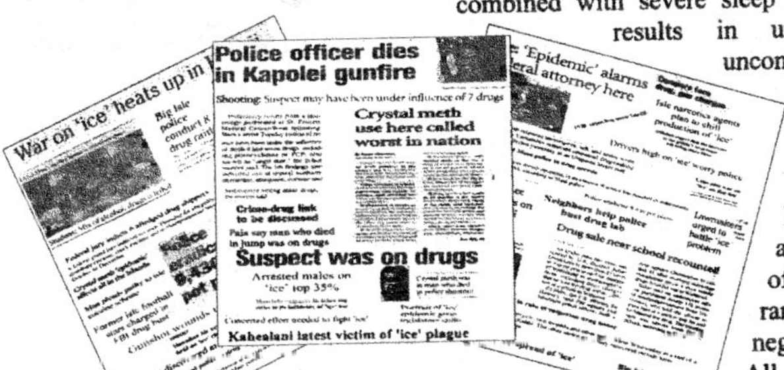
War on 'ice' heats up in
Police officer dies in Kapolei gunfire
Crystal meth use here called worst in nation
Suspect was on drugs
Kahealani latest victim of 'ice' plague

Sources: Honolulu Advertiser & Star Bulletin

Drug abuse has been linked to violent crimes in Hawaii, including an alarming number of domestic crimes ranging from child neglect to homicide. All of the federal, state, and local law enforcement agencies that responded to the 2003 National Drug Threat Survey (NDTS) indicated that crystal methamphetamine abuse contributed more to violent crime and property crime throughout Hawaii than all other illicit drugs.

Marijuana-related violence in Hawaii is associated with protection of marijuana plots. According to the Hawaii County Police Department, officers occasionally encounter growers who resort to violent methods such as pipe guns, barb wire fences, bear traps, and "bungee sticks" to injure law enforcement, along with others who come upon the site. Hawaii has also experienced homicides relating to drug debts associated with marijuana trafficking and disputes over ownership of the harvested drug.

Section V.

Summary of Threat & Needs Assessment

The State of Hawaii and U.S. Territories of the Pacific are currently under attack from crystal methamphetamine. The abuse and the violence associated with it have reached epidemic proportions. This is the single most significant drug problem facing the region and cannot be over emphasized.

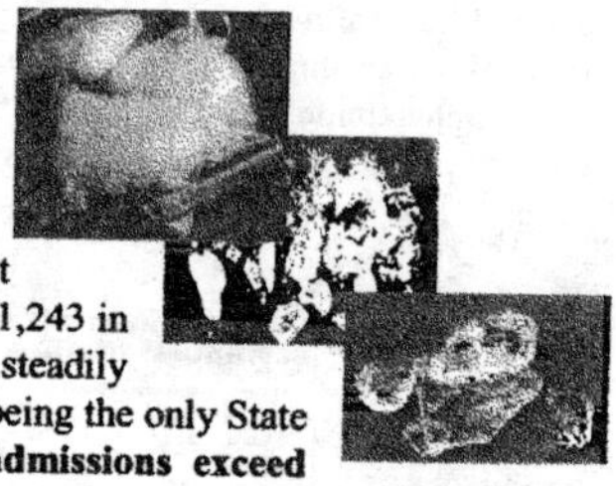

Crystal methamphetamine is the most significant drug threat in Hawaii. High purity crystal methamphetamine, ranging from 95-100 percent pure, is readily available, and is commonly abused throughout the State. According to Treatment Episode Data Sets (TEDS), treatment admissions for amphetamine abuse increased from 1,243 in 1998 to 2,238 in 2002[8]. This rate has increased steadily and in 2003 Hawaii had the dubious distinction of being the only State to have **crystal methamphetamine treatment admissions exceed alcohol abuse treatment admissions**. Estimates run as high as 90 percent of the property crimes committed in the State being drug-related. In 2001, the latest year for which national data is available, Hawaii ranked 10th for burglaries, 1st for larceny-thefts, and 6th for motor vehicle thefts. Overall Hawaii has risen from 6th highest in the nation to **3rd highest total crime rate** per 100,000 resident population in just one year[9].

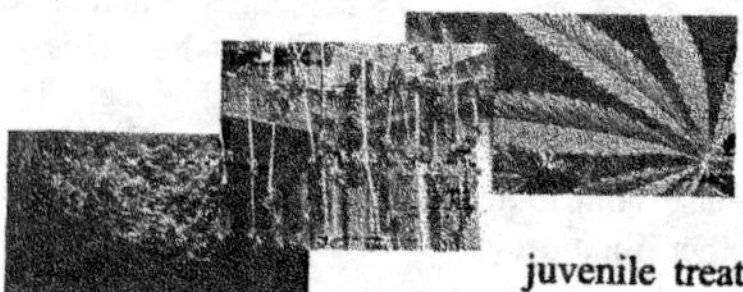

Hawaii's second most significant drug threat is marijuana. This drug is widely available, and abuse is increasing among Hawaii's juveniles. Health care professionals indicate that high rates of juvenile treatment admissions result from the addictive properties of the high-potency marijuana available in the State. Hawaiian grown marijuana is commonly cultivated and contains some of the highest tetrahydrocannabinol (THC) in the nation. Although most of the marijuana available in Hawaii is produced locally, BC Bud is occasionally smuggled into the state from Canada, via domestic flights and parcels.

Hawaii is seeing an emergence of violence and death related to marijuana. In July 2003, a 53-year old Kahuku man was charged with killing his partner in a 700 marijuana plant

[8] This category includes methamphetamine and other amphetamines including Benzedrine, Dexedrine, preludin, Ritalin and any other amines and related drugs (SAMSHA description of drug categories).

[9] Source: Hawaii Attorney General's Office, Crime Prevention and Justice Assistance Division, 2002 Crime in Hawaii

growing operation. Likewise, in September, a Manoa man was charged with killing his partner over a marijuana cultivation scheme gone bad. In November 2003, three subjects were arrested after shooting two victims during a marijuana dispute. Add to this, senseless acts like a man who jumped off a 150-foot cliff into a waterfall pool after drinking alcohol and smoking marijuana, and a contradictory picture surfaces from those who would legalize marijuana. Whereas marijuana is promoted by legalization advocates as a nonviolent, harmless drug, these incidents are perfect examples of the dangers associated with this drug.

Cocaine is Hawaii's third most significant drug threat. Cocaine prices indicate that sufficient quantities of cocaine and crack cocaine are available to meet user demand in Hawaii, and Honolulu Police Department arrest statistics indicate that cocaine arrests (182) occur approximately 6 times more often than heroin arrests (29). The distribution and abuse of powdered and crack cocaine are associated with criminal activities such as homicides, assaults, and child abuse/neglect cases.

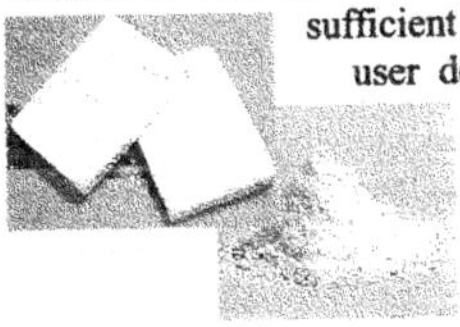

Heroin is commonly abused in Hawaii and decreasing heroin prices indicate that sufficient quantities of the drug are readily available. According to TEDS, heroin abuse is decreasing as indicated by the lower number of heroin treatment admissions to publicly funded treatment facilities.

Use of predatory drugs, including MDMA, GHB, and LSD, is increasing among Hawaii's youth (which is contrary to a decline among youth on the continental U.S.) and the large military population stationed in Hawaii. These drugs are readily available and typically consumed by military personnel, teenagers, and young adults attracted to dance clubs, raves, and bars.

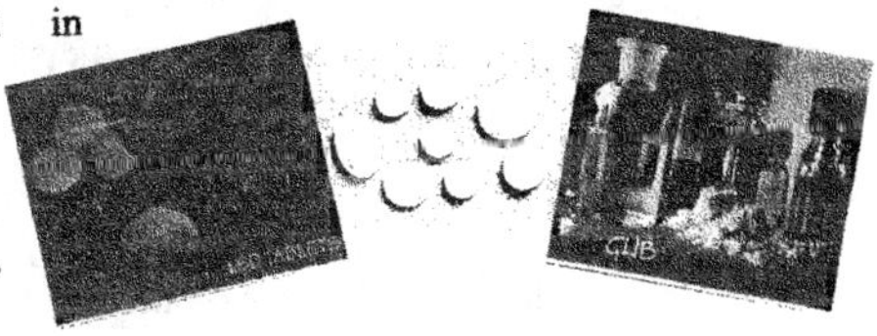

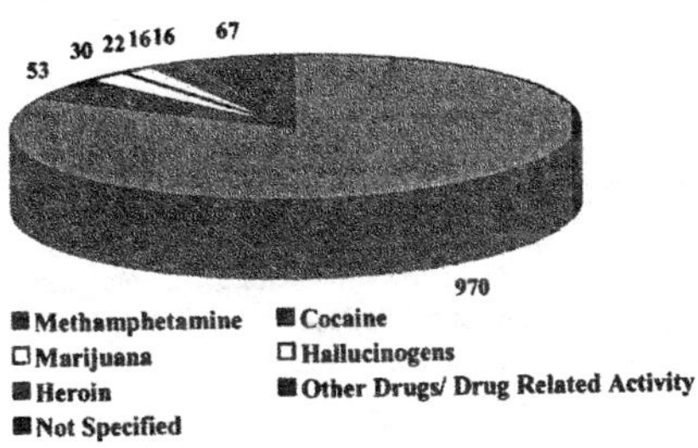

Western States Information Network (WSIN) deconfliction shows that methamphetamine (including amphetamines and crystal methamphetamine) accounted for 83 percent of critical event activity reported in Hawaii for CY2003. Although marijuana is still a top priority for drug enforcement, the decreasing arrest statistics are likely a result of drained law enforcement resources diverted to crystal methamphetamine cases.

THREAT POSED BY DRUG TRAFFICKING ORGANIZATIONS.

Drug trafficking organizations and their related criminal activities remain a constant concern for Hawaii's law enforcement agencies and are a major threat throughout Hawaii. Drug trafficking is big business, and like any business seeks to increase its customer base and profitability. Drug trafficking organizations (DTOs) undermine efforts of community groups, treatment providers, prevention/education efforts, and law enforcement by pushing their illegal products in Hawaii's cities and neighborhoods.

International DTOs produce high volumes of illegal drugs and use foreign countries as platforms from which to control their empires. These traffickers maintain control of their workers through highly compartmentalized cell structures that separate production, shipment, distribution, money laundering, communications and security. They use corruption and intimidation to protect their activities. Because of the ethnic diversity of Hawaii's population, International DTOs have easy access to the drug trade in Hawaii. International DTOs are made up of ethnic Japanese, Chinese, Korean, Filipino, and other Asian groups from Thailand, Laos, Cambodia, and Vietnam. These international DTOs are linked with their ethnic counterparts in Hawaii.

Consolidated Priority Organization Targets (CPOTs) are national priority targets set by the Department of Justice. CPOTs are linked to Hawaii's local and Pacific Islander drug trafficking organizations through high level Mexican polydrug traffickers. Most of the crystal methamphetamine, cocaine, and heroin destined for distribution in Hawaii is sent from the West Coast, primarily Los Angeles, Las Vegas and San Diego to local, Mexican, and Pacific Islander DTOs. However, while cocaine and heroin typically originates from South America and Mexico the methamphetamine is mostly produced in California or Mexican labs controlled by Mexican CPOTs. During CY2003 there were six CPOT linked investigations identified in Hawaii.

Regional Priority Organizational Targets (RPOTs) are organizations that conduct operations over an expanded area, including two or more of Hawaii's, ocean separated, island counties. Intelligence reporting indicates that there are several Asian RPOTs and DTOs operating in Hawaii. These Asian RPOTs and DTOs remain highly cohesive and difficult for law enforcement authorities to penetrate because of their strong ethnic, family and/or tribal ties. Hawaii's RPOTs are prosecuted in conjunction with the Organized Crime Drug Enforcement Task Force (OCDEFT).

Local DTOs are responsible for the majority of *mid-level & retail distribution* of crystal methamphetamine, cocaine, and heroin in Hawaii. They are typically supplied through loose connections or links to International DTOs, RPOTs, and/or CPOTs. Local DTOs are difficult for law enforcement agencies to dismantle and disrupt because they are fluid organizations with tight family/ethnic relationships. The ability to easily grow marijuana in Hawaii has also allowed some local DTOs to become wholesalers and distributors within the state and exporters of marijuana to other parts of the world.

Independent distributors without a structured distribution network are mostly associated with the lesser threat of predatory drugs such as ecstasy, GHB, and GBL as well as diverted pharmaceuticals.

THREAT POSED BY FUGITIVES REMAINING AT LARGE IN COMMUNITIES.

Hawaii's drug laws and Constitution form gaps and divergence when matched against federal statutes. (See – Need for Amendment to State and Local Law – later in chapter) This and other factors have led to a disproportionate share of individuals having multiple felony arrests and/or felony fugitives remaining free in communities and neighborhoods. This circumstance is particularly worrisome, with regard to those wanted on violent offenses, drug trafficking offenses, weapons offenses and money laundering. This threat impacts on the safety and well-being of citizens and families, and allows arrested traffickers to continue drug related crime, aided by this revolving door policy.

THREAT POSED BY ARMED VIOLENT DRUG TRAFFICKING OFFENDERS.

Crystal methamphetamine and cocaine abusers have been linked to violent crimes in Hawaii, including an alarming number of domestic crimes such as child neglect, hostage situations, and homicides. Although heroin abuse has been associated with the high rate of property crimes, there have been limited reports on violence associated with heroin distribution and abuse.

THREAT POSED BY TRANSPORTATION AND/OR TRANSSHIPMMENT OF ILLICIT DRUGS VIA COURIER, COMMERCIAL SHIPMENT, AND PARCEL.

Since 9-11 airborne package delivery services such as FedEx, UPS, and the U.S. Postal Service have been the primary transportation method for drugs entering the State of Hawaii. In 2003, the U.S. Postal Service delivered 18 million packages to the state. In addition, FedEx receives approximately 10,000 express delivery packages a day. This translates to approximately 25 million packages entering Hawaii each year just between these two delivery services. This transportation method, although significant, makes it difficult to determine the actual volume of illegal drugs transported into Hawaii. It has been estimated by some local law enforcement agencies that more than 50 percent of illegal narcotics transported to Hawaii come via package delivery services.

Package delivery services are the most common transportation methods encountered in Hawaii since they are fast and inexpensive. The same tracking system that allows individuals and businesses to follow their packages across the country also alerts drug traffickers if there is a delay along the route that could be caused by law enforcement interception. DTOs can easily transport multi-pound or multi-kilogram quantities of drugs on a weekly basis. The same services are also used to send illegal drug proceeds back to the continental U.S.

International drug smuggling is common and many seizures at the U.S. Postal Service's International Mail Branch have been made involving opium, steroids, pharmaceutical drugs, as well as other illicit drugs, such as crystal methamphetamine. The International Mail Branch in Hawaii reported that poppies typically are smuggled from Laos to Hawaii and then on to the continental U.S. Hawaii is also an international transshipment point for crystal methamphetamine and heroin from the west coast to other Pacific Basin locations. The many diverse methods of transporting illicit drugs into Hawaii make it difficult to quantify actual numbers. DTOs have couriers who make multiple trips from Hawaii to the continental U.S. and transport the drugs using the body carry technique or by simply mailing the drugs to Hawaii using parcel delivery services. Neither method permits the trafficking of large amounts; however, the practice of making frequent trips assures an adequate supply for their distribution networks.

THREAT POSED BY MONEY LAUNDERING.

The same package delivery services used to transport drugs into Hawaii are used to mail illegal drug proceeds back to the Continental U.S to the sources of supply.

Money laundering is the act of hiding the source and/or destination of illegally obtained funds. Money laundering is usually performed so that the profits of criminal activity - be it theft, drug sales, or some other crime - will appear to have originated from a legitimate transaction. It is estimated that nationally about $500 billion in illegally obtained funds are laundered annually. Money that is laundered and sent from Hawaii poses a significant economic threat, in that it is not used to pay taxes, build schools or roads, and it leaves the state with no benefit to the local economy.

CPOT linked DTOs commonly send the majority of their proceeds back to Mexico, using parcels, mail, cash couriers, money orders, wire transfers, and remittance services. Funds are often transported from points throughout Hawaii directly to Mexico or through major collection points in California, Texas, and Arizona where the funds are used to pay suppliers. International DTOs typically send their proceeds to their countries of origin, where the money is used to purchase businesses or real property. Authorities are aware of money laundering involving the purchase of expensive residential real estate on all the islands by individual drug traffickers associated with continental U.S. and Asian DTOs.

Local DTOs typically do not use sophisticated money laundering techniques. They purchase items such as cars, motorcycles, and personal watercraft. A majority of local DTOs will simply mail the money back to the source of supply via package delivery services or transport the money via couriers.

THREAT POSED BY CULTIVATION AND PRODUCTION OF MARIJUANA.

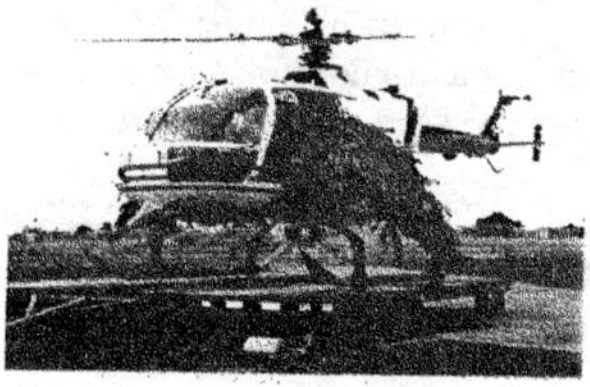

High-potency Hawaiian grown marijuana as well as BC bud is readily available in Hawaii. Marijuana prices indicate that availability remains stable with wholesale and retail prices remaining the same or slightly higher from 1992 to 2003. Wholesale quantities of marijuana sold for $400–$800 per ounce in 1992 and $400–$800 in 2003. In CY2003 retail quantities sold for $100-175 per 1/4 ounce[10].

Aided by abundant sunshine and warm afternoon rains Hawaii's weather makes for optimal growing conditions. The National Institute on Drug Abuse Marijuana Potency Monitoring Program states the average THC level of samples supplied to them from Hawaii has shown a decline in potency from 11.9 percent in 1998, 11.1 percent in 1999, and 6.2 percent in 2000, to 5.0 in 2001. This decline is contradicted by the Hawaii County Police Department which reported THC levels in the Hilo area have risen as high as 19-20 percent in 2003.

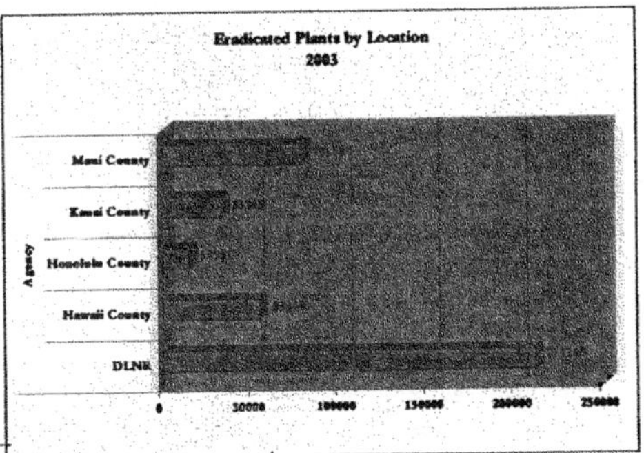

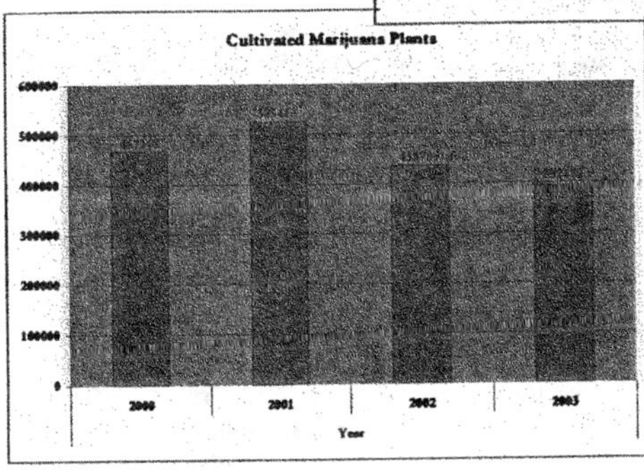

Marijuana cultivators often use public lands such as national forests and state parks. The state Department of Land and Natural Resources accounted for nearly 58% of eradicated marijuana plants in 2003[11]. The majority of marijuana is cultivated at remote sites located in Hawaii County (Big Island), although it is cultivated throughout the State. Typically, indoor marijuana grows are small and located in private residences. The marijuana from these indoor grows is usually for local distribution or personal use.

The percentage of marijuana-related federal sentences in Hawaii was approximately one-fourth of the national average in FY2001. According to the United States Sentencing Commission 9.7 percent of drug-related federal sentences in Hawaii were marijuana-related, compared with the national average of 32.8 percent. The number of marijuana-related federal sentences in Hawaii was the lowest of all illicit drug federal sentences from FY1997 through FY2001. Hawaii had 7 marijuana-related federal sentences in FY1997, 9 in FY1998, 14 in FY1999, 12 in FY2000, and 17 in FY2001[12].

---

[10] Source: 2004 Hawaii HIDTA Threat Assessment and NDIC Narcotics Digest Weekly, Volume 2, Number 50

[11] Source: Drug Enforcement Administration, Domestic Cannabis Eradication/Suppression Program, Honolulu District Office

[12] Source: United States Sentencing Commission, FY2001 Federal Sentencing Statistics by State

NEED FOR AMENDMENT TO STATE AND LOCAL LAWS

Hawaii's drug laws and Constitution form gaps when matched against federal statutes.

Hawaii's electronic surveillance laws were originally adopted in 1978 and have not been significantly amended since 1989. Technology has changed substantially in the intervening 14 years leaving Hawaii's law hopelessly outdated and restrictive. The most serious problem with the electronic surveillance law is its challenger provision. The challenger provision, which is not in the federal statutes, requires that before an order authorizing or approving the interception of wire, oral or electronic communications can be issued, an in-camera adversarial hearing must be held before a judge. A *defense attorney* is appointed for the purpose of the hearing and is provided with the application for the wiretap as well as all supporting documents. At the hearing, the defense attorney has the right to cross-examine all witnesses.

The philosophy behind the "challenger provision" is that an adversarial hearing would protect against rubber stamping by judges or decisions based on a distorted view of evidence and arguments supporting the application. However, this argument is flawed in that judges grant search warrants, which are more invasive than electronic surveillance, yet no adversarial hearing is required. The challenger provision creates many problems for local law enforcement. The additional dissemination of information regarding potential targets, witnesses, and evidence increases the risk that the target of the investigation will find out about the investigation and increases potential danger to any informants and witnesses. ***Furthermore, evidence obtained from federal wiretaps is inadmissible in Hawaii's courts, since it lacks the "challenger provision."*** As a result many "down-line" dealers who do not meet federal thresholds go unprosecuted in State Courts. It is not uncommon to find individuals with 30 plus arrests still free on city streets.

Consensual encounters, commonly referred to as "walk and talk" are not permited under the Hawaii State Constitution. In 1996 the Hawaii Supreme Court ruled in ***State v. Trainor***, 83 Hawaii 250 (1996), that simply approaching someone in the airport violated the Hawaii Constitution. Even if an investigator informed the person being approached that a drug investigation was being conducted; and they were talking to a police officer; and that they were free to leave at any time; that person could not be prosecuted in State Court for any drugs discovered pursuant to the state law governing consensual encounters.

It is interesting to note that consensual encounters are currently being conducted at Hawaii airports. Local law enforcement officers are cross-designated with federal authority to conduct encounters. The problem faced by law enforcement here is that any evidence of an offense that is discovered through this technique can only be used in Federal Court, which has a limited number of attorneys available to prosecute the offenses. ***Therefore, evidence obtained from federal consensual encounters is inadmissible in Hawaii State Court, since it lacks constitutional standing.*** As with the wiretap law, federal thresholds prohibit prosecution and repeat offenders remain free.

Medical Marijuana
In 2000, the State of Hawaii passed a law that allowed qualified patients and their caregivers to possess an "adequate supply" of marijuana not to exceed three mature marijuana plants, four immature marijuana plants, and one ounce of usable marijuana per each mature plant[13]. The law states that medical use of marijuana by a patient is permitted if they have been diagnosed by a physician as having a debilitating medical condition that the patient's physician has certified in writing that the potential benefit of medical marijuana would likely outweigh the health risk for the patient.

This law has caused many problems for law enforcement agencies. Changes are needed to help law enforcement personnel differentiate between allowances under state law and illegal marijuana use. Stricter guidelines on record keeping are needed. Clarification of state law is also needed to address the cultivation of medical marijuana.

Training Needs
The Hawaii HIDTA has identified the need for training that improves the ability of participating agencies to counter drug trafficking and related criminal activity. Coordinated effort is needed to fulfill the training needs of personnel assigned to the Hawaii HIDTA. By providing on-site training, coordinating other agency and/or out-source training, and disseminating information about training opportunities the Hawaii HIDTA is able to increase the knowledge, skills, and abilities of investigative and analytical personnel directly involved in the drug suppression effort. Appropriate in-service training also needs to be provided to improve the efficiency of HIDTA management and support operations. Other criminal activities conducted by CPOTs and other DTOs are hard to track because the State of Hawaii does not specifically report drug-related crimes. HIDTA and law enforcement officials believe the number of clandestine labs operating in Hawaii is significantly underreported due to lack of training on proper identification of a lab.

[13] Source: Hawaii State Legislature, 2003 Hawaii Revised Statutes, Part IX Medical Use of Marijuana

HIDTA Goals

Section VI.

*The overall objective of the HIDTA Program is to reduce drug availability by creating intelligence driven drug task forces aimed at eliminating or reducing domestic drug trafficking and its harmful consequences through enhancing and helping to coordinate drug trafficking control efforts among federal, state and local law enforcement agencies.**

HIDTA HAS IDENTIFIED THREE GOALS TO ACCOMPLISH THE MISSION.

GOAL ONE. REDUCE DRUG AVAILABILITY BY ELIMINATING OR DISRUPTING DRUG TRAFFICKING ORGANIZATIONS

The illegal drug market in the United States is one of the most profitable in the world. Prices in Hawaii and the Pacific Region are two to four times as high as the continental US, creating an attractive market for drug traffickers and organizations from both the continental US and Asian countries.

	matrix – goal 1 (consolidated) - desired outcomes
COMBINED HAWAII HIDTA GOALS	TARGET 10 OF IDENTIFIED DRUG DISTRIBUTION ORGANIZATIONS AND DISMANTLE OR DISRUPT 10 OF THOSE TARGETED
	TARGET 6 OF IDENTIFIED DRUG MANUFACTURING ORGANIZATIONS AND DISMANTLE OR DISRUPT 5 OF THOSE TARGETED
	CLEAR 250 WARRANTS FOR DRUG CHARGES
	ARREST 50 ARMED VIOLENT DRUG OFFENDERS WITH A NARCOTICS NEXUS
	ARREST 50 INDIVIDUALS WHO SMUGGLE NARCOTICS THROUGH THE AIRPORT
	INSPECT 750 PARCELS AND SEIZE 500 PARCELS
	SECURE 25 HIDTA-ASSISTED FEDERAL INDICTMENTS AGAINST STATE/LOCAL DRUG TRAFFICKERS
	TARGET 1 MONEY REMITTANCE ESTABLISHMENT FOR MONEY LAUNDERING CHARGES
	SEIZE $1,000,000 IN ILLICIT DRUG RELATED ASSETS
	FORFEIT $1,000,000 IN ILLICIT DRUG RELATED ASSETS
	ERADICATE 50,000 MARIJUANA PLANTS
	SEIZE 50 FIREARMS

Section 3 HIDTA Matrix – consolidated goals for all Investigative Initiatives

The Hawaii HIDTA's primary goal is to dismantle, disrupt, arrest, and prosecute drug trafficking organizations, drug gangs and organized crime groups involved in drug distribution, drug manufacturing, money laundering, and other drug related crimes. The team and task force concepts advance the National Drug Control Strategy and the

* Source: Revised HIDTA Program Policy and Budget Guidance, Section XIII Performance Management, page 3

National Gang Strategy by emphasizing collocated/commingled, multi-agency investigations and promotes cooperative efforts among HIDTA participants.

Part of the HIDTA's goal is to have an effective airport, marine and parcel interdiction program targeting both domestic and international drug traffickers. It is designed to identify persons and organizations utilizing commercial airports, US mail facilities, and private mail/cargo/container companies within the State of Hawaii to facilitate the movement of illegal drugs and drug proceeds throughout the State. The goal is to assist narcotic interdiction teams nationwide in their attempt to identify and arrest drug traffickers and prosecute those persons involved in the transportation of illegal drugs.

HIDTA also targets individuals and rogue chemical suppliers that are providing chemicals and lab equipment used in the illicit manufacturing of methamphetamine. Interdiction efforts are made to intercept shipments of precursor chemicals that often come from international sources in Asia. Law enforcement personnel are trained to identify chemicals and equipment that are used to manufacture methamphetamine and to convert it to crystal methamphetamine.

Money laundering is another aspect of the drug trade that is a concern to law enforcement. HIDTA personnel gather and analyze intelligence that can be used to identify, criminally investigate and prosecute organizations utilizing various means to facilitate drug trafficking activities and launder illicit drug proceeds. The goal is to dismantle these organizations through the proactive use of federal and state seizure and forfeiture laws; to target suspicious money transmitting organizations, both internationally and domestically; and to identify and monitor the methods used by drug organizations and money launderers to transport drug proceeds in and out of the State of Hawaii.

To accomplish this goal HIDTA focuses participating agencies on conducting long term, complex, multi-jurisdictional investigations. HIDTA brings federal, state and local narcotics law enforcement resources within Hawaii together under one task force "umbrella" that is collocated on all county islands, where possible.

GOAL TWO. REDUCE THE HARMFUL CONSEQUENCES OF DRUG TRAFFICKING

Drug trafficking causes various problems in the community and negatively impacts the quality of life.

- Crystal methamphetamine use affects nearly 30,000 people in the State of Hawaii. The state's total population is 1,224,398[14]. This means that 1 in 40 people or approximately 2.5% of the population is affected.

[14] Source: US Census Bureau

- Hawaii ranks number two in the nation for property crime, and it is estimated that 90% of these crimes are drug related[15].

- 62.4% of male arrestees tested positive for drug use. [16]

- 46% of arrestees in Honolulu for any crime tested positive for methamphetamine use[16a].

- Statewide there are approximately 3500 active warrants for drug charges[17].

- 90% of child abuse cases stem from drug and/or alcohol abuse[18]

COMBINED HAWAII HIDTA GOALS	matrix – goal 2 (consolidated) - desired outcomes
	SEIZE 100 FIREARMS FROM VIOLENT DRUG TRAFFICKERS
	APPREHEND 100 DRUG FUGITIVES
	PROPOSE MODEL LEGISLATION TO INCREASE INVESTIGATIVE METHODS

Section 3 HIDTA Matrix – consolidated goals and outcomes for community consequences

In addition to the effects of drug trafficking on the quality of life in the community, Hawaii state law impedes the ability of law enforcement to effectively combat drug traffickers. Evidence obtained from federal wiretap and consensual encounters is not admissible in Hawaii State Courts. Therefore, any evidence of a crime found during a federal investigation can only be used in federal court but not state court. Because the federal threshold for drug possession is higher than that at the state level, persons are currently being released without prosecution.

Goal Three. Improve the Efficiency and Effectiveness of Law Enforcement Organizations

The guiding theme of the HIDTA Program is to attack drug trafficking from all angles by combining all available resources from federal, state and local law enforcement organizations.

The main goal of the support initiatives, including the Management and Coordination initiative is to facilitate the efficient operation of all investigative and case support activities by providing oversight, administrative, and budgetary support, in accordance with ONDCP and Hawaii HIDTA Executive Board policy and directives. The support

[15] Source: Honolulu Police Department, published Honolulu Advertiser
[16] Source: ADAM website, Honolulu branch
[16a] Source: ADAM website, Honolulu branch
[17] Source: United States Marshall Service, District of Hawaii
[18] Source: Child Protective Services, published Honolulu Star Bulletin October 8, 1998 Day 1: Downward Spiral - The Lure Of Ice

initiatives coordinate resources and promote and encourage information sharing. The Hawaii HIDTA also provides a strong training program to enhance the knowledge and skills of participating personnel and staff.

	matrix – goal 3 (consolidated) - desired outcomes
COMBINED HAWAII HIDTA GOALS	ACHIEVE AND MAINTAIN 100% PARTICIPATION BY LAW ENFORCEMENT AGENCIES IN THE WSIN DECONFLICTION SERVICES
	SUBMIT 9000 CASE/SUBJECT DECONFLICTIONS AMONG HIDTA INITIATIVES AND PARTICIPATING AGENCIES
	SUBMIT 1400 EVENT DECONFLICTIONS AMONG HIDTA INITIATIVES AND PARTICIPATING AGENCIES
	ISC TO CONDUCT 4000 DATABASE QUERIES & PROVIDE 100 INTELLIGENCE REPORTS
	PROVIDE ANALYTICAL CASE SUPPORT TO 20 CASES
	PROVIDE 3000 ANALYTICAL PRODUCTS (TOLL ANALYSES, LINK ANALYSES, GRAPHS, CHARTS, PROFILES, ETC)
	PROVIDE ELECTRONIC LINK FROM ISC TO NEIGHBOR ISLANDS VIA WSIN SECURE INTRANET
	SHARE INTELLIGENCE DATA WITH OTHER HIDTAS/LEAS OUTSIDE OF HAWAII
	DEVELOP AN ACTIVE MEANS OF COMMUNICATING WITH PACIFIC BASIN/RIM LAW ENFORCEMENT
	SPONSOR QUARTERLY TRAINING PROGRAMS FOR REGIONAL AND/OR SPECIALIZED TRAINING
	SPONSOR QUARTERLY CLANDESTINE LAB TRAINING PROGRAMS
	DISSEMINATE EXISTING TRAINING OPPORTUNITIES FROM OTHER AGENCIES TO HIDTA PERSONNEL
	DEVELOP & MAINTAIN HIDTA TRAINING DATABASE
	ESTABLISH CORRDINATION WITH CLAN LAB RESPONSE COORDINATORS AT FEDERAL, STATE, AND LOCAL AGENCIES
	PROVIDE COLLOCATION FOR HIDTA INITIATIVES
	DEVELOP PARTNERSHIPS WITH EXISTING TRAINING COORDINATORS AT FEDERAL, STATE, AND LOCAL AGENCIES
	MEET IN EXECUTIVE SESSION A MINIMUM OF 6 TIMES TO COORDINATE HAWAII HIDTA ACTIVITIES
	CONDUCT MONTHLY MEETINGS WITH HIDTA INITIATIVES
	ATTAIN 100% OF DEVELOPMENTAL STANDARDS
	COMPLETE AND TRACK A FULL INVENTORY OF ACCOUNTABLE EQUIPMENT PURCHASED WITH HIDTA FUNDS
	MONITOR, REVIEW, AND TRACK FISCAL EXPENDITURES BY HIDTA INITIATIVES TO ENSURE COMPLIANCE WITH POLICIES
	CONDUCT FISCAL AUDITS OF ALL INITIATIVES
	IMPLEMENT & CONDUCT HAWAII HIDTA'S INTERNAL REVIEW PROGRAM
	HOLD QUARTERLY MEETINGS WITH INITIATIVE AND PARTICIPATING AGENCY SUPERVISORS
	PREPARE THE ANNUAL REPORT, THREAT ASSESSMENT, STRATEGY, AND BUDGET

Section 3 HIDTA Matrix – consolidated goals and outcomes for oversight and support

Among the HIDTA Program's goals is providing subject and event deconfliction to ensure officer and citizen safety during law enforcement activities; and providing a secure electronic link to neighbor islands via WSIN intranet. Another goal is providing analytical support, intelligence, enhanced case support, and access to open-source and closed-source information for participating agencies.

Hawaii historically has long served as a crossroad for international narcotics planning, staging and as a transit point. By focusing drug intelligence from the Pacific Rim/Basin into the ISC, participating agencies can obtain timely, useful information to coordinate and synchronize efforts to reduce drug trafficking. This cooperative information is available nowhere else.

The HIDTA has established a goal to coordinate and support all "first responders" to clandestine laboratory calls ensuring that all island teams are fully outfitted and have completely certified and operational equipment; to share personnel resources, providing certified personnel for clandestine laboratory operations and also support personnel in the sampling and recovery of lab evidence. In pursuit of unification, personnel certification and management, equipment maintenance and team function, each county team will be part of a single Hawaii Clandestine Laboratory Response Team coordinated by a full time dedicated Manager.

Because of Hawaii's unique island makeup, HIDTA initiatives on the islands of Maui, Hawaii, and Kauai maintain separate office facilities that justify their operational needs. Through the ISC LAN/WAN and WSIN, HIDTA initiatives can communicate and exchange information among the various facilities. This infrastructure is important to fulfilling the investigative, intelligence, and administrative needs of these initiatives.

The Hawaii HIDTA Fiscal Officer ensures compliance with ONDCP and the NHPO policy of expenditure tracking. Each initiative is required to provide a detailed quarterly report identifying their respective budget and documenting their expenses. The information is then imported into a spreadsheet used to track the overall Hawaii HIDTA budget.

In order to achieve and exceed developmental standards, the Hawaii HIDTA has implemented an annual internal audit and self-review policy as directed by ONDCP and NHPO. The reviews address the following areas: support of the National Drug Control Strategy through the Hawaii HIDTA strategy and initiatives; effectiveness of the Hawaii HIDTA's efforts in accomplishing its missions; efficiency in the use of Hawaii HIDTA resources; accountability in the use of Hawaii HIDTA resources; and compliance with Hawaii HIDTA and ONDCP/NHPO policies and directives.

Hawaii HIDTA Strategy

Section VII.

The Hawaii HIDTA accomplishes its mission through a coordinated strategy and wide participation by Federal, State and Local law enforcement agencies. During CY2003 law enforcement organizations contributed 123 full-time officers, 120 part-time officers and/or non-collocated officers on neighbor islands, for a total of 243 law enforcement personnel organized into 9 initiatives. Each HIDTA initiative develops a mission statement to focus their efforts on one or more of the HIDTA Program's three goals.

Each of the initiatives and the investigative task forces target identified drug threats from the current HIDTA Threat Assessment. Each Hawaii HIDTA element is required to accomplish one or more of the following goals:

- Disrupt/dismantle International, CPOT, RPOT, and Local drug trafficking organizations.
- Interdict illicit drugs destined for Hawaii, or transiting Hawaii's airports and seaports, for the continental U.S. and other foreign destinations.
- Reduce drug trafficking of methamphetamine, marijuana, heroin, cocaine and predatory drugs by major drug trafficking organizations engaged in smuggling, transportation, supply or distribution.
- Reduce the number of firearms connected with drug trafficking and the number of drug fugitives operating within the Hawaii HIDTA.
- Reduce money laundering crime related to drug trafficking.
- Provide drug intelligence and investigative support to HIDTA initiatives.
- Provide event deconfliction and electronic communication links among the island counties.
- Provide administrative support and oversight for program coordination, planning, development, performance, and fiscal accountability of HIDTA resources.
- Provide training that will advance the knowledge and coordinate the skills of HIDTA participating personnel.

Hawaii Interagency Mobile Police Apprehension Crime Task Force (HI-IMPACT)
The strategy behind the HI-IMPACT initiative is to organize a large part of HIDTA resources into efficient, interlocked task forces that target the most significant DTOs operating within the state. HI-IMPACT's mission is to use advanced investigative techniques to disrupt and dismantle these DTOs, gangs and organized crime groups involved in drug distribution, manufacturing, money laundering and other drug related crimes. Priorities include crystal methamphetamine, cocaine, heroin, marijuana, ecstasy and other drugs. The HI-IMPACT initiative advances the National Drug Control Strategy and the National Gang Strategy by emphasizing collocated/commingled, multi-agency investigations targeting CPOT/RPOT linked investigations and promotes cooperative efforts among HIDTA participants.

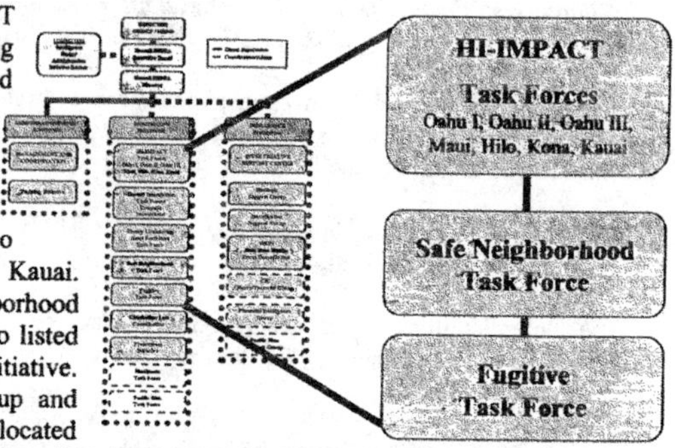

There were nine HI-IMPACT groups for CY2003 consisting of three groups on Oahu and collocated within HIDTA-funded space, one group on Maui, two groups on the "Big Island" of Hawaii County in the cities of Hilo and Kona, and one group on Kauai. For CY2003 the Safe Neighborhood and Fugitive groups were also listed under the HI-IMPACT initiative. The Safe Neighborhood group and the Fugitive group were both located on Oahu, but served all counties. The HI-IMPACT initiative is comprised of 102 full-time and part-time members. Participating agencies include Drug Enforcement Administration (DEA), Federal Bureau of Investigation (FBI), Immigration and Customs Enforcement (ICE), Bureau of Alcohol, Tobacco & Firearms (ATF), United States Marshall Service (USMS), United States Postal Service (USPS), Hawaii State Narcotics Enforcement Division (NED), Honolulu Police Department (HPD), Maui Police Department (MPD), Hawaii County Police Department (HCPD), Kauai County Police Department (KCPD), Hawaii National Guard (HNG), and Naval Criminal Investigative Service (NCIS).

Hawaii Interdiction Task Force (HITF)
Two interdiction groups constitute an airport, marine and parcel interdiction program targeting both domestic and international drug traffickers. This strategy is designed to identify persons and organizations utilizing commercial airports, US mail facilities and private mail/cargo/container firms within the State of Hawaii to facilitate the movement of illegal drugs and drug proceeds throughout the state. The interdiction groups target all levels and types of drug trafficking organizations attempting to utilize Hawaii's commercial airports, harbors, and parcel distribution centers for illicit purposes. The groups assist narcotics interdiction teams nationwide in their attempts to identify and arrest individuals involved in the transportation of illegal drugs.

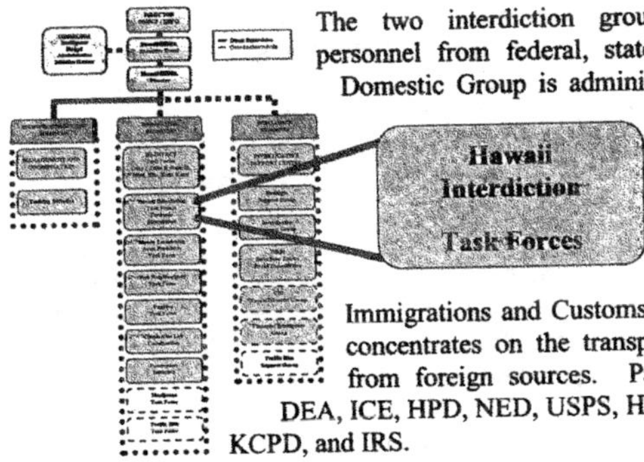

The two interdiction groups are commingled with personnel from federal, state and local agencies. The Domestic Group is administered by a DEA supervisor and focuses its efforts on drugs entering Hawaii from other U.S. locations.

The International Group is administered by an Immigrations and Customs Enforcement supervisor and concentrates on the transportation of drugs to Hawaii from foreign sources. Participating agencies include DEA, ICE, HPD, NED, USPS, HNG, FBI, ATF, MPD, HCPD, KCPD, and IRS.

Money Laundering Asset Forfeiture Task Force (MLAF)

The task of the Money Laundering Asset Forfeiture (MLAF) Task Force is to detect, disrupt and dismantle drug organizations that launder proceeds from illegal activities by tracing assets and the flow of drug money both internationally and nationally into and out of Hawaii. The task force also targets and penetrates suspicious money transmitting organizations. This initiative dismantles these organizations through the proactive use of federal and state seizure and forfeiture laws.

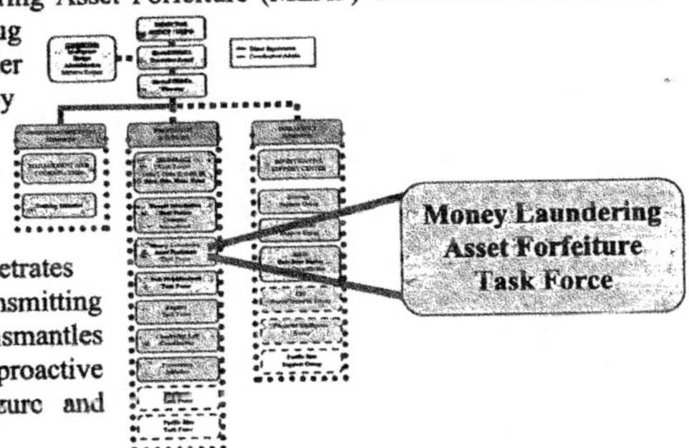

During CY2003 the Money Laundering Asset Forfeiture Task Force had a total of eight personnel from the following agencies: ICE, IRS, FBI, HPD, MPD, HCPD, KCPD.

Clandestine Laboratory Coordination Initiative

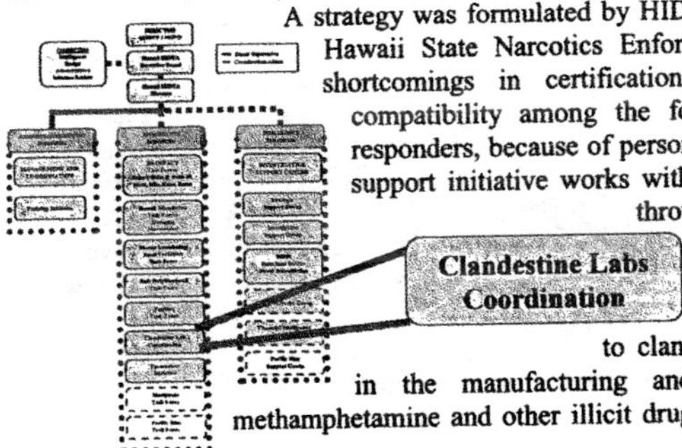

A strategy was formulated by HIDTA and implemented by the Hawaii State Narcotics Enforcement Division to address shortcomings in certification, training, and equipment compatibility among the four counties' clan lab first responders, because of personnel rotations. The Clan Lab support initiative works with law enforcement personnel throughout the State of Hawaii to provide oversight, consolidated training and to coordinate a first response to clandestine laboratories involved in the manufacturing and/or conversion of crystal methamphetamine and other illicit drugs. The purpose is to ensure that statewide first response teams are compliant with Occupational Safety and Health Administration (OSHA) certification and equipment requirements.

This strategy involves federal, state, and local law enforcement personnel from each of the state's four counties. Individual counties take the lead in identifying their own needs and organizing operations within their jurisdiction. The teams share personnel and equipment resources to process and dismantle illicit labs.

The Clan Lab Initiative is coordinated by the Hawaii State Narcotics Enforcement Division. It has a total of 15 primary response team members and 18 alternate response members from the following agencies: NED, DEA, State of Hawaii Department of Health, Hazard Evaluation and Emergency Response, HNG, HPD, MPD, HCPD, KCPD.

Prosecutorial Initiative

The primary objectives of the Hawaii HIDTA Prosecutorial Initiative are to increase coordination among prosecutors across the State of Hawaii, to provide legal guidance to HIDTA initiatives through the investigative stage, and to effectively and efficiently prosecute the cases developed by HIDTA initiatives. The Prosecutorial Initiative has designated prosecutors collocated at the Hawaii HIDTA who may provide legal support for subpoenas, arrest and search warrants, electronic surveillance, undercover operations and other related issues to Hawaii HIDTA initiatives . The Prosecutorial Initiative collaborates with prosecutors statewide to develop and implement coordinated strategies that address certain statewide drug enforcement problems including input supporting enactment and modification of state drug laws.

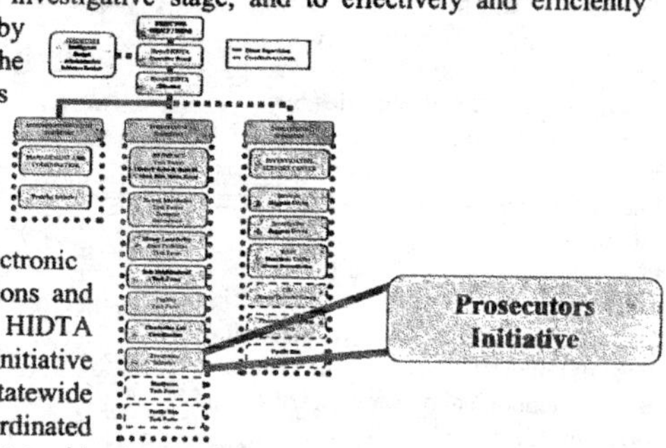

The Department of the Prosecuting Attorney for the City and County of Honolulu and the United States Attorney's Office provided initiative personnel for CY2003.

Investigative Support Center

The Hawaii HIDTA Investigative Support Center (ISC) provides tactical and strategic intelligence support to enforcement and interdiction initiatives in an effort to reduce drug trafficking in the State of Hawaii. To facilitate the availability and exchange of information, the ISC is collocated with several HIDTA initiatives and links electronically to other initiatives through the Western States Information Network (WSIN). Operation of the ISC provides full support to all HIDTA task forces and other law enforcement within the HIDTA region to achieve an intelligence-based approach to all counter-drug operations.

The ISC consists of two intelligence groups. The Investigative Support Group focuses on supporting on-going drug trafficking investigations primarily in the areas of communications analysis, association/link analysis, post seizure analysis, and event/subject deconfliction. The Strategic Support Group focuses on money laundering investigations and strategic reporting. The group collects, assembles, and disseminates data for the Hawaii HIDTA Threat Assessment and Annual Report, Trafficking Trends reports and other intelligence bulletins. Groups outlined by a dashed line do not currently exist, but have been planned by the Executive Board.

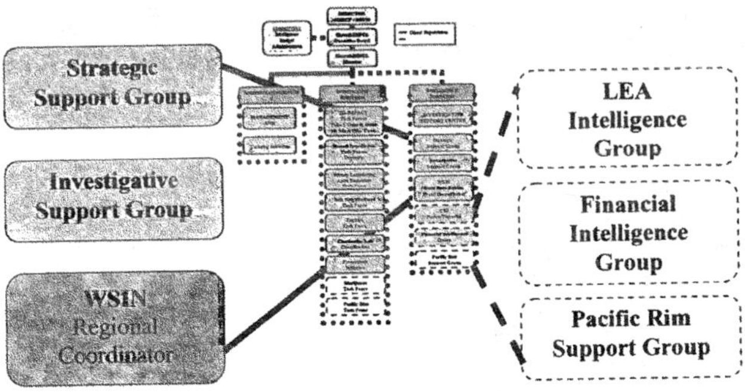

The collocated and commingled office space is configured to provide open access between investigative task forces and the intelligence component. This encourages free exchange of information between law enforcement officers and intelligence analysts. Because of Hawaii's unique island makeup, task forces and intelligence components on the outer islands maintain separate office facilities that justify their operational needs. Although there are separate facilities located on the outer islands they do maintain contact with the other initiatives through the ISC LAN/WAN, WSIN and various modes of communications (i.e., telephone, meeting, documents, etc.).

The Investigative Support Center is jointly managed by a DEA supervisor and a Honolulu PD supervisor and has sixteen personnel from the following agencies: DEA, HPD, HNG, ICE, FBI, United States Bureau of Prisons (USBOP), USCG, HCPD, MPD, KCPD, and WSIN. In addition, the ISC has three contract intelligence analysts.

Management and Coordination Initiative (MCI)

The Hawaii HIDTA Management and Coordination initiative provides day-to-day administrative support and oversight through its Director and staff. The initiative is responsible for administrative activities supporting the implementation of the HIDTA Performance Management System. Through the Director and staff, the initiative serves as liaison between ONDCP, the Hawaii HIDTA Executive Board, and participating agencies. The Management and Coordination initiative oversees preparation of administrative and fiscal reports required by ONDCP, coordinates programmatic and fiscal accountability of HIDTA resources, and oversees the progression of Hawaii HIDTA developmental standards.

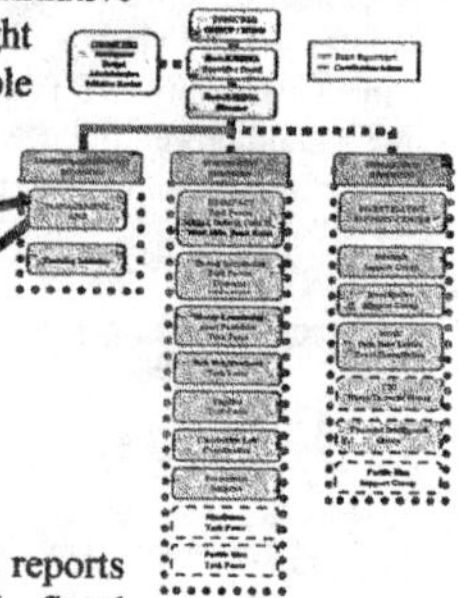

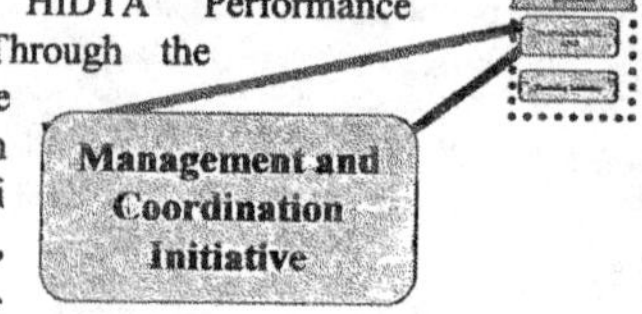

The Management and Coordination Initiative coordinates the collocation/commingling of task force members and the Investigative Support Center in a central office facility.

During the reporting period the Management and Coordination Initiative had a total of three contract personnel: Director, Financial Officer, and Administrative Assistant.

Training Initiative

The strategy of the Hawaii HIDTA Training Initiative is to improve the ability of participating agencies to counter drug trafficking and related criminal activity by providing pertinent, comprehensive training opportunities. The Training Initiative coordinates on-site and out-source training to enhance the knowledge, skills, and abilities of investigative and analytical personnel and provides in-service training to management and support personnel. In addition, the initiative tracks training and associated costs to determine effectiveness and eliminate duplication.

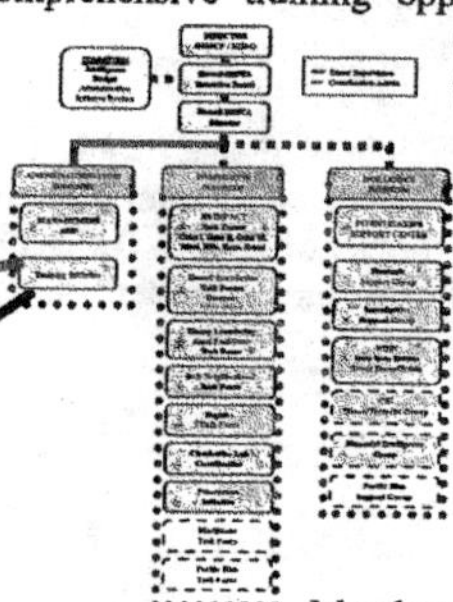

Members of the Training Initiative include the Training Coordinator and others who conduct the Training Program. It does not include personnel who receive training. Oversight is provided by: DEA, HPD, HNG.

Outcomes For Goal One

Section VIII.

Goal One. Reduce Drug Availability by Eliminating or Disrupting Drug Trafficking Organizations

INVESTIGATIVE SUBSYSTEM

	matrix – goal 1 (initiative specific)	Goal	Actual	%
HI-IMPACT, HITF, MLAF	TARGET DRUG DISTRIBUTION ORGANIZATIONS AND DISMANTLE OR DISRUPT THOSE TARGETED	10	34	340%
	TARGET DRUG MANUFACTURING ORGANIZATIONS AND DISMANTLE OR DISRUPT THOSE TARGETED	4	4	100%
	CLEAR WARRANTS FOR DRUG CHARGES	100	290	290%
	ARREST ARMED VIOLENT OFFENDERS WITH A NARCOTICS NEXUS	45	95	211%
	ARREST INDIVIDUALS WHO SMUGGLE NARCOTICS THROUGH AIRPORTS	50	47	94%
	INSPECT PARCELS	1000	10,000	1000%
	SEIZE PARCELS	100	60	60%
	TARGET DTOs FOR MONEY LAUNDERING CHARGES	1	1	100%
	SEIZE ILLICIT DRUG RELATED ASSETS	$1,000,000	2,510,906	251%
	ERADICATE MARIJUANA PLANTS	50,000	392,276	784.5%
	SEIZE FIREARMS	110	162	147.2%

Hawaii Interagency Mobile Police Apprehension Task Force (HI-IMPACT)
The HI-IMPACT Initiative is the main investigative arm of the Hawaii HIDTA whose focus is to disrupt and dismantle drug trafficking organizations. Statewide HI-IMPACT initiated **2137 drug cases** during CY2003. Hawaii HIDTA policy and procedures dictate that OCDETF designation be routinely sought for all investigations. HI-IMPACT cases resulted in **1605 arrests** on charges of possessing, manufacturing, and distributing illicit drugs. During the year HI-IMPACT groups coordinated with the Investigative Support Center to identify each group's top 10 drug trafficking organizations. By the end of 2003, **34 organizations had been disrupted or dismantled.**

Operation Shave Ice was a HI-IMPACT OCDETF investigation that involved a large

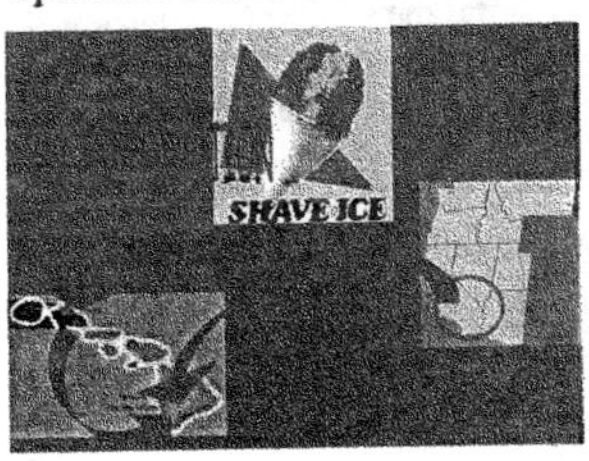

crystal methamphetamine and cocaine trafficking network operating on the Islands of Hawaii, aka "Big Island", and Oahu. The network was made up of five local drug trafficking organizations and three drug trafficking organizations on the continental U.S. These groups were responsible for distributing multi-kilo quantities of crystal methamphetamine and cocaine throughout the State of Hawaii from sources in California, Las Vegas and Arizona. They used store front auto detailing businesses to facilitate the flow of drugs and money. Drugs would be sent to Oahu via parcels and body carry and then forwarded to the Big Island concealed in cargo such as stereo speakers, cleaning supplies and auto parts. This investigation led to the initiation of 16 wiretaps which revealed links to two Mexican CPOTS. In October 2003 agents and officers in Hawaii, California, Nevada, and Arizona simultaneously executed over 60 arrest warrants and 50 search warrants on this network. Items seized during the takedown include 15 firearms and assets worth nearly $600,000. This coordinated effort dismantled the five local DTOs and severely disrupted the regional network. Subsequent leads have resulted in significant spin-off investigations and approximately 13 additional arrests of significant targets that transport drugs into Hawaii.

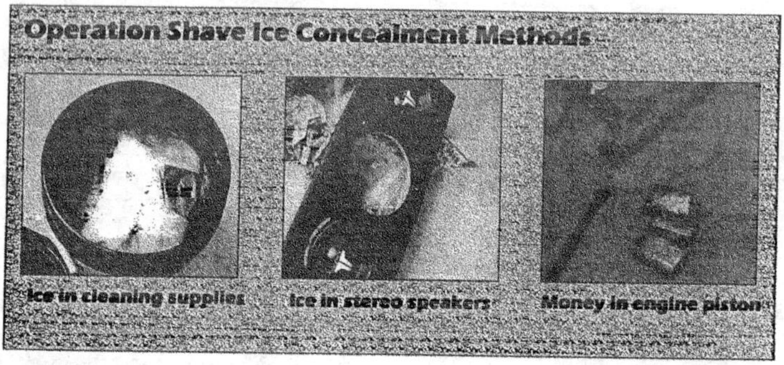
Operation Shave Ice Concealment Methods
Ice in cleaning supplies
Ice in stereo speakers
Money in engine piston

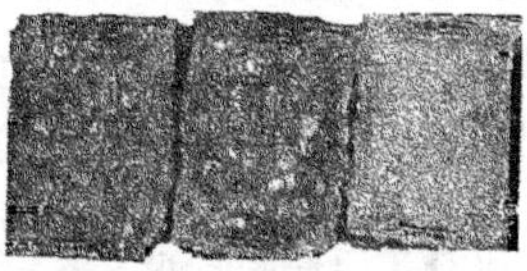

HI-IMPACT also received information that a subject was distributing crystal methamphetamine through a travel agency. Using confidential informants and undercover officers it was soon determined that the subject was one of several crystal methamphetamine lines leading to organized crime groups on Oahu. Further investigation, including the use of electronic surveillance, revealed drug sources in Las Vegas and Los Angeles. Beginning in March 2003, law enforcement began the first of several takedowns in an effort to dismantle the entire network from the street level dealer to the sources on the continental U.S. So far over 30 people have been indicted and several more indictments are expected. As of the reporting date, this operation has resulted in the seizure of 10 pounds of crystal methamphetamine valued at $1,359,000, 39 firearms, thousands of rounds of ammunition, $354,700 US currency, a boat, automobiles, and other assets totaling over $800,000.

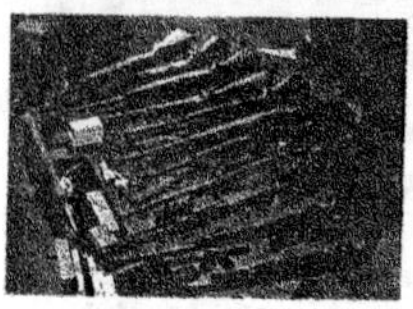

HAWAII INTERDICTION TASK FORCE (HITF)
The Hawaii Interdiction Task Force stops the transport of illicit drugs as they enter through Hawaii's airports and harbors. Since the majority of illicit drugs entering the State of Hawaii come through its airports, HITF plays a significant role in reducing drug trafficking throughout the state. This initiative was responsible for inspecting over 10,000 parcels from domestic and international mail which resulted in the seizure of nearly 100 kilograms of drugs. In addition, HITF arrested 47 drug couriers attempting to conceal drugs. Interceptions resulted in seizures of the following:

- ♦ Crystal methamphetamine: 55 pounds
- ♦ Marijuana: 38 kilograms
- ♦ Cocaine: 10 kilograms
- ♦ Opium: 19 kilograms
- ♦ Pharmaceuticals: 25,000 tablets
- ♦ $1,267,548 US currency

In two related investigations, controlled deliveries of parcels resulted in the identification of an organization supplying crystal methamphetamine to Hawaii-based distribution organizations. In the first case, a parcel controlled delivery of 454 grams of crystal

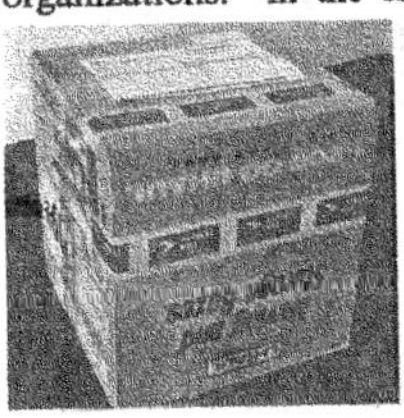

methamphetamine resulted in the arrest of 4 Mexican males who took delivery of a FedEx parcel at a residential address. The organization learned and adapted to law enforcement techniques of controlled delivery and sent a second parcel via US Mail to a post office box. The recipient then led the Task Force on a 1 hour and 45 minute journey from one end of the island to the other in an attempt to lose surveillance. That attempt failed and the subject was arrested. A related controlled delivery conducted by HITF resulted in the identification of a Hawaii-based organizer and controller. This combination of investigations disrupted and then dismantled a transportation organization responsible for the delivery of 50 to 100 pounds of crystal methamphetamine to Hawaii over the past two years.

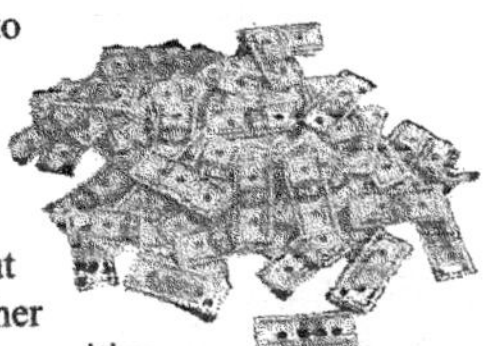

A female subject attempted to board a flight from Honolulu to Las Vegas with $235,700 cash in her luggage. The subject aroused the suspicion of TSA screeners when she told them she had $9,000.00 in cash after currency was observed in her carry-on luggage at the checkpoint. Members of HITF were called to investigate. The subject was inconsistent about the origin of the money and left the cash behind to catch her flight. The currency was seized for federal forfeiture after a positive alert by a narcotic detection canine. This was the largest cash seizure in the past 3 years at any airport in Hawaii. As of March 2004 no claim has been filed for this cash.

The Hawaii Airport Task Force was notified by the Ottawa, Canada Country Office of the seizure of 2268 grams of crystal methamphetamine concealed inside a mini-refrigerator bound for Hawaii. DEA and ICE conducted a controlled delivery that resulted in the arrest of 2 defendants. Two additional defendants were subsequently arrested after delivering 3140 grams of crystal methamphetamine to an undercover agent.

The supplier of this methamphetamine was identified and arrested as he arrived in Honolulu. A total of 5 arrests were made in this case.

Concealment Methods
"I Want my MTV"
In July 2003 members of HATF seized 9.6 pounds of crystal

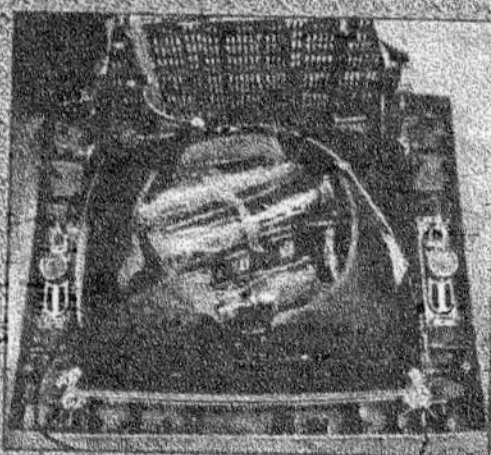

methamphetamine. The group's narcotic canine alerted to a parcel sent as next day air through UPS. When investigators opened the box they found a Philips television. Upon further inspection they noticed inconsistencies with the packaging. Original tape and packing materials were removed and there were smudges on the inside of the screen. Investigators removed the rear panel to find duct tape covering bundles of crystal methamphetamine inside the picture tube. The estimated street value totaled $1.2 million.

Money Laundering Asset Forfeiture Task Force (MLAF)
Dismantling and disrupting drug trafficking organizations is not only a matter of seizing drugs and arresting those individuals involved in their distribution. Making an effective impact on the ability of DTOs to function requires seizing the money they use to operate and the assets they acquire with illicit drug proceeds. The Hawaii HIDTA Money Laundering Asset Forfeiture Task Force is the choke point for identifying and seizing proceeds gained through illegal operations.

On December 10, 2003 members of the Money Laundering Asset Forfeiture Group arrested a video store owner indicted on 91 counts of money laundering. The individual was charged with managing and controlling a building that facilitated drug trafficking and drug use. For a $20 fee dealers were allowed to sell crack cocaine out of the video store which operated 24 hours a day 7 days a week. It was estimated that as many as 20,000 transactions occurred each day. This investigation led to the seizure of 2 condominiums, 2 cars, and various bank accounts. In addition, the video store was closed along with a service station owned by the offender that had been paid for with drug proceeds. The estimated worth of all of the seized assets exceeds $1 million. As part of the investigation, DEA arrested 38 alleged dealers and users in the state and elsewhere with connections to cocaine and methamphetamine suppliers in California and Arizona. If convicted of managing a drug trafficking house, the offenders face up to 20 years in prison for managing a drug trafficking house as well as a maximum 20-year sentence for each of the 91 money laundering charges.

Outcomes For Goal Two

Section IX.

Goal Two. Reduce the Harmful Consequences of Drug Trafficking

INVESTIGATIVE SUBSYSTEM

PSN/ HIFTF	matrix – goal 2 (initiative specific)	Goal	Actual	%
	SEIZE FIREARMS FROM VIOLENT DRUG TRAFFICKERS	110	162	147.2%
	CLEAR WARRANTS FOR DRUG CHARGES	100	290	290%

Safe Neighborhoods Initiative

The HIDTA Executive Board approved the addition of the Safe Neighborhoods Initiative for FY2003. It is a joint effort with the Department of Justice's Project Safe Neighborhoods (PSN) initiative that targets gun crime and violent offenders to remove guns from the street and keep communities safe. HIDTA supplements the Project Safe Neighborhoods endeavor with resources needed to reduce the harmful consequences of drug trafficking by taking a hard line against armed criminals.

According to Project Safe Neighborhoods, there were 6,990 firearms permits issued in Hawaii in 2002 under which a total of 15,822 firearms were registered. This brings the total number of firearms registered in the State of Hawaii to over one million.

Since the beginning of Project Safe Neighborhoods in February 2002, 214 investigations have been initiated in the State of Hawaii and have resulted in 155 criminal indictments. Over 90% of these investigations are narcotics related. In fact, the United States Attorney's Office for the District of Hawaii reviewed the criminal histories of the first 150 defendants charged under PSN and found these individuals were responsible for a combined total of over 3000 arrests and 1000 misdemeanor and felony convictions.

Month	Number of Cases	Number of Firearms Seized	Number of Drug-Related Cases	Number of Offenders Previously Arrested for Drugs	Number of Offenders Previously Convicted for Drugs
January	7	9	5	3	1
February	11	19	10	8	1
March	8	9	7	4	3
April	13	57	12	6	4
May	10	11	9	5	1
June	12	16	11	7	1
July	3	3	3	2	0
August	9	10	7	4	1
September	6	9	6	3	1
October	5	5	4	3	2
November	7	10	7	5	0
December	4	4	5	2	0
TOTALS	95	162	86	52	15

2003 ATF/PSN statistics submitted by ATF Honolulu Field Office

The number of crimes committed by a few people is staggering. With the majority of PSN investigations having a narcotic nexus removing chronic offenders has a significant impact on the amount of crime occurring in the State of Hawaii.

PSN also works closely with Operation Weed and Seed, a U.S. Department of Justice initiative that aims to reclaim, restore, and rebuild neighborhoods, by "weeding" out the criminal element, then "seeding" the community with services that support neighborhood revitalization[19]. As part of the "weeding", police officers are assigned to Crime Reduction Units (CRU) in neighborhoods with high occurrences of drug sales. Officers conduct numerous sting operations to remove drug dealers from the area. Increased police activity creates leads for Project Safe Neighborhoods by arresting individuals who are in possession of drugs and firearms and passing them on for federal prosecution.

One example of the work of PSN involved a known crystal methamphetamine dealer on the island of Hawaii. The subject was at his residence with another individual when a third subject attempted to rob the house. All three subjects were carrying a firearm and a shootout ensued. Concern over witness credibility prohibited the state from filing charges. Instead the case was adopted under the Project Safe Neighborhood initiative. All three subjects were charged with possession of a firearm with intent to distribute. Each was convicted and sentenced to between 2 and 4 years in federal prison.

Hawaii Fugitive Task Force (HFTF)

The Hawaii Fugitive Task Force is one of 28 HIDTA Fugitive Task Forces across the nation. The task force kicked off on March 7, 2003, with the arrest of a fugitive who had been on the run for ten years. Although not officially funded as a HIDTA initiative until FY2004, the task force was organized and functioned throughout 2003 because of a need to reduce drug-related crimes by fugitives involved in the drug trade or who have a criminal history involving drugs and/or drug related violence.

In 2003, based on specific criteria, HFTF arrested 175 State fugitives and cleared 204 warrants. These individuals had a combined criminal history of:

1,442 felony arrest - 427 felony convictions
1,535 misdemeanor arrest – 646 misdemeanor convictions
(note: all pending felony cases, i.e. drugs, homicide, etc., are not included)

In 2003, HFTF executed 115 federal felony arrest warrants:

93 primary warrants, 21 ATF warrants, 9 collateral/UFAP warrants.

Noteworthy accomplishments:

1) The arrest of state fugitives has lead to the indictment of over 20 individuals for federal violations involving narcotic and/or weapons.

2) HFTF was directly involved in the seizure over 72.0 ounces of crystal methamphetamine.

3) HFTF was directly involved in the seizure/recovery of 25 weapons.

[19] Source: U.S. Department of Justice, Office of Justice Programs, Weed and Seed, Hawaii Initiative

4) In August 2003, HFTF conducted Operation Kaulike on the island of Maui, resulting in a noticeable decrease in criminal activity during and post operation.

SUPPORT SUBSYSTEM

PROSECU-TORIAL	matrix – goal 2 (initiative specific)	Goal (Pieces of Legislation)	Actual	%
	PROPOSE MODEL LEGISLATION	2	2	100%

Prosecutorial Initiative
As mentioned earlier in the report, Hawaii state laws impede the ability of local law enforcement agencies to effectively counter drug trafficking. The lack of investigative methods available has allowed career criminals to remain free on the streets and repeat their offenses with no recourse. The Hawaii HIDTA Prosecutorial Initiative has supported legislation to amend the law and provide law enforcement the tools to aid in convicting those individuals who are responsible for numerous offenses.

The purpose of proposed legislation is to conform the state's electronic surveillance and consensual encounter laws to federal laws, facilitate law enforcement activities to curtail drug trafficking and update the laws to keep up with current technology while providing adequate constitutional safeguards that protect individual rights and liberties. With crystal methamphetamine use at an all time high, the People of Hawaii have opened up to the idea that reducing the problems associated with drugs requires not only treatment and prevention among drug users but meaningful consequences for those providing the drugs. Limitations on law enforcement techniques do not send a message to drug traffickers that Hawaii is serious about combating the crystal methamphetamine epidemic.

The City and County of Honolulu prosecutor assigned to the Hawaii HIDTA has been actively engaged in testifying in support of this legislation. He is a conduit for the interests of the Hawaii HIDTA and the United States Attorney's Office to enhance the ability of the law enforcement community in the State of Hawaii to effectively battle the crystal methamphetamine epidemic.

Outcomes for Goal Three

Section X.

Goal Three. Improve the Efficiency and Effectiveness of Law Enforcement Organizations

INTELLIGENCE SUBSYSTEM

INVESTIGATIVE SUPPORT CENTER / WSIN	matrix – goal 3 (initiative specific)	Goal	Actual	%
	ACHIEVE AND MAINTAIN 100% PARTICIPATION BY LAW ENFORCEMENT AGENCIES IN THE WSIN DECONFLICTION SERVICES	100%	100%	100%
	SUBMIT CASE/SUBJECT DECONFLICTIONS AMONG HIDTA INITIATIVES AND PARTICIPATING AGENCIES	9000	9393	104.3%
	SUBMIT EVENT DECONFLICTIONS AMONG HIDTA INITIATIVES AND PARTICIPATING AGENCIES	1400	1333	95.2%
	ISC TO CONDUCT DATABASE QUERIES & PROVIDE INTELLIGENCE REPORTS	4000 100	3202 390	80% 390%
	COMPLETE REQUESTS FOR CASE ASSISTANCE	20	24	120%
	PROVIDE ANALYTICAL PRODUCTS (TOLL ANALYSES, LINK ANALYSES, GRAPHS, CHARTS, PROFILES, ETC)	3,000	4,030	134.3%
	DEVELOP AN ACTIVE MEANS OF COMMUNICATING WITH PACIFIC BASIN/RIM LAW ENFORCEMENT	100%	25%	25%
	PROVIDE ELECTRONIC LINK FROM ISC TO NEIGHBOR ISLANDS VIA WSIN SECURE INTRANET	100%	100%	100%
	SHARE INTELLIGENCE WITH HIDTAS/LEAS OUTSIDE OF HAWAII	*	*	*

*All three HIDTA subsections shared intelligence with HIDTAs/LEAs on the continental U.S. relating to controlled deliveries and joint investigations. Contacts with continental U.S. counterparts occur on a daily basis. This 2003 goal does not lend itself to measurement under the Matrix system.

Investigative Support Center (ISC)

The ISC creates a communication infrastructure for the Hawaii HIDTA. The ISC facilitates information sharing, intelligence collection, analysis and dissemination, technical and strategic support to HIDTA initiatives and participating agencies. Near the end of 2002, the Hawaii HIDTA became fully operational to support Title III investigations through the addition of a wire room. During CY2003 this gave all initiatives easy access to intelligence and analytical support because of proximity to the ISC. It also allowed the ISC to develop and provide operational support to investigations being conducted by HIDTA initiative personnel or their agencies. This support included, but was not limited to, time sensitive analysis of Dialed Number Recorder (DNR) information, subpoenaed TOLL information, pager and clone pager data, post seizure analysis of documents and financial investigative analysis.

The ISC Strategic Unit provides strategic analysis to ONDCP and law enforcement organizations domestically. The initiative is electronically linked, via Western States Information Network (WSIN) and the Regional Information Sharing System (RISS), to all other HIDTA enforcement initiatives nation wide. ISC personnel can interact with the

WSIN Watch Center located in Sacramento, California, and all other enforcement initiatives located on the islands of Kauai, Maui, and Hawaii. The ISC serves as the clearing house of intelligence information obtained by the various initiatives.

The ISC currently comprises of 18 full-time collocated federal, state and local personnel and three non-collocated part-time state and local personnel. The three non-collocated personnel are on the Islands of Maui, Kauai, and Hawaii. Personnel are connected to the ISC via a secure Internet connection and have direct access to WSIN.

The Hawaii HIDTA is unique to all other HIDTA's in that the Hawaii ISC is sponsoring the development of an intelligence/enforcement outreach program that provides direct narcotics law enforcement links with countries in the Pacific Basin and Pacific Rim. The ISC, through its Be On the Lookout (BOLO) developmental component, will be able to provide first hand, timely, actionable information from Pacific Rim/Basin countries for methodical investigation, targeting, and establishment of joint intelligence pools. Partnered with Australia and New Zealand, this information is available to all law enforcement agencies operating within the Hawaii HIDTA and HIDTAs across the country that are destination points for Asia/pacific manufactured drugs.

Investigative Support Center/Intelligence Center Activity	Quantity			
	2001	2002	2003	% +/- 2002-2003
Event/Subject Deconfliction Inquiries	0	450	420	-6.7%
Charts/Graphs	2	71	644	907%
Telephone Tolls	3	216	2185	1011.5%
Document Analysis	1	62	502	809.6%
Geo-mapping	1	2	105	5250%
Link Analysis	3	51	578	1133.3%
Statistical Analysis	0	2	16	800%
Intelligence Profiles	0	550	390	-29.1%
Photographs	150	215	827	384.7%
Data Base search	152	6344	3202	-49.5%
Power Point presentations	6	8	25	312.5%

The ISC has recently begun using the WSIN Master Telephone Index as another analytical tool to provide law enforcement personnel with the most up-to-date intelligence. Telephone tolls, pen register information and other telecommunications information is indexed and compared to identify links among cases throughout the state and the Pacific region.

Western States Information Network (WSIN)

The Hawaii HIDTA is part of the Regional Information Sharing System (RISS) through WSIN. WSIN allows law enforcement agencies to share information and coordinate efforts against criminal networks that operate across jurisdictional boundaries. The WSIN region also includes the states of Alaska, California, Oregon, and Washington, and has member agencies in Canada, Australia, and Guam.

WSIN provides the Hawaii HIDTA with subject/event deconfliction services, access to an automated criminal intelligence sharing database, and a secure intranet for electronic networking among participating agencies. The WSIN Watch Center, located in Sacramento, California, maintains and operates an intelligence database that is populated through subject inquiries and critical events (operations) submissions. Each of the Hawaii HIDTA initiatives has developed protocol to ensure submission to WSIN for event and subject deconfliction. Submissions can be made by contacting the Watch Center via phone or fax, or through remote access via the secure riss.net Intranet. Since the standardization of WSIN participation by HIDTA initiatives submissions have consistently been on the rise.

Total Critical Event (Operation) Submissions
January 1st through December 31st 2003

WSIN posted a total of 1,333 law enforcement critical events (operations) for deconfliction purposes in the State of Hawaii for 2003. Monthly critical event submissions increased significantly during the last half of the year. The average number of operations submitted per month in 2003 was 112. This is twice as high as the average from 2002 (56 per month).

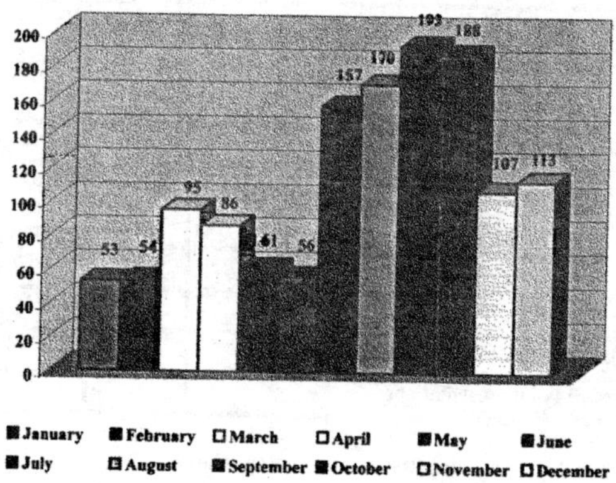

Critical Event Submissions by Drug Types
January 1st through December 31st 2003

Methamphetamine (including amphetamines and crystal methamphetamine) accounted for approximately 83 percent of drug related critical event activity reported in Hawaii for 2003. Cocaine (including rock/crack cocaine), the second most reported drug, accounted for approximately 5 percent. Drugs not specified represented approximately 6 percent.

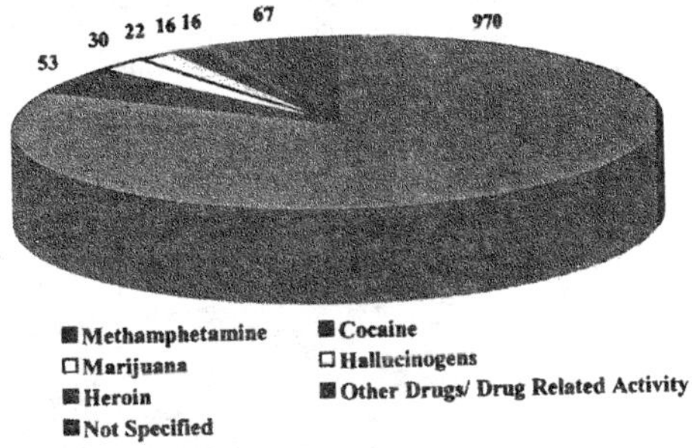

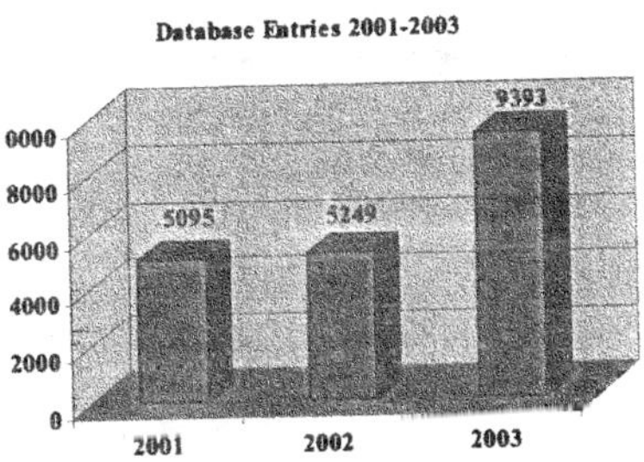

WSIN Database Entries
2001 through 2003

WSIN database entries remained consistent from 2001 through 2002. However, for CY2003 the amount of entries dramatically increased by approximately 79 percent.

WSIN Database Hit Rates
2001 through 2003

There was approximately a 10 percent increase in hit rates from 2001 to 2002. This could be due the increasing amount of entities from Hawaii being entered into the WSIN database, thus improving the odds of a hit. CY2003 continues the rise in hit rates.

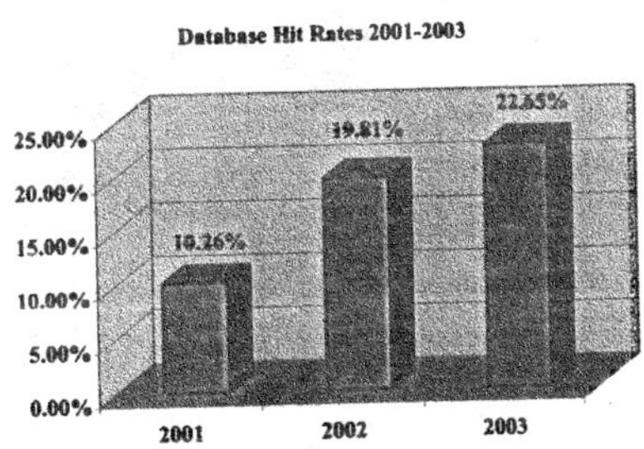

WSIN Database Inquiries and Entries by Agencies

January 1st through December 31st 2003

As with critical event submissions, Honolulu Police Department continues to be the significant contributor of database entries. FBI, DEA, and Hawaii County Police Department (Kona) also showed a lot of activity.

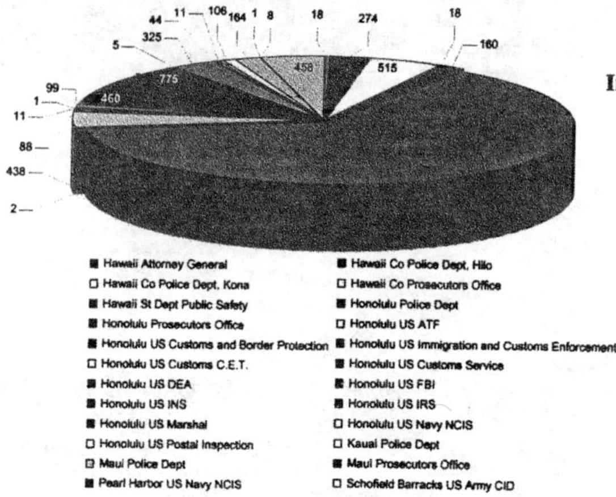

Inquiries

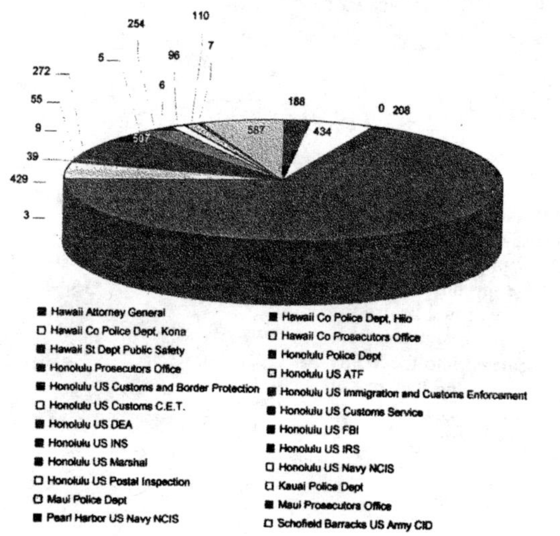

Entries

ADMINISTRATIVE SUPPORT SUBSYSTEM

Management and Coordination Initiative

The Management and Coordination Initiative's success is measured by its ability to facilitate greater efficiency, effectiveness and cooperation among and between external participating agencies at the local, state and federal level.

By design, significant effort is made to collocate and commingle Hawaii HIDTA resources. In fostering interagency cooperation and sharing of strategic and tactical information, the Hawaii HIDTA provides a comprehensive response to illicit drug activity by bringing together all available law enforcement resources in a united front.

The Management and Coordination initiative facilitates efficient operation of all Hawaii HIDTA initiatives by providing oversight, administrative, and budgetary support in accordance with ONDCP and Hawaii Executive Board policy and directives. The initiative is responsible for administrative activities supporting the implementation of the HIDTA strategy, through program guidance, policy compliance, budget analysis, collocation/integration of effort, and information sharing between the participating agencies. This initiative, through the Director and staff, serves as liaison between ONDCP, the Hawaii HIDTA Executive Board, and participating agencies. The Management and Coordination initiative oversees the preparation of administrative and fiscal reports, including threat assessments, strategies, initiatives, budgets, and annual reports required by ONDCP. It coordinates the programmatic and fiscal accountability of HIDTA resources, and oversees the progress of Hawaii HIDTA's development standards.

MANAGEMENT AND COORDINATION TRAINING	matrix – goal 3 (Initiative Specific)	Goal	Actual	%
	ACHIEVE AND MAINTAIN 100% PARTICIPATION BY LAW ENFORCEMENT AGENCIES IN THE WSIN DECONFLICTION SERVICES	100%	100%	100%
	SPONSOR QUARTERLY TRAINING PROGRAMS FOR REGIONAL AND/OR SPECIALIZED TRAINING	4	10	250%
	DEVELOP PARTNERSHIPS WITH EXISTING TRAINING COORDINATORS AT FEDERAL, STATE AND LOCAL AGENCIES	100%	100%	100%
	DEVELOP & MAINTAIN HIDTA TRAINING DATABASE	100%	100%	100%
	DISSEMINATE EXISTING TRAINING OPPORTUNITIES FROM OTHER AGENCIES & OUT-SOURCES TO HIDTA PERSONNEL	100%	100%	100%
	PROVIDE COLLOCATION FOR HIDTA INITIATIVES	*	*	*
	MEET IN EXECUTIVE SESSION TO COORDINATE HAWAII HIDTA ACTIVITIES	6	6	100%
	ATTAIN ONDCP/NHPO DEVELOPMENTAL STANDARDS	100%	89%	89%
	TRACK FISCAL EXPENDITURES OF INITIATIVES TO ENSURE COMPLIANCE WITH POLICIES	100%	100%	100%
	CONDUCT FISCAL AUDITS OF ALL INITIATIVES	100%	100%	100%
	IMPLEMENT & CONDUCT HAWAII HIDTA INTERNAL REVIEW PROGRAM	100%	100%	100%
	MEET QUARTERLY WITH INITIATIVE AND PARTICIPATING AGENCY SUPERVISORS	4	4	100%
	PREPARE THE ANNUAL REPORT, THREAT ASSESSMENT, STRATEGY AND BUDGET	100%	100%	100%

*ONDCP exemptions apply to 4 task forces because of Hawaii's island makeup and costly office rental market.

During the course of CY2003 the HIDTA was successful in presenting a supplemental request and receiving $1,000,000 for Title III and ISC expansion. The CY2002 Annual Report was prepared; as was the CY2004 Threat Assessment and the CY2004 Strategy. Accomplishments include the completion of the Hawaii HIDTA's Administrative and Policy Manual as well as acquiring and implementing the Quarter Master Inventory System. The Fiscal Officer conducted a 100% internal audit of all HIDTA funded agencies and departments, including HPD as the fiduciary. Significant progress was made in Hawaii HIDTA's performance measurements by attaining 50 out of 56 developmental standards. Five new initiatives were solicited and reviewed by the management and coordination team and these initiatives were presented to the Executive Board for final review.

Training Initiative

Training is a key element in improving the efficiency and effectiveness of law enforcement. The need for skills and resources to get ahead of drug traffickers is always a concern to law enforcement.

During CY2003 the Hawaii HIDTA Training Initiative coordinated 8,024 hours of training for 15 federal, state and local agencies and departments throughout the state. A large part was the Clandestine Lab and Designer Drugs course which provided 960 hours of training to 40 law enforcement personnel. In addition, the following courses were conducted:

i2 Analyst's Notebook
Clandestine Lab and Designer Drugs
Federal Law Enforcement Analysis Training
Conspiracy Investigations
NDIC COMEX Training
Domestic Money Laundering Investigations
Clandestine Laboratory Seizure System
19th Annual Pacific Basin Customs Conference
Annual WSIN Training/Conference
California DOJ 17th Annual Organized Crime, Gang, Criminal Intelligence & Terrorism Training Conference

The Hawaii HIDTA Training Initiative exceeded its expected number of training courses by 250% for CY2003. In addition, it coordinated 10 courses, which is 3 more than the 7 coordinated in CY2002. Throughout the year, the Training Coordinator, through the National HIDTA Assistance Center, was successful at building relationships with coordinators throughout the nation. The initiative has made great strides in informing law enforcement personnel in the State of Hawaii of existing training opportunities and facilities available to meet their needs.

Conclusion

Section XI.

During Calendar Year 2003 the Hawaii HIDTA initiatives worked hard to achieve their respective missions. Each initiative played an important role in the effort to accomplish the three general goals established by the National HIDTA Program.

Through a combined effort among federal, state, and local law enforcement agencies 3 initiatives under the Investigative Subsystem, HI-IMPACT, HITF, and MLAF, reduced drug availability by disrupting and/or dismantling 34 drug trafficking/money laundering organizations. Several of these organizations operated internationally, nationally, and statewide across multiple island counties. Six organizations were linked to Consolidated Priority Organization Targets (CPOTs). A total of 1664 arrests were affected by all investigative initiatives combined.

Two new investigative initiatives, PSN and HFTF, focused on reducing the harmful consequences associated with drug trafficking. They were charged with lessening gun violence and a crime rate that is 3rd highest in the nation. During CY2003 290 federal and state fugitives were apprehended. These individuals represent career criminals whose removal from the community improved public safety. In addition, PSN removed 162 firearms from Hawaii's neighborhoods, lessening the chance for homicides, armed robberies, domestic violence, and child endangerment.

During CY2003 the Clandestine Lab Coordination Initiative verified that personnel assigned to clandestine lab response teams were properly trained and certified under OSHA health screening requirements. It coordinated and standardized clandestine lab response procedures for all agencies statewide. Policies and procedures were established to standardize respirators and other equipment to ensure interagency operability.

The Prosecutors Initiative was actively engaged in testifying in support of two pieces of legislation that would drastically change state law to match federal wiretap statute. The initiative coordinated with the United States Attorney's Office to enhance the ability of the law enforcement community in the State of Hawaii to effectively battle the crystal methamphetamine epidemic.

The Intelligence Subsystem is the heart of the HIDTA effort. The ISC and WSIN promote effective and efficient operations by providing tools and resources to conduct successful investigations, and developing the intelligence needed to identify the drug threat by which HIDTA resources are allocated. The ISC generated 8,474 intelligence products during CY2003. WSIN processed 1,333 critical event deconflictions, 10,880 database inquiries, and 9,393 database entries for law enforcement in the State of Hawaii.

The Administrative Subsystem provided oversight to Hawaii HIDTA activities ensuring effective and efficient operations of its initiatives. The Administrative Subsystem brought law enforcement agencies throughout the state together in a cooperative effort to address the issue of drug trafficking in Hawaii. It provided 178,728 hours of training for participating federal, state and local agencies.

In relation to the ONDCP general goals actual outputs exceeded expectations and clearly shows consistency by all Hawaii HIDTA participating agencies.

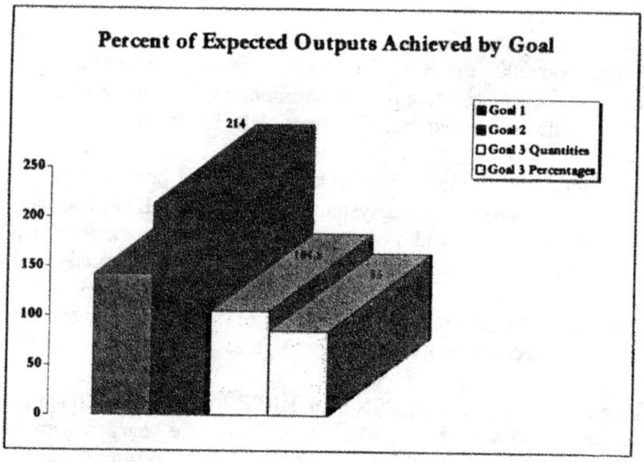

2003 Annual Report
Source Notes

The following sources of information can be found as footnotes throughout this report:

[1] Source: United States Census Bureau, State and County Quick Facts 2000
[2] Source: 2002 State of Hawaii Data Book, State Department of Business, Economic Development & Tourism, Table 10.03
[3] Source: 2002 State of Hawaii Data Book, State Department of Business, Economic Development & Tourism, Tables 13.04 and 7.03, respectively
[4] Source: 2002 State of Hawaii Data Book, State Department of Business, Economic Development & Tourism, Table 13.01
[5] Source: National Agriculture Statistics Service, Hawaii Agriculture Statistics Service, Agriculture Contributions to Hawaii's Economy, 2000
[6] Source: US Census Bureau, Poverty:1999, Table 3 State and Regional Poverty Rates, issued May 2003
[7] Source: State of Hawaii, Department of Transportation, Report to the Governor 2002
[8] This category includes methamphetamine and other amphetamines including Benzedrine, Dexedrine, preludin, Ritalin and any other amines and related drugs (SAMSHA description of drug categories).
[9] Source: Hawaii Attorney General's Office, Crime Prevention and Justice Assistance Division, 2002 Crime in Hawaii
[10] Source: 2004 Hawaii HIDTA Threat Assessment and NDIC Narcotics Digest Weekly, Volume 2, Number 50
[11] Source: Drug Enforcement Administration, Domestic Cannabis Eradication/Suppression Program, Honolulu District Office
[12] Source: United States Sentencing Commission, FY2001 Federal Sentencing Statistics by State
[13] Source: Hawaii State Legislature, 2003 Hawaii Revised Statutes, Part IX Medical Use of Marijuana
[*] Source: Revised HIDTA Program Policy and Budget Guidance, Section XIII Performance Management, page 3
[14] Source: US Census Bureau
[15] Source: Honolulu Police Department, published Honolulu Advertiser
[16] Source: ADAM website, Honolulu branch
[16a] Source: ADAM website, Honolulu branch
[17] Source: United States Marshall Service, District of Hawaii
[18] Source: Child Protective Services, published Honolulu Star Bulletin October 8, 1998 Day 1: Downward Spiral - The Lure Of Ice
[1] Source: United States Census Bureau, State and County Quick Facts 2000
[1] Source: 2002 State of Hawaii Data Book, State Department of Business, Economic Development & Tourism
[3] Source: 2002 State of Hawaii Data Book, State Department of Business, Economic Development & Tourism, Tables 13.04 and 7.03, respectively
[4] Source: 2002 State of Hawaii Data Book, State Department of Business, Economic Development & Tourism, Table 13.01

[5] Source: National Agriculture Statistics Service, Hawaii Agriculture Statistics Service, Agriculture Contributions to Hawaii's Economy, 2000
[6] Source: US Census Bureau, Poverty:1999, Table 3 State and Regional Poverty Rates, issued May 2003
[7] Source: State of Hawaii, Department of Transportation, Report to the Governor 2002
[8] This category includes methamphetamine and other amphetamines including Benzedrine, Dexedrine, preludin, Ritalin and any other amines and related drugs (SAMSHA description of drug categories).
[9] Source: Hawaii Attorney General's Office, Crime Prevention and Justice Assistance Division, 2002 Crime in Hawaii
[10] Source: 2004 Hawaii HIDTA Threat Assessment and NDIC Narcotics Digest Weekly, Volume 2, Number 50
[11] Source: Drug Enforcement Administration, Domestic Cannabis Eradication/Suppression Program, Honolulu District Office
[12] Source: United States Sentencing Commission, FY2001 Federal Sentencing Statistics by State
[13] Source: Hawaii State Legislature, 2003 Hawaii Revised Statutes, Part IX Medical Use of Marijuana
[14] Source: US Census Bureau
[15] Source: Honolulu Police Department, published Honolulu Advertiser
[16] Source: ADAM website, Honolulu branch
[16a] Source: ADAM website, Honolulu branch
[17] Source: United States Marshall Service, District of Hawaii
[18] Source: Child Protective Services, published Honolulu Star Bulletin October 8, 1998 Day 1: Downward Spiral - The Lure Of Ice
[19] Source: U.S. Department of Justice, Office of Justice Programs, Weed and Seed, Hawaii Initiative
[*] Source: Revised HIDTA Program Policy and Budget Guidance, Section XIII Performance Management, page 3
Front cover credit- Douglas Peebles

In addition, the following agencies and departments provided information to support this report:

Bureau of Alcohol, Tobacco and Firearms

Bureau of Immigration and Customs Enforcement

Community Epidemiology Work Group

Department of Defense

Department of Public Safety, Narcotics Enforcement Division

Drug Enforcement Administration

Federal Bureau of Investigation

Hawaii County Police Department

Hawaii National Guard

Honolulu City & County Prosecutor's Office

Honolulu Police Department

Honolulu Weed and Seed Program

Internal Revenue Service

Kauai County Police Department

Maui Police Department

National Drug Intelligence Center

Naval Criminal Investigative Service

United States Attorney's Office

United States Coast Guard

United States Marshall Service

United States Postal Inspection Service

Western States Information Network

Appendix I
Hawaii HIDTA
Table of Organization

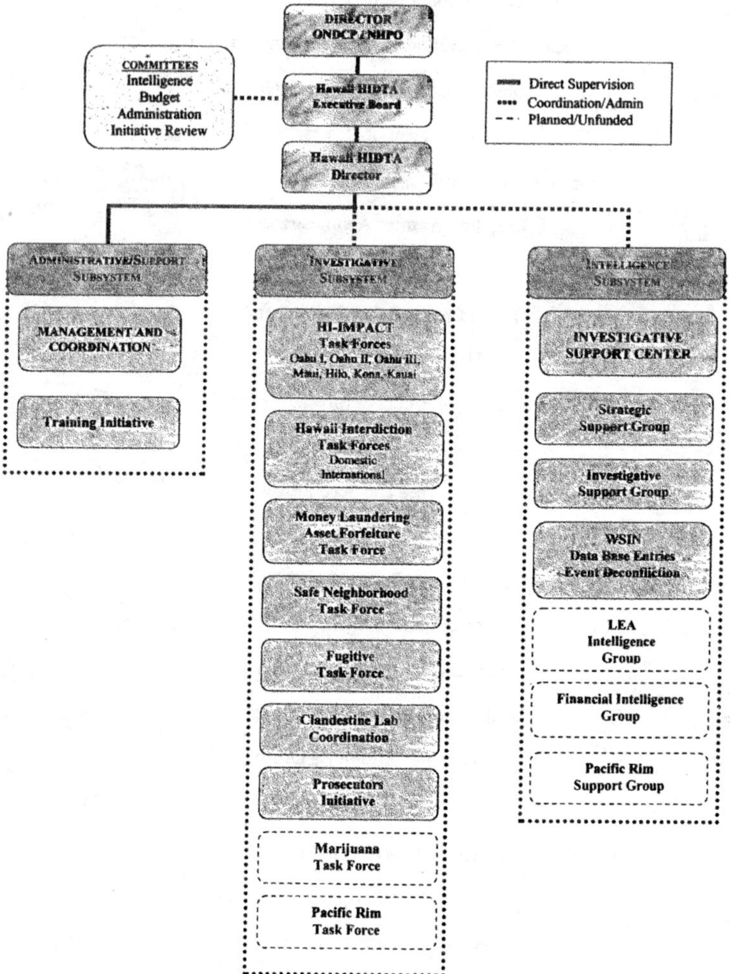

Appendix II
Hawaii HIDTA
CY2003 Executive Board Listing

Name	Agency	Title	Status
Peter Carlisle	Honolulu City & County Prosecutor's Office	Prosecuting Attorney	State/Local Voting
Paul Ciccarelli	Naval Criminal Investigative Service	Special Agent in Charge	Federal Non-voting
Kathryn Derwey	U.S. Postal Inspection Service	Postal Inspector/Projects Coordinator	Federal Voting
Charles Goodwin	Federal Bureau of Investigation	Special Agent in Charge	Federal Voting
Tracy Elder	Bureau of Alcohol, Tobacco and Firearms	Resident Agent in Charge	Federal Voting
Willy Ihu	Kauai Police Department	Acting Chief of Police	State/Local Voting
Briane Grey	Drug Enforcement Administration	Assistant Special Agent in Charge	Federal Voting – VICE CHAIR
Cathy Cowley	Internal Revenue Service	Group Supervisor	Federal Voting
Keith Kamita	Department of Public Safety	Deputy Director Law Enforcement	State/Local Voting – CHAIR
Henry Lau	Honolulu Police Department	Assistant Chief of Police	State/Local Voting
Ed Kubo	U.S. Attorney's Office	United States Attorney	Federal Voting
Tamah-Lani Noh	Hawaii National Guard	Major, Counterdrug Unit	State/Local Voting
Lawrence Mahuna	Hawaii County Police Department	Chief of Police	State/Local Voting
Thomas Phillips	Maui Police Department	Chief of Police	State/Local Voting
Mark Hanohano	U.S. Marshals Service	U.S. Marshal	Federal [redacted]-Voting
Mardelle Tamashiro Wayne Wills	Bureau of Immigration and Customs Enforcement	Assistant Special Agent in Charge Associate Special Agent in Charge	Federal Voting
Ken Tano	Western States Information Network	Regional Director	State/Local Voting
Charles D. Wurster	U.S. Coast Guard	Rear Admiral	Federal Non-Voting

Appendices III & IV
Hawaii HIDTA
Personnel & Participating Agencies

AGENCY	FULL-TIME	PART-TIME	TOTAL (FULL-TIME PLUS PART-TIME)
Bureau of Alcohol, Tobacco and Firearms	7	2	9
Bureau of Immigration and Customs Enforcement	13	11	24
Department of Public Safety	6	6	12
Drug Enforcement Administration	8	4	12
Federal Bureau of Investigation	12	1	13
Federal Bureau of Prisons	1	0	1
Fisheries Service	0	1	1
Hawaii County Police Department	4	28	32
Hawaii HIDTA Contract Personnel	6	0	6
Hawaii National Guard	10	1	11
Honolulu City & County Prosecutor's Office	5	0	5
Honolulu Police Department	27	23	50
Internal Revenue Service	4	1	5
Kauai Police Department	2	8	10
Maui Police Department	3	30	33
Naval Criminal Investigative Service	1	0	1
U.S. Attorney's Office	1	0	1
U.S. Coast Guard	1	0	1
U.S. Inspector General	0	1	1
U.S. Marshals Service	6	0	6
U.S. Postal Inspection Service	1	3	4
Western States Information Network	5	0	5
TOTALS	**123**	**120**	**243**

Appendix V
Hawaii HIDTA
Developmental Standards

Basic	Intermediate	Optimal
Event Deconfliction Services		
A.1.1☒service to all HIDTA task forces A.1.2☒work week availability A.1.3☒same day service	A.1.4☒service to all drug control agencies within HIDTA	A.1.5☒service to all law enforcement in HIDTA region A.1.6☒24 hours/7 day availability A.1.7☒immediate service
2. Case/Subject Deconfliction		
A.2.1☒criminal subject deconfliction to all HIDTA task forces	A.2.2☒pointer index service to the HIDTA region A.2.3☒connectivity of all HIDTA task forces to the intelligence center and each other	A.2.4☒connectivity to national pointer index A.2.5☒pointer index service to other HIDTA and HIDTA agencies
3. Post Seizure Analysis		
A.3.1☒ad hoc post seizure analysis	A.3.2☒post seizure analysis and dissemination for HIDTA task forces and participating agencies	A.3.3☒post seizure analysis and national dissemination
4. Analytical Case Support		
A.4.1☒case support for most significant cases	A.4.2☒specific analytical support to HIDTA task forces (e.g. toll, Title III, and document analysis)	A.4.3☒full-service case support to all HIDTA cases upon request (complete analysis including prosecution stage)
5. Connectivity to Other Databases		
A.5.1☒collocated access to major databases A.5.2☒access to regional intelligence	A.5.3☒access to unique databases A.5.4☒access to domestic intelligence	A.4.3☒access to global intelligence
6. Strategic Intelligence		
A.6.1☒collection of trend and pattern analysis	A.6.2☒full trend & pattern analysis, special assessments produced	A.6.3☐predictive analysis (strategic intelligence products)

Basic	Intermediate	Optimal
1. Task Force Operations		
B.1.1☒multi-jurisdictional, collocated task forces (exceptions must be approved)	B.1.2☒joint OCDETF level investigations, HIDTA region multi-task force operations (information exchange, case coordination)	B.1.3☒routine/institutional multi-task force OCDETF operations B.1.4☒task force operations with other HIDTAs
2. Training		
B.2.1☒joint training for HIDTA task forces	B.2.2 ☒joint training for HIDTA region	B.2.3☐export specialized training to requesting HIDTAs

Basic	Intermediate	Optimal
1. Planning		
C.1.1☒develop available HIDTA region Threat Assessment, Strategy, and Annual Report C.1.2☒correlate Strategy to Threat C.1.3☒identify measurable objectives	C.1.4☒produce measurable outputs and outcomes	C.1.5☒achieve targeted (articulated) outputs and outcomes C.1.6☒establish evaluation capacity C.1.7☒integrated planning with other HIDTAs
2. Initiative Execution		
C.2.1☒ implement initiatives which execute Strategy	C.2.2☒integrated systems approach among HIDTA task forces (investigation, intelligence, interdiction, prosecution)	C.2.3☒integrated systems approach within HIDTA region (parole, courts, probation, corrections, testing, sanctions)
3. Resource Management		
C.3.1☒correlate budget to Strategy (Initiatives)	C.3.2☒periodically review and reallocate resources	C.3.3☒continuous review and reallocation of resources

Basic	Intermediate	Optimal
1. Fiscal Controls		
D.1.1☒establish sound fiscal/ programmatic management including shared fiscal reports among EXCOM members D.1.2☒identify and implement resource saving systems, eliminate duplication	D.1.3☒implement scheduled self-inspection program to monitor HIDTA resources D.1.4☒share successes, failures with all HIDTAs (recommend best practices)	D.1.5☒implement self-review process to evaluate initiatives and recommend programming needs to EXCOM D.1.6☒adapt efficiencies developed by other HIDTAs
2. Inventory Controls		
D.2.1☒establish and maintain HIDTA equipment inventory and control system	D.2.2☒system allows sharing of equipment between initiatives	D.2.3☐sharing of equipment with other HIDTAs
3. Information Management		
D.3.1☒establish an information management system		

REMARKS: D.2.3 No request from other HIDTAs was received, however, due to geographic isolation timely sharing of equipment will be difficult.

3. Summary

a) Using the milestone identifying numbers, indicate the milestones specifically achieved during this reporting year. A.3.3, B.1.3 and D.1.4.

b) What percentage of the National HIDTA Developmental Standards has been accomplished to date by this HIDTA?

Total number of milestones accomplished to date	=	53	=	95%
56 (total number of milestones)		56		

Appendix VI
Hawaii HIDTA
Initiative Outputs in CY2003 Format

HAWAII IMPACT (State-Wide) CY2003 Expected Outputs:	HAWAII IMPACT (State-Wide) CY2003 Actual Outputs:
Dismantle/disrupt 10 major drug distribution organizations.	Dismantled/disrupted 24 drug distribution organizations.
Dismantle/disrupt 4 drug manufacturing organizations.	Dismantled/disrupted 4 drug manufacture organizations.
Seizure and process of 2 production clandestine labs.	Seized and processed 15 clandestine labs.
Arrest 50 persons for manufacturing and/or distribution of drugs.	Arrests 1605 subjects on drug charges.
Seize 10 pounds of finished methamphetamine and/or methamphetamine solution.	Seized 16 pounds of crystal methamphetamine.
Prepare and serve 50 search warrants in support of investigations of manufacturing and/or distribution of methamphetamine.	Served 113 search warrants.
Identify 10 organization cells engaged in methamphetamine manufacturing and/or distribution.	Identified each counties top 10 drug distribution organizations.
Identify 50 persons actually engaged in manufacturing and/or distribution of methamphetamine.	Identified 250 persons.
Conduct 3 reverse sting operations targeting persons purchasing methamphetamine or precursor chemicals.	Conducted 12 reverse sting operations.
Attempt to seize and forfeit all drug-related assets and proceeds identified by the task force during the course of their investigation.	Seized over $1 million in drug related assets to include U.S. currency, vehicles, a boat, and jewelry.
Conduct 6 wiretaps in support of investigations of manufacturing and/or distribution of methamphetamine.	Conducted 16 wiretaps in support of drug manufacturing/distribution investigations.

Hawaii Airport Task Force CY2003 Expected Outputs:	Hawaii Airport Task Force CY2003 Actual Outputs:
Arrest a total of 50 narcotic couriers who enter the State via commercial air facilities.	Arrested 47 narcotics couriers.
Examine 750 high-risk parcels entering the parcel sorting facilities, including the international mail facility.	Examined 10,000 parcels.
Seize a total of 60 kilograms of illegal narcotics and drugs.	Seized 60 kilograms of drugs.
Seize $600,000 in narcotics proceeds.	Seized $1,009,916.

Foreign Interdiction Task Force CY2003 Expected Outputs:	Foreign Interdiction Task Force CY2003 Actual Outputs
Conduct six (6) controlled deliveries of controlled substances seized as result of border interdiction.	Conducted 13 controlled deliveries.
Identify two (2) major drug smuggling organization.	Identified two drug smuggling organizations.
Dismantle one internet based illicit drug organization.	Seized numerous internet-based shipments of pharmaceuticals.
Develop two new sources of information/informants to furnish intelligence and other information concerning importation of controlled substances into Hawaii.	Developed four new sources of information.
Attend training conferences on airport and maritime interdiction operations.	Attended Jetway training and gave presentations on interdiction operations.
Support requests from county police departments for training on Oahu and the continental U.S.	Supported all requests from county police departments for training.
Initiate requests to county police departments to participate in interdiction operations conducted on Oahu.	Maui, Hawaii, Kauai counties all participated in interdiction operations conducted throughout the state and region.
Conduct interdiction and outreach operations on the Islands of Hawaii, Maui, and Kauai.	Conducted controlled deliveries on the islands of Hawaii, Maui, and Kauai.
Support requests from State and Local law enforcement for equipment needed to conduct controlled deliveries, surveillance, and law enforcement operations.	Supported intelligence and operational requests. No equipment requested.
Travel to Guam to conduct intelligence exchange with Guam Customs and Police.	Funded travel of Postal Inspector to Guam to conduct intelligence exchange.
Support requests from law authorities on Guam to travel to Hawaii in furtherance of drug smuggling investigations	No travel requests received.
Support travel to the U.S. mainland in furtherance of other HIDTA's drug smuggling investigations.	Traveled to CA and Texas in furtherance of HIDTA drug investigations.

Money Laundering/Asset Forfeiture Task Force CY2003 Expected Outputs:	**Money Laundering/Asset Forfeiture Task Force CY2003 Actual Outputs:**
Target one clandestine money remittance house/establishment suspected of wiring/transporting narcotics proceeds internationally.	One money remittance house has been targeted and the investigation is on-going.
Conduct an undercover operation at a money remittance house and/or nontraditional financial institution.	One money remittance house has been targeted and the investigation is on-going.
Conduct five outreach programs with local financial institutions on money laundering trends, SAR activity and BSA reporting	There have been more than five contacts of various banking and other financial institutions.
Pursue the identification and forfeiture of at least five assets acquired by defendants charged with federal and state narcotics violations.	In two separate HIDTA financial investigations, assets totaling over $1 million have been identified and seized.
Provide support to state and local police departments with funding, personnel and equipment in conjunction with investigations and initiatives.	Funding and equipment has been provided to NED and county police departments.
Provide financial investigative support and asset forfeiture assistance to other Hawaii HIDTA initiatives.	All of HIDTA money laundering cases have connections to or originated out of other HIDTA initiatives except the money remittance house investigation.
Conduct quarterly meetings with FITF designees concerning case activity and intelligence.	Meetings are held on a continuing basis.

Clan Lab Initiative CY2003 Expected Outputs:	Clan Lab Initiative CY2003 Actual Outputs:
Select and staff the Clandestine Laboratory Response Coordinator position.	Response Coordinator position staffed by NED investigator.
Provide in-service training for Clandestine Laboratory Response Coordinator.	The Clan Lab response coordinator has and is continuing to provide training.
Conduct assessment survey of HIDTA clandestine laboratory response needs.	An initial assessment of the four local police departments was conducted.
Identify and establish coordination with clandestine laboratory response Coordinators at major Federal, State, and Local agencies.	This CY2003 output has been finalized.
Sponsor one training program each quarter for regional and/or specialized training.	Training sessions conducted. Annual Safety Recertification; Precursor Extraction Training; Confined Space Training.
Contribute clandestine laboratory response information to the Hawaii HIDTA newsletter.	This initiative has worked with HIDTA analysts to provide basic information about the Clan Lab initiative.
Develop and populate a clandestine laboratory response database in conjunction with the Hawaii HIDTA ISC.	The initiative has begun to develop a local standard database for statistical purposes.

Prosecutor Initiative CY2003 Expected Outputs:	Prosecutor Initiative CY2003 Actual Outputs:
Fill county prosecutor position, including completion of all necessary background and security checks.	This position has been filled by a deputy prosecutor from the City and County of Honolulu Prosecutors Office.
Obtain all necessary cross-designations.	The deputy prosecutor is designated as a SAUSA.
Obtain clerical support and office space for the HIDTA prosecutors in the Hawaii HIDTA Center.	The deputy prosecutor has been assigned office space at the HIDTA facility.
Conduct a monthly meeting with the existing Hawaii HIDTA interdiction and investigative initiatives and task forces.	No monthly meetings have been held.
Assist in the investigation, indictment and prosecution of at least two (2) drug trafficking and/or money laundering organization multi-defendant cases.	The deputy prosecutor has not assisted in any drug trafficking and/or money laundering cases.

Investigative Support Center CY2003 Expected Outputs:	Investigative Support Center CY2003 Actual Outputs:
Provide analytical case support to 10 Title III new/ongoing cases.	ISC has provided analytical support to 14 new/on-going cases.
Provide technical case support to 10 new/ongoing cases.	ISC has provided technical support to 10 new cases.
Continue to provide investigative intelligence support to all requests from HIDTA Law Enforcement Initiatives within the State of Hawaii.	This output has been finalized for CY2003. The ISC has provided 390 intelligence profiles; 105 geo-mapping reports; and 827 photographs.
Continue to perform time-sensitive analysis for all law enforcement requests, to include specialized communications analysis of Title III, DNR data, subpoenaed tolls, pager and clone pager data, seized documents and financial data.	This output has been finalized for CY2003. ISC has provided document analysis for 502 documents; 2,158 telephone tolls; and 3,202 database searches.
Continue to share/provide "Cross Border" investigative intelligence data with other HIDTA, Federal, State and local Law Enforcement Agencies outside of Hawaii's area of responsibility as they develop.	This output has been finalized for CY2003.
Maintain and expand databases in standard use within the national HIDTA program.	This has been finalized via the riss.net WSIN.
Continue to interview and hire contract personnel as stated in this report.	This output has been finalized for CY2003.
Obtain security clearance for all personnel assigned to the ISC.	The ISC analysts obtained their security clearances via DEA.
Provide 'real time' ISC connectivity to all satellite Initiatives (neighbor Islands).	This output has been finalized for CY2003.
Complete all i2, Pen-Link, and RAID training of all analysts assigned to the ISC.	All ISC analysts have received i2 and Pen-Link training. The RAID program has not yet been adopted for use in the ISC.
Procure T-III equipment.	This has been finalized.
Provide analytical and technical support to at least 1 Title III intercept investigation.	This CY2003 output has been finalized. The ISC has provided support to at least three investigations which included 8 separate telephone lines.
Continue subject and case 'de-confliction' with WSIN.	This CY2003 output is continuing with the reported 420 WSIN subject/event deconfliction inquiries.
Complete installation of all neighbor island WAN computer equipment.	This has been finalized via the riss.net/HIDTA.net network.
Coordinate/Provide training for initiative participant and ISC personnel as needed. (FLEAT, RAID, i2, Pen-Link etc.)	The ISC has coordinated and provided training to the initiative participants and ISC personnel. These training classes were i2, money laundering, conspiracy, NDIC training, HASH Keeper, and Arc View.
Produce the Hawaii HIDTA CY 2004 Threat Assessment.	The Hawaii HIDTA CY2004 Threat Assessment has been finalized.

Management & Coordination Initiative CY2003 Expected Outputs:	Management & Coordination Initiative CY2003 Actual Outputs:
Prepare the CY2002 Annual Report.	Prepared and submitted.
Prepare the FY2003 Threat Assessment Summary, Strategy and Initiative/Budgets.	Prepared and submitted.
Provide other ONDCP requested reports and surveys in a timely manner.	Prepared all requested reports.
Continue to upgrade and modify the Hawaii HIDTA's administrative and policy manual.	Policy and Procedure manual completed and will be updated as necessary.
Upgrade and modify the Hawaii HIDTA's property and inventory control system to conduct a 100% annual audit of equipment and property using Quarter Master inventory control system.	Inventory control system in place and audits have been performed on all initiatives and annual audits will continue.
Establish internal review teams to track initiative development and progress towards stated objectives (goals). Utilize Internal Audit and Self-Review Policy.	Annual reviews have been completed and will continue.
Schedule and conduct an annual internal program review of all initiatives, to include a self-inspection and an initiative accomplishment report.	Annual internal program reviews of all initiatives have been completed and will continue.
Provide efficient and accurate financial management, to include 100% expenditure tracking.	The Fiscal Officer has tracked all expenditures and they are current and accurate.
Solicit resource contributions from participating agencies that keeps involvement at current or higher levels.	Participating levels have increased from FY2002.
Meet with initiative supervisors quarterly.	Meetings regularly scheduled.
Meet with participating agency initiative managers regarding reprogramming issues.	Meetings occur as needed for reprogramming issues.
Implement 10% additional HIDTA development standards above 2002 level.	Development standards reached by 89%.
Meet with ISC and Task Force supervisors to ensure the continued flow of information between the ISC and the field initiatives.	Meeting regularly scheduled.
Attend required HIDTA Director meetings and seminars as approved by the Executive Board.	Attended all required HIDTA Director meetings in CY2002.

Training Initiative CY 03 Expected Outputs:	Training Initiative CY 03 Actual Outputs:
Select and staff the Training Coordinator position.	The Training Coordinator position has been assigned as a collateral duty of the DEA ISC Supervisor and is assisted by 1 National Guardsman.
Provide in-service training for Training Coordinator.	The Training Coordinator has attended the National HIDTA Training Coordinators meeting(s).
Conduct assessment survey of HIDTA training needs.	This is done annually at the beginning of the calendar year.
Identify and establish coordination with Training Coordinators at major Federal, State, and Local agencies.	Coordination occurs through the National HIDTA Assistance Center, newsletters, and meetings with law enforcement personnel.
Disseminate existing training opportunities from other agencies and out-sources to Hawaii HIDTA personnel.	100% dissemination of training opportunities.
Sponsor one training program each quarter for regional and/or specialized training.	Sponsored and/or coordinated 10 training programs.
Contribute training information to the Hawaii HIDTA newsletter.	A Hawaii HIDTA newsletter has not yet been produced.
Develop and populate HIDTA training database.	The Training Initiative has developed a spreadsheet to track training.